The Metaverse for the Healthcare Industry

Chiranji Lal Chowdhary
Editor

The Metaverse for the Healthcare Industry

Springer

Editor
Chiranji Lal Chowdhary
School of Computer Science Engineering &
Information Systems
Vellore Institute of Technology
Vellore, Tamil Nadu, India

ISBN 978-3-031-60072-2 ISBN 978-3-031-60073-9 (eBook)
https://doi.org/10.1007/978-3-031-60073-9

This Springer imprint is published by the registered company Springer Nature Switzerland AG
The registered company address is: Gewerbestrasse 11, 6330 Cham, Switzerland

Chiranji Lal Chowdhary dedicates this book volume with profound gratitude to his esteemed research guide, Prof. (Dr.) D.P. Acharjya. Throughout the Ph.D. journey, Dr. Acharjya's invaluable guidance and unwavering support have been the cornerstone of this scholarly endeavor. His wisdom and encouragement have played a pivotal role in shaping the contents of this work.

Special appreciation is extended to Vellore Institute of Technology (VIT), Vellore, for providing an enriching academic environment. The culture of academic excellence fostered at VIT has significantly contributed to laying the solid foundation of knowledge that is reflected in the pages of this book volume.

In a heartfelt tribute, Chiranji Lal Chowdhary remembers the late Dr. V.K. Ananthashyana, his esteemed guide during MTech at Ramaiah Institute of Technology, Bangalore. Dr. Ananthashyana's profound guidance and mentorship have left an indelible mark on the academic journey, influencing the trajectory of knowledge and research encapsulated within this comprehensive volume.

Preface

In transforming healthcare, obtaining awareness and actionable perspectives from diverse, high-dimensional, and heterogeneous biomedical data have been a constant challenge. In modern biomedical research, data generated are in various forms, including electronic health records, imaging, omics, sensor data, and text, which are nuanced, heterogeneous, poorly annotated, and typically unstructured. In the healthcare domain, traditional machine learning methods have been found to be efficiently managing learning tasks when domains are limited to small datasets. However, large datasets from hospital management systems and other healthcare informatics are increasingly used in the healthcare domain. Healthcare informatics is one among the primary focus of researchers and industry experts due to its significant effects on society and has emerged as a growing area of interest among researchers worldwide. The emergence of digital healthcare solutions has enabled hospitals, clinics, and other healthcare facilities to greatly enhance the delivery of medical services and products to their patients. Digital health management combines technological innovation with transformation services to give people the support they need, when and where they need it.

The metaverse has gained "eye-catching" attention in literal sense since the concept promises to leapfrog the confluence of physical world into an evolved virtual space to eventually deliver an immersive end-user experience. Despite being in its early stages, the metaverse is constantly developing. The technology, which combines Artificial Intelligence (AI), Augmented Reality (AR), Virtual Reality (VR), and web 3.0 technologies, has enormous potential in healthcare. The Internet of Medical Devices, quantum computing, and robotics are all poised to completely transform the healthcare ecosystem. The metaverse is likely to change the paradigm of the healthcare system, improving surgical precision, therapeutic usage, and more. The metaverse promotes health 4.0 by combining AI, AR, and VR, improving patient safety outcomes, and allowing patients to interact and gain a clear understanding of their health condition. It is essentially the next version of the internet that uses AI, AR, VR, and ever-increasing connectivity such as 5G networks to create more immersive, interactive, and experiential online environments.

In the current healthcare system, the management of chronic diseases still faces challenges, such as uneven distribution of medical resources, and difficulty in follow-up, overburdening of specialists, and so on. However, the metaverse medical platforms incorporating advanced AI technologies, such as industrial-scale digital twins, may address these issues. In this volume, we are going to present several topics under the current status of research in the metaverse for healthcare industry as stated below.

Chapter "Fundamentals of the Metaverse for the Healthcare Industry" introduces the foundational elements of the metaverse and explores its transformative potential in healthcare. It highlights the dynamic fusion of virtual, augmented, and real environments, emphasizing the positive impact on remote diagnosis, diagnostic processes, and healthcare education.

Chapter "Intelligent Healthcare Systems in the Metaverse: Architecture, Applications, Challenges, and Opportunities" delves into the architecture of intelligent healthcare systems within the metaverse. It covers real-time case studies, ethical considerations, and the integration of Web3-based metaverse healthcare systems, showcasing the potential for revolutionizing healthcare access and quality.

Chapter "The Metaverse in Healthcare: The Emerging Future of the Next Generation" explores the metaverse's rise in healthcare amid the COVID-19 pandemic. It discusses virtual medical consultations, research, and training, emphasizing the potential in entertainment and education. The chapter also addresses emerging ethical, legal, and technological challenges associated with the metaverse.

Chapter "The Social and Ethical Challenges of the Metaverse" examines the potential consequences of the metaverse technology on human life, focusing on user privacy and security. The discussion provides insights to guide the formulation of new laws and empower users with information about their rights in the evolving the metaverse environment.

Chapter "Harnessing the Potential of the Metaverse in Medical Education and Training" explores the transformative potential of the metaverse in medical education. It highlights personalized patient engagement and inclusive learning experiences, presenting case studies that showcase the rich impact of the metaverse on medical training and education.

Chapter "The Metaverse in Medicine: Medical Internet of Things (MIoT)" explores the secure integration of biosensors, wearable sensors, and medical devices within the metaverse. The chapter addresses privacy concerns through blockchain technology and underscores the pivotal role of the metaverse in timely decision-making, diagnosing, and predicting diseases.

Chapter "The Metaverse and Mental Well-Being" uncovers the potential benefits of the metaverse in mental health treatment and education. It explores virtual reality therapy and online support groups while addressing challenges like the surge in fake news, emphasizing the delicate balance between positive potential and associated risks.

Chapter "The Metaverse-Enabled Medical Internet of Things (IoMT)" reveals a new paradigm for personalized and precision medicine. It explores the integration of IoT in clinical applications and wireless body area networking, showcasing the potential to revolutionize healthcare through innovative technologies like virtual reality and augmented reality.

Chapter "The Metaverse in Prevention and Treatment of Disease" explores the transformative role of the metaverse in disease prevention and treatment. It showcases immersive educational experiences, real-time data sharing, and innovative avenues for telemedicine and remote patient monitoring. The chapter examines ethical and privacy concerns, emphasizing careful integration for unprecedented opportunities and challenges.

Chapter "The Metaverse in Healthcare 4.0" delves into the technical aspects of the metaverse-based healthcare systems. It highlights the integration of cutting-edge technologies and their potential to empower individuals in monitoring their health, expanding access to healthcare services, and offering innovative solutions to evolving challenges.

Chapter "A Revolution in Healthcare Using the Metaverse for the Elderly" focuses on the transformative potential of the metaverse for elderly care. It explores how 3D virtual reality capabilities can enhance the quality of life for the elderly, addressing their unique needs and turning cherished memories into immersive experiences.

Chapter "The Metaverse Game" immerses readers into the dynamic universe of the metaverse games, exploring social interaction, personalization, and innovative features like blockchain integration, cryptocurrencies, NFTs, and AR technology.

Chapter "The Metaverse and Its Related Technologies in Telesurgery in Healthcare 5.0: A Case Study" delves into the intersection of the metaverse and healthcare, with a focus on Telesurgery. It explores the amalgamation of mixed reality, IoT, AI, and blockchain within the metaverse, highlighting its application in Telesurgery and remote patient monitoring.

Chapter "Challenges, Ethics, and Limitations of the Metaverse for the Healthcare Industry" critically examines the integration of the metaverse into the healthcare industry, exploring ethical considerations and inherent limitations. It provides valuable insights into the delicate balance required to harness the full potential of the metaverse for healthcare, emphasizing the need for careful consideration and ethical frameworks.

The intended audience includes academicians, researchers in the fields of AI, specifically from the domain of the metaverse, Digital Twins, Augmented Reality, Virtual Reality, Web 3.0, Deep Learning, Data Science, and Healthcare Informatics; Postgraduate Students, Professional Data Analysts, Healthcare System Designers and Practitioners, and people associated with personalized healthcare sector.

The book is designed so that it can be a preferred reference in libraries of academic institutions, research and development centers, departments of business, computer and information sciences, organizations dealing with healthcare informatics, and IT firms developing products in the domain of health industries.

Vellore, Tamil Nadu, India Chiranji Lal Chowdhary

Contents

Fundamentals of the Metaverse for the Healthcare Industry

Chiranji Lal Chowdhary, Siva Rama Krishnan Somayaji, Vijay Kumar, and Sandeep Singh Sengar

1 Introduction to the Metaverse

1.1 Defining the Metaverse

The metaverse represents a groundbreaking integration of physical and virtual realities, creating a digital universe where users interact in real time. Figure 1 depicts the interaction between the metaverse and physical world by the usage of mixed reality headsets. This section provides a detailed exploration of the metaverse's fundamental concepts, delving into the technologies that underpin this innovative space, including augmented reality (AR), virtual reality (VR), and 3D computer-generated environments [1, 2] (Table 1).

C. L. Chowdhary (✉) · S. R. K. Somayaji
School of Computer Science Engineering and Information Systems, Vellore Institute of Technology, Vellore, Tamil Nadu, India
e-mail: chiranji.lal@vit.ac.in; siva.s@vit.ac.in

V. Kumar
Department of Information Technology, Dr. B R Ambedkar National Institute of Technology, Jalandhar, Punjab, India
e-mail: vijaykumarchahar@gmail.com

S. S. Sengar
Senior Lecturer, Department of Computer Science, Cardiff Metropolitan University, Cardiff, UK
e-mail: SSSengar@cardiffmet.ac.uk

C. L. Chowdhary (ed.), *The Metaverse for the Healthcare Industry*,
https://doi.org/10.1007/978-3-031-60073-9_1

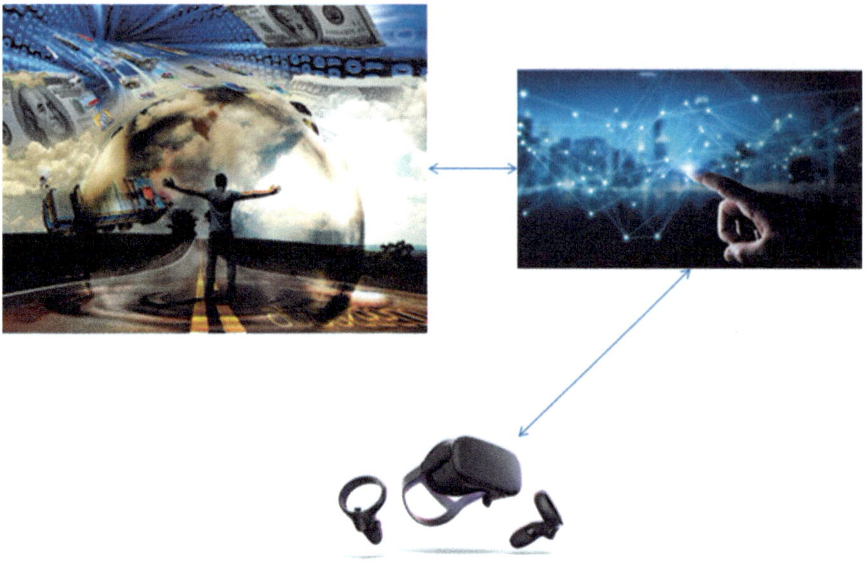

Fig. 1 The metaverse – bridging physical and virtual realities

Table 1 Key technologies underpinning the metaverse [3]

Technology	Description
Augmented reality (AR)	Overlays digital content onto the real-world view
Virtual reality (VR)	Immerses users in a computer-generated environment
3D environments	Three-dimensional simulated spaces for interaction

1.2 Historical Evolution and Technological Foundations

Tracing the evolution of the metaverse from its conceptual origins to contemporary advancements, this subsection sheds light on the historical context. Additionally, it explores the technological foundations that make the metaverse possible, such as blockchain, artificial intelligence, and advanced networking protocols [4].

The historical evolution and technological foundations of the metaverse for the healthcare industry highlight a journey from speculative fiction to tangible reality. As technologies such as virtual and augmented reality, artificial intelligence, blockchain, and advanced networking converge, the healthcare sector stands on the brink of a transformative era. Subsequent chapters will explore the practical applications, benefits, and challenges of integrating the metaverse into healthcare practices [5].

Table 2 outlines the historical evolution and technological foundations that have paved the way for the metaverse's integration into the healthcare industry.

Table 2 Outline of the historical evolution and technical fundamentals

Evolution stage	Key technological milestones
Emergence of the metaverse concept	Depicted in science fiction works like "snow crash" and "Neuromancer"
Early virtual and augmented reality	Development of head-mounted displays and interactive 3D environments
Evolution of networking and connectivity	Advancements in the internet and high-speed, low-latency networks
Convergence of technologies	Integration of powerful GPUs, spatial computing, and blockchain
Virtual and augmented reality in healthcare	Applications in medical education, surgery, and diagnostics
Artificial intelligence and machine learning	Utilization for data analysis, diagnostics, and personalized care
Blockchain for data security and interoperability	Ensuring secure, decentralized transactions and data integrity
Advanced networking and 5G	Propelling the potential of the metaverse in healthcare through improved connectivity

1.3 Emergence of the Metaverse Concept

The concept of the metaverse has its roots in science fiction and speculative fiction, with early visions depicted in works such as Neal Stephenson's "Snow Crash" (1992) [6] and William Gibson's "Neuromancer" (1984) [7]. These fictional depictions laid the conceptual groundwork for a shared, immersive virtual space that could transcend physical limitations [8].

1.4 Early Virtual Reality and Augmented Reality Technologies

The practical realization of the metaverse began with the development of early virtual reality and augmented reality technologies. In the 1960s and 1970s, pioneering efforts by Ivan Sutherland and his student, Jaron Lanier, led to the creation of the first head-mounted displays and interactive 3D environments [9]. These early developments laid the foundation for the immersive experiences that define the metaverse.

1.5 Evolution of Networking and Connectivity

As computing power and networking capabilities advanced, the idea of a connected virtual space gained momentum. The evolution of the Internet and the rise of high-speed, low-latency networks became crucial enablers for creating seamless, real-time interactions within the metaverse [10]. The transition from text-based communication to multimedia-rich content paved the way for a more immersive digital environment.

1.6 Convergence of Technologies

The late twentieth and early twenty-first centuries witnessed a convergence of technologies that would be integral to the metaverse. The development of powerful GPUs, spatial computing, and advanced sensors contributed to more realistic and interactive virtual experiences. Additionally, the emergence of blockchain technology introduced new possibilities for secure, decentralized transactions within the metaverse [11].

1.7 Virtual and Augmented Reality in Healthcare

In the healthcare industry, the adoption of virtual and augmented reality technologies has been transformative. Virtual reality simulations allow medical professionals to practice complex procedures in a risk-free environment, enhancing their skills and reducing the likelihood of errors. Augmented reality overlays digital information onto the physical world, offering applications in medical education, surgery, and diagnostics [12].

1.8 Artificial Intelligence and Machine Learning

The integration of artificial intelligence (AI) and machine learning (ML) plays a pivotal role in the metaverse for healthcare. AI algorithms can analyze vast amounts of medical data, assist in diagnostics, and personalize treatment plans. Machine learning models enhance the responsiveness and adaptability of virtual environments, making them more realistic and tailored to individual user interactions [13].

1.9 Blockchain for Data Security and Interoperability

Blockchain technology addresses critical issues of data security and interoperability within the metaverse for healthcare. By providing a decentralized and tamper-resistant ledger, blockchain ensures the integrity of medical records, protects patient privacy, and facilitates secure sharing of data across different healthcare entities [14]. This is particularly crucial in a sector where sensitive information must be handled with the utmost care.

1.10 Advanced Networking and 5G

The metaverse's seamless operation depends on advanced networking capabilities, and the advent of 5G technology further propels its potential in healthcare. High-speed, low-latency connectivity is essential for real-time communication, remote patient monitoring, and the delivery of immersive healthcare experiences. The combination of 5G and edge computing enhances the responsiveness of the metaverse applications, ensuring a smooth and latency-free user experience [15].

2 The Metaverse in the Healthcare System and Challenges

As the healthcare industry undergoes a transformative journey with the integration of the metaverse, understanding both its applications and the associated challenges is crucial. Striking a balance between technological innovation and ethical considerations will be pivotal in maximizing the positive impact of the metaverse technologies in healthcare. Subsequent chapters will further explore case studies, best practices, and emerging trends in this dynamic intersection [16].

2.1 Integration of the Metaverse in Healthcare

This section explores various applications where the metaverse is impacting healthcare practices, focusing on patient care, medical education, and research. Figure 2 shows the various applications of the metaverse in the healthcare process.

The integration of the metaverse technologies in the healthcare sector represents a paradigm shift, introducing innovative solutions to longstanding challenges [17]. This section delves into the various applications where the metaverse is making a significant impact on healthcare practices (Table 3).

2.2 Patient Care Applications

Telemedicine and Remote Consultations

The metaverse facilitates telemedicine by creating immersive virtual environments where patients can consult with healthcare professionals remotely. This is particularly valuable for individuals in remote locations or those with mobility challenges [19].

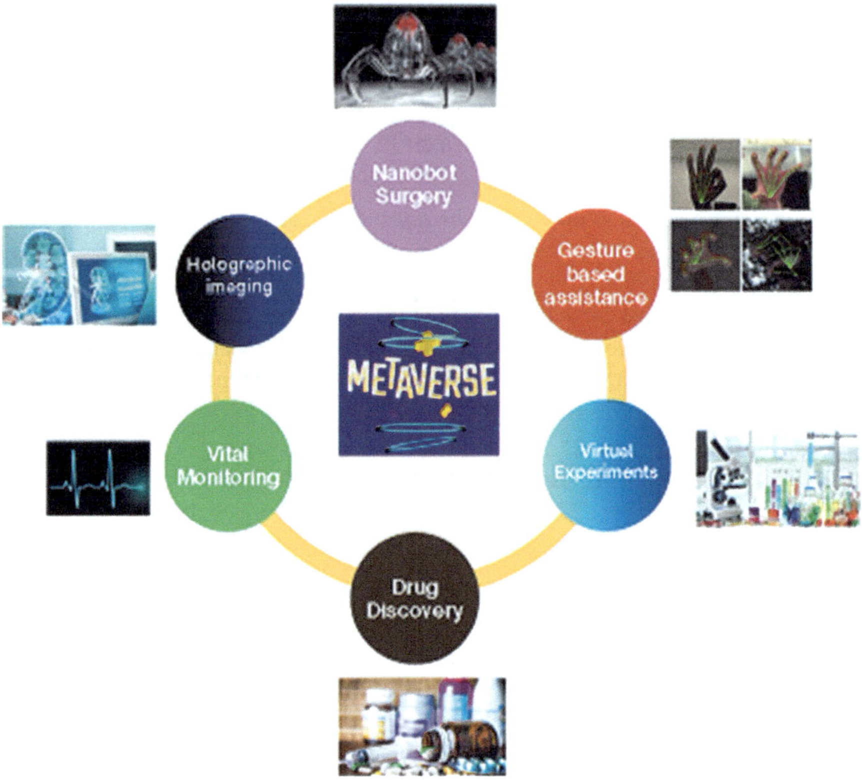

Fig. 2 Applications of the metaverse in healthcare

Table 3 Impact areas of the metaverse in healthcare [18]

Impact area	Description
Patient care applications	Enhancing accessibility through telemedicine and remote monitoring
Medical education and training	Simulation-based training for healthcare professionals
Research and development	Accelerating drug discovery and collaborative research environments

Remote Patient Monitoring

The metaverse technologies enable real-time monitoring of patients through wearable devices and sensors integrated into virtual environments. Healthcare providers can track vital signs, medication adherence, and other health metrics in a virtual setting [20].

Personalized Healthcare Experiences

By leveraging the metaverse, healthcare providers can offer personalized and interactive experiences for patients. Virtual reality (VR) environments can be tailored to individual patient needs, providing a more engaging and effective approach to healthcare delivery [21].

2.3 Medical Education and Training

Simulation-Based Training
The metaverse plays a crucial role in medical education by providing realistic simulation environments for training healthcare professionals. Virtual simulations allow medical students and practitioners to hone their skills in a risk-free and controlled setting [22].

Surgical Planning and Simulation
Surgeons can use virtual reality to plan and simulate complex surgical procedures. This application enhances surgical precision, reduces errors, and offers a platform for collaborative surgical training [23].

2.4 Research and Development

Drug Discovery and Testing
The metaverse technologies support virtual simulations for drug discovery, allowing researchers to explore molecular structures and test potential medications in a virtual space. This accelerates the drug development process and reduces the need for physical experiments [24].

Collaborative Research Environments
Virtual collaboration spaces within the metaverse enable researchers from different geographical locations to work together seamlessly. This fosters innovation and accelerates the pace of healthcare research [25].

3 Challenges and Ethical Considerations

Figure 3 outlines the key challenges and ethical considerations in integrating the metaverse into healthcare, emphasizing the importance of data security, regulatory frameworks, and ethical implications.

The integration of the metaverse in healthcare, while promising, brings forth a set of challenges and ethical considerations that necessitate careful examination [26] (Table 4).

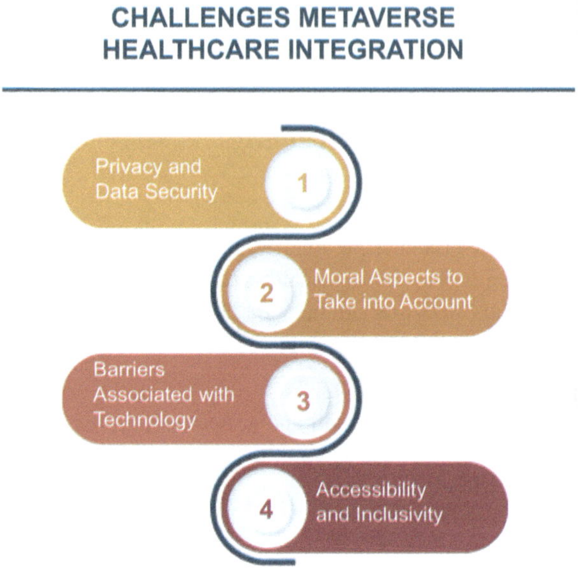
CHALLENGES METAVERSE
HEALTHCARE INTEGRATION
Privacy and
Data Security
1
2
Moral Aspects to
Take into Account
Barriers
Associated with
Technology
3
4
Accessibility
and Inclusivity

Fig. 3 Challenges and ethics in the metaverse healthcare integration

Table 4 Addressing challenges and ethical concerns

Challenge/concern	Mitigation strategies
Data security and privacy concerns	Implementation of robust encryption, decentralized solutions, and secures access controls
Regulatory frameworks and compliance	Development and implementation of standardized regulations and compliance with existing healthcare standards
Ethical implications	Establishment of ethical guidelines for informed consent in virtual environments and efforts toward digital inclusion

3.1 Data Security and Privacy Concerns

Protection of Sensitive Health Data

The metaverse involves the collection and storage of sensitive health data in virtual environments. Ensuring the security and privacy of this information is paramount to prevent unauthorized access and protect patient confidentiality [27].

Encryption and Decentralization

Addressing data security concerns involves implementing robust encryption mechanisms and exploring decentralized solutions, such as blockchain, to safeguard patient information and maintain data integrity [27].

3.2 *Regulatory Frameworks and Compliance*

Lack of Standardization
The absence of standardized regulations for the metaverse applications in healthcare poses a challenge. Developing and implementing regulatory frameworks is essential to ensure the responsible and ethical use of the metaverse technologies [28].

Compliance with Healthcare Standards
The metaverse applications must comply with existing healthcare standards to guarantee the quality and safety of healthcare services. Adhering to standards such as Health Insurance Portability and Accountability Act (HIPAA) is crucial for protecting patient rights [29].

3.3 *Ethical Implications*

Informed Consent in Virtual Environments
The immersive nature of the metaverse raises questions about obtaining informed consent from patients, especially in virtual clinical trials or treatment scenarios. Ethical guidelines must be established to address this challenge [30].

Digital Inclusion and Accessibility
Ensuring that all individuals, including those with disabilities or limited access to technology, can benefit from the metaverse-enabled healthcare services is a pressing ethical consideration. Efforts should be made to prevent the exacerbation of existing healthcare disparities [31].

4 Benefits of the Metaverse in the Healthcare Industry

The benefits of incorporating the metaverse into the healthcare industry are multifaceted, ranging from enhanced patient care experiences to revolutionary training opportunities for healthcare professionals. As technology continues to evolve, the metaverse stands as a transformative force, contributing to improved healthcare delivery, increased accessibility, and the continuous advancement of medical knowledge and skills. Subsequent chapters will explore case studies, implementation strategies, and emerging trends within this dynamic intersection of the metaverse and healthcare [19, 32].

4.1 Enhanced Patient Care

The integration of the metaverse technologies into healthcare practices brings forth a myriad of benefits, particularly in enhancing patient care. This section explores the applications and advantages of the metaverse in improving the overall patient experience.

4.2 Telemedicine and Remote Consultations

Accessibility and Reach
The metaverse-enabled telemedicine extends healthcare services to remote and underserved areas. Patients can access consultations with healthcare professionals, specialists, or mental health practitioners without geographical constraints.

Real-Time Monitoring
Virtual environments allow for real-time monitoring of patients' health conditions, enabling timely interventions and personalized care plans. Wearable devices and sensors in the metaverse contribute to continuous health tracking.

4.3 Personalized Healthcare Experiences

Tailored Treatment Plans
The metaverse enables the creation of personalized healthcare experiences, tailoring treatment plans to individual patient needs. VR environments can simulate therapeutic activities and exercises, enhancing engagement and adherence to treatment regimens.

Patient Education
Patients can access immersive educational content within the metaverse to better understand their health conditions, treatment options, and self-care practices. This contributes to increased health literacy and empowers patients to actively participate in their care.

4.4 Virtual Rehabilitation

Physiotherapy and Rehabilitation
The metaverse applications offer virtual rehabilitation programs, providing interactive exercises and simulations for patients undergoing physical therapy. This aids in the recovery process and promotes consistent engagement in rehabilitation activities.

Pain Management
Virtual reality environments can be used as distraction therapy for patients experiencing pain. By immersing patients in soothing or engaging virtual landscapes, the metaverse becomes a valuable tool for managing pain and discomfort.

4.5 Training and Simulation

The metaverse plays a pivotal role in revolutionizing medical education and training, offering realistic simulations and interactive learning experiences for healthcare professionals [33].

Simulation-Based Training: Realistic Scenarios
The metaverse-enabled simulations replicate real-world medical scenarios, allowing healthcare professionals to practice and refine their skills in a risk-free environment. This is particularly beneficial for high-stakes situations such as surgical procedures.

Team-Based Training
Virtual simulations in the metaverse facilitate team-based training scenarios, fostering collaboration among healthcare professionals. This enhances communication, coordination, and teamwork, which are critical aspects of delivering quality patient care.

4.6 Surgical Planning and Skill Enhancement

Precision in Surgical Procedures
Surgeons can use the metaverse for detailed surgical planning and practice, improving precision and reducing the likelihood of errors during actual procedures. Virtual reality simulations offer a platform for refining intricate surgical skills.

Continuous Professional Development
Healthcare professionals can engage in continuous learning and skill development through the metaverse-based training modules. This ensures that practitioners stay updated with the latest medical advancements and techniques.

5 Role of the Metaverse in Healthcare 4.0

The integration of the metaverse into Healthcare 4.0 represents a powerful convergence of technologies that holds the potential to revolutionize healthcare delivery [34]. The combination of immersive virtual experiences, advanced data analytics, and interconnected healthcare processes creates a synergistic ecosystem that enhances patient care, training, and overall healthcare outcomes. As the journey into this transformative intersection continues, future chapters will explore practical implementations, case studies, and emerging trends within this dynamic landscape.

5.1 *Healthcare 4.0 Overview*

The emergence of Healthcare 4.0 represents a transformative era in healthcare, driven by the integration of advanced technologies for improved efficiency, accessibility, and patient-centric care. This section provides a comprehensive overview of Healthcare 4.0 and its key components [35].

Digitization of Healthcare Processes: Electronic Health Records (EHRs)
Healthcare 4.0 emphasizes the digital transformation of patient records through the adoption of electronic health records. EHRs enable seamless data sharing among healthcare providers, leading to more informed decision-making and coordinated care [21, 36, 37].

Interconnected Devices and IoT
The integration of Internet of Things (IoT) devices facilitates real-time monitoring of patients, collecting data on vital signs, medication adherence, and other health metrics. This interconnected ecosystem enhances preventive care and early intervention [21, 36, 37].

5.2 *Artificial Intelligence and Data Analytics*

Predictive Analytics
Healthcare 4.0 leverages predictive analytics powered by artificial intelligence to forecast disease outbreaks, patient outcomes, and resource requirements. This proactive approach enhances the efficiency of healthcare delivery [38].

Personalized Medicine
Advanced data analytics enable the customization of treatment plans based on individual patient data, genomics, and lifestyle factors. This shift towards personalized medicine optimizes therapeutic outcomes and minimizes adverse effects [39].

5.3 *Telehealth and Remote Monitoring*

Remote Consultations
Telehealth services have become integral to Healthcare 4.0, allowing patients to access medical consultations remotely. This approach improves access to healthcare services, especially for individuals in rural or underserved areas [40].

Continuous Remote Monitoring
Healthcare 4.0 emphasizes continuous remote monitoring through wearable devices and sensors, enabling healthcare providers to track patient health in real time and intervene as needed [12].

5.4 Synergy Between the Metaverse and Healthcare 4.0

The integration of the metaverse with Healthcare 4.0 creates a synergistic relationship, amplifying the impact of both technologies and ushering in a new era of intelligent and immersive healthcare experiences [37, 41].

Virtual Health Records and Environments: Immersive Health Records
The metaverse enhances the visualization of health records by creating immersive and interactive virtual environments. Healthcare professionals can navigate through patient data in three-dimensional spaces, facilitating a more comprehensive understanding of medical information.

Virtual Consultation Spaces
The metaverse technologies complement Healthcare 4.0 by providing virtual spaces for remote consultations. Patients can engage with healthcare professionals in realistic virtual environments, fostering a sense of presence and enhancing the overall telehealth experience.

5.5 Training and Professional Development

Virtual Training Modules
The synergy between the metaverse and Healthcare 4.0 extends to training and professional development. Virtual reality simulations, augmented by Healthcare 4.0 data, offer realistic scenarios for continuous learning and skill enhancement among healthcare professionals.

Data-Driven Decision-Making
By integrating the metaverse technologies with Healthcare 4.0's data analytics, healthcare professionals can make informed, data-driven decisions. Virtual simulations can incorporate real-world patient data, improving the accuracy and relevance of training scenarios.

6 Conclusion

This chapter serves as a comprehensive exploration of the fundamental concepts surrounding the integration of the metaverse into the healthcare industry. By examining its historical evolution, technological foundations, challenges, benefits, and role in Healthcare 4.0, readers gain a nuanced understanding of the transformative potential the metaverse holds for shaping the future of healthcare. Subsequent chapters will delve deeper into specific applications, case studies, and emerging trends within this dynamic intersection.

References

1. Dolata, M., & Schwabe, G. (2023). What is the Metaverse and who seeks to define it? Mapping the site of social construction. *Journal of Information Technology, 9*, 02683962231159927.
2. Nevelsteen, K. J. (2018). Virtual world, defined from a technological perspective and applied to video games, mixed reality, and the metaverse. *Computer Animation and Virtual Worlds, 29*(1), e1752.
3. Knox, J. (2022). The metaverse, or the serious business of tech frontiers. *Postdigital Science and Education, 4*(2), 207–215.
4. Avsar, B. (2023). Historical process and theoretical foundations of metaverse starting from Web 1.0. In *Metaverse: Technologies, opportunities and threats* (pp. 1–18). Springer Nature.
5. Lv, Z., Shang, W. L., & Guizani, M. (2022). Impact of digital twins and Metaverse on cities: History, current situation, and application perspectives. *Applied Sciences, 12*(24), 12820.
6. Boehm, C. (2004). Hiro of the platonic: Neal Stephenson's snow crash. *Journal of the Fantastic in the Arts, 14*(56), 394–408.
7. Yadav S. *Cyberpunk's not dead: The enduring relevance of technological and spiritual motifs in William Gibson's Sprawl trilogy*. Doctoral dissertation, Birkbeck, University of London.
8. Barrera, K. G., & Shah, D. (2023). Marketing in the metaverse: Conceptual understanding, framework, and research agenda. *Journal of Business Research, 155*, 113420.
9. McLellan, H. (1996). Virtual realities. In *Handbook of research for educational communications and technology* (pp. 457–487).
10. Zhang, S., Lim, W. Y., Ng, W. C., Xiong, Z., Niyato, D., Shen, X. S., & Miao, C. (2023). Towards green metaverse networking: Technologies, advancements and future directions. *IEEE Network*.
11. Mystakidis, S. (2022). Metaverse. *Encyclopedia., 2*(1), 486–497.
12. Bhugaonkar, K., Bhugaonkar, R., & Masne, N. (2022). The trend of metaverse and augmented & virtual reality extending to the healthcare system. *Cureus., 14*(9).
13. Rospigliosi, P. A. (2022). Adopting the metaverse for learning environments means more use of deep learning artificial intelligence: This presents challenges and problems. *Interactive Learning Environments., 30*(9), 1573–1576.
14. Li, T., Yang, C., Yang, Q., Lan, S., Zhou, S., Luo, X., Huang, H., & Zheng, Z. (2023). Metaopera: A cross-metaverse interoperability protocol. *IEEE Wireless Communications., 30*(5), 136–143.
15. Kim, D. S., Lee, J. M., Nwakanma, C. I., & Tran-Dang, H. (2023). Campus-based test-bed implementation of 5G+ networks at the 28GHz band: Challenges and opportunities. *한국통신학회논문지, 48*(8), 1031–1048.

16. Musamih, A., Yaqoob, I., Salah, K., Jayaraman, R., Al-Hammadi, Y., Omar, M., & Ellahham, S. (2022). Metaverse in healthcare: Applications, challenges, and future directions. *IEEE Consumer Electronics Magazine*.
17. Ali, S., Abdullah, A. T. P., Athar, A., Hussain, A., Ali, M., Yaseen, M., Joo, M. I., & Kim, H. C. (2023). Metaverse in healthcare integrated with explainable ai and blockchain: Enabling immersiveness, ensuring trust, and providing patient data security. *Sensors, 23*(2), 565.
18. Li, J. (2022). Impact of metaverse cultural communication on the mental health of international students in China: Highlighting effects of healthcare anxiety and cyberchondria. *American Journal of Health Behavior, 46*(6), 809–820.
19. Tan, T. F., Li, Y., Lim, J. S., Gunasekeran, D. V., Teo, Z. L., Ng, W. Y., & Ting, D. S. (2022). Metaverse and virtual health care in ophthalmology: Opportunities and challenges. *The Asia-Pacific Journal of Ophthalmology, 11*(3), 237–246.
20. Sharma, M., & Sharma, S. (2023). A holistic approach to remote patient monitoring, fueled by ChatGPT and Metaverse technology: The future of nursing education. *Nurse Education Today, 131*, 105972.
21. Song, Y. T., & Qin, J. (2022). Metaverse and personal healthcare. *Procedia Computer Science*, (1), 189–197.
22. Rabotin, A., Glick, Y., Gelman, R., Ketko, I., Taran, B., Fink, N., & Furer, A. (2023). Practicing emergency medicine in the Metaverse: A novel mixed reality casualty care training platform. *Surgical Innovation, 30*(5), 586–594.
23. Pregowska, A., Osial, M., Dolega-Dolegowski, D., Kolecki, R., & Proniewska, K. (2022). Information and communication technologies combined with mixed reality as supporting tools in medical education. *Electronics, 11*(22), 3778.
24. Yang, D., Zhou, J., Chen, R., Song, Y., Song, Z., Zhang, X., Wang, Q., Wang, K., Zhou, C., Sun, J., & Zhang, L. (2022). Expert consensus on the metaverse in medicine. *Clinical eHealth, 5*, 1–9.
25. Schaf, F. M., Pereira, C. E., & Müller, D. (2010). Collaborative Environment Architecture Proposal: A study of virtual environments for learning purposes in control engineering. In *Proceedings of the international conference on remote engineering and virtual instrumentation (REV 2010)*. Stockholm.
26. Bang, J., & Kim, J. Y. (2023). Metaverse ethics for healthcare using AI technology: Challenges and risks. In *International conference on human-computer interaction* (pp. 367–378). Springer Nature.
27. Wylde, V., Prakash, E., Hewage, C., & Platts, J. (2023). Post-Covid-19 metaverse cybersecurity and data privacy: Present and future challenges. In *Data protection in a post-pandemic society: Laws, regulations, best practices and recent solutions* (pp. 1–48). Springer.
28. Uzun, M. M. (2023). Metaverse governance. In *Metaverse: Technologies, opportunities and threats* (pp. 231–244). Springer Nature.
29. Veras, M., Labbé, D. R., Furlano, J., Zakus, D., Rutherford, D., Pendergast, B., & Kairy, D. (2023). A framework for equitable virtual rehabilitation in the metaverse era: Challenges and opportunities. *Frontiers in Rehabilitation Sciences, 4*, 1241020.
30. Papagiannidis, S., Bourlakis, M., & Li, F. (2008). Making real money in virtual worlds: MMORPGs and emerging business opportunities, challenges and ethical implications in metaverses. *Technological Forecasting and Social Change, 75*(5), 610–622.
31. Kumar, V. (2023). Fintech. In *The economic value of digital disruption: A holistic assessment for CXOs* (pp. 111–229). Springer Nature.
32. Aljumaie, M., Chi Nguyen, H., Chu, N. H., Nguyen, C. T., Nguyen, D. N., Thai Hoang, D., & Dutkiewicz, E. (2023). Potential applications and benefits of metaverse. In *Metaverse communication and computing networks: Applications, technologies, and approaches* (pp. 17–37).
33. Holloway, D. (2012). Virtual worlds and health: Healthcare delivery and simulation opportunities. In *Virtual worlds and metaverse platforms: New communication and identity paradigms* (pp. 251–270). IGI Global.

34. Kumar, V., Joshi, K., Kumar, R., Anandaram, H., Bhagat, V. K., & Baloni, D. (2023). Multi modalities medical image fusion using deep learning and metaverse technology: Healthcare 4.0 a futuristic approach. *Biomedical and Pharmacology Journal, 16*(4).
35. Mozumder, M. A., Armand, T. P., Imtiyaj Uddin, S. M., Athar, A., Sumon, R. I., Hussain, A., & Kim, H. C. (2023). Metaverse for digital anti-aging healthcare: An overview of potential use cases based on artificial intelligence, blockchain, IoT technologies, its challenges, and future directions. *Applied Sciences, 13*(8), 5127.
36. Ullah, H., Manickam, S., Obaidat, M., Laghari, S. U., & Uddin, M. (2023). Exploring the potential of metaverse technology in healthcare: Applications, challenges, and future directions. *IEEEAccess*.
37. Dang, V. A., Vu Khanh, Q., Nguyen, V. H., Nguyen, T., & Nguyen, D. C. (2023). Intelligent healthcare: Integration of emerging technologies and internet of things for humanity. *Sensors, 23*(9), 4200.
38. Al Kuwaiti, A., Nazer, K., Al-Reedy, A., Al-Shehri, S., Al-Muhanna, A., Subbarayalu, A. V., Al Muhanna, D., & Al-Muhanna, F. A. (2023). A review of the role of artificial intelligence in healthcare. *Journal of Personalized Medicine, 13*(6), 951.
39. Koebe, P., & Bohnet-Joschko, S. (2023). The impact of digital transformation on inpatient care: Mixed methods study. *JMIR Public Health and Surveillance, 9*(1), e40622.
40. Mohamed, R. A., Mohammed, K. K., Darwish, A., & Hassanien, A. E. (2023). The use of metaverse in the healthcare sector: Analysis and applications. In *The future of metaverse in the virtual era and physical world* (pp. 77–91). Springer.
41. Liu, Z., Ren, L., Xiao, C., Zhang, K., & Demian, P. (2022). Virtual reality aided therapy towards health 4.0: A two-decade bibliometric analysis. *International Journal of Environmental Research and Public Health, 19*(3), 1525.

Intelligent Healthcare Systems in the Metaverse: Architecture, Applications, Challenges, and Opportunities

D. Lakshmi, Isha Kondurkar, Raj Kumar, and Roshni Banerjee

1 Introduction to the Metaverse

COVID-19 is poised to expedite and usher in a new era within the landscape of healthcare systems, with some of the transformative changes encompassing real-time monitoring, digital therapeutics, and remote health solutions [1, 2]. The healthcare industry has achieved significant breakthroughs through the development of technologies such as the metaverse, Medical Internet of Things (MIoT), real-time health monitoring, remote monitoring, cyber-physical systems (CPS), artificial intelligence of things (AIoT), augmented reality, virtual reality, Web 3.0, digital twin, big data analytics, blockchain, quantum computing, cloud computing, and robotics. A combination of these technologies can be termed a "Smart Healthcare System." Although these cutting-edge technologies enable precise and value-driven healthcare solutions, the metaverse enhances connectivity with physicians and healthcare experts worldwide, regardless of geographical distances [3, 4].

The term "metaverse" was coined and initially introduced in Neal Stevenson's 1992 science fiction novel "Snow Crash." It represented an alternate virtual reality universe constructed through computer-generated graphics, accessible to people

D. Lakshmi (✉) · I. Kondurkar
School of Computing Science and Engineering, VIT Bhopal University, Bhopal, Madhya Pradesh, India

R. Kumar
Data Science and Business Systems, School of Computing, SRM Institute of Science and Technology, Kattankulathur, Tamil Nadu, India
e-mail: rajkumar2@srmist.edu.in

R. Banerjee
School of Computing, SRM Institute of Science and Technology, Kattankulathur, Tamil Nadu, India
e-mail: rb9857@srmist.edu.in

C. L. Chowdhary (ed.), *The Metaverse for the Healthcare Industry*,
https://doi.org/10.1007/978-3-031-60073-9_2

worldwide through specialized goggles and headphones. The metaverse's infrastructure relied on a protocol known as the "Street," which interconnected various virtual neighborhoods and locations, analogous to the information superhighway. Within the metaverse, users could manifest themselves in customizable digital forms called "avatars." Although Stevenson's metaverse was digital and synthetic, the experiences within it had tangible effects on one's physical self. A forerunner to the metaverse in literature is William Gibson's VR cyberspace, referred to as the "Matrix," from his 1984 science fiction novel "Neuromancer." In the realm of virtual reality, the metaverse was conceived as the 3D Internet or "Web 3.0." [5–8].

The integration of the metaverse into the healthcare system holds the promise of addressing substantial healthcare disparities resulting from a lack of specialized medical professionals and geographical obstacles to traditional healthcare access. Moreover, it can offer patients rapid personalized care that is highly accessible and minimizes concerns related to stigma and privacy [9].

There are three primary therapeutic categories based on treatment methods. Cognitive behavioral therapy delivered through digital platforms has proven effective in addressing central nervous system disorders, including conditions like sleep disorders, depression, anxiety, post-traumatic stress disorder, addiction (alcohol and drugs), pain management, and panic disorders. For systemic diseases like diabetes, cancer, and hypertension, where lifestyle improvements play a significant role, as well as for illnesses that require effective management of seriously ill patients, a lifestyle modification approach is applied. Digital therapies focused on medication management are utilized for chronic diseases that necessitate long-term, consistent medication use, such as asthma, chronic obstructive pulmonary disease, and schizophrenia. Furthermore, digital therapies are in development for conditions like amblyopia, neurological damage resulting from stroke and traumatic injuries, and attention deficit hyperactivity disorder, utilizing neuro-rehabilitation techniques [10–12].

"Meridius" stands as a healthcare research platform rooted in the metaverse. It was established in 2015 by a team of medical professionals. The primary function lies in enabling the collaborative sharing of healthcare data among researchers, aiming to harness collective efforts in the search for innovative treatment options. Solve.Care, a global frontrunner in Web3 and metaverse-driven healthcare solutions, is dedicated to revolutionizing healthcare systems on a worldwide scale. Recognizing the inherent challenges and inadequacies of the existing healthcare infrastructure, they embarked on the journey to create Solve.Care. In times of illness, patients and their loved ones often find themselves trapped in an unending cycle of attempting to coordinate medical care. This realization inspired Solve.Care to pioneer a patient-centric system that fosters seamless communication among individuals, empowering them to take control of their health insurance, healthcare, and financial matters [13].

In the age of the metaverse, digital twins play a pivotal role in patient-specific modeling, medical education, remote monitoring, drug development, healthcare system efficiency, surgical preparation, rehabilitation, chronic disease management, behavioral health, staffing, patient care models, and operational strategies. Some notable platforms for implementing digital twin solutions include AWS IoT Twin-Maker, Azure Digital Twins, Google Supply Chain Twin, and NVIDIA Omniverse Enterprise, as mentioned in Ref. [14].

2 The Architecture of Web3-Based Metaverse Healthcare System

The architectural framework of a healthcare system within the metaverse operates on a Web3-based platform. The entire framework is segmented into multiple phases.

To gather, transmit, and analyze information on patient's health and well-being, the medical Internet of Things (MIoT) incorporates Internet-connected devices and sensors into healthcare and medicine. By allowing data processing to take place on or close to the devices, edge computing reduces the demand on the network's capacity. IoT and AI are combined to create AIoT, which improves data analysis and decision-making skills. Additionally, employing healthcare data standards like HL7 and simple encryption methods like AES, data standardization, and encryption assure interoperability.

Now, creating a bidirectional cloud-based healthcare data gateway makes it easier for patients, healthcare practitioners, and cloud-based systems to exchange information. A patient's medical history is digitally represented in an electronic health record (EHR), and authentication and authorization are essential for limiting access to resources.

A promising approach to improving data security and integrity inside the healthcare system is blockchain technology. The ability to connect to blockchain networks and communicate with decentralized applications is provided by Web3 interfaces. Stakeholder interactions, alarm systems, and data visualization can all help to improve patient outcomes, the healthcare experience, and the security and safety of virtual healthcare settings. Figure 1 illustrates the architectural framework.

1. **Data Acquisition System**

Systems using the Internet of Things (IoT) often have a complicated architecture that connects several sorts of devices to offer the user a particular service [15]. The Medical Internet of Things (MIoT) [16] refers to the integration of Internet-connected devices and sensors into the field of healthcare and medicine. These devices, often referred to as "smart" or "IoT-enabled" medical devices, are designed to collect, transmit, and analyze data related to patients' health and well-being. MIoT encompasses a wide range of devices, including wearable fitness trackers, smartwatches, blood pressure monitors, glucose meters, implantable medical devices, and even smartphone applications that can collect health-related data.

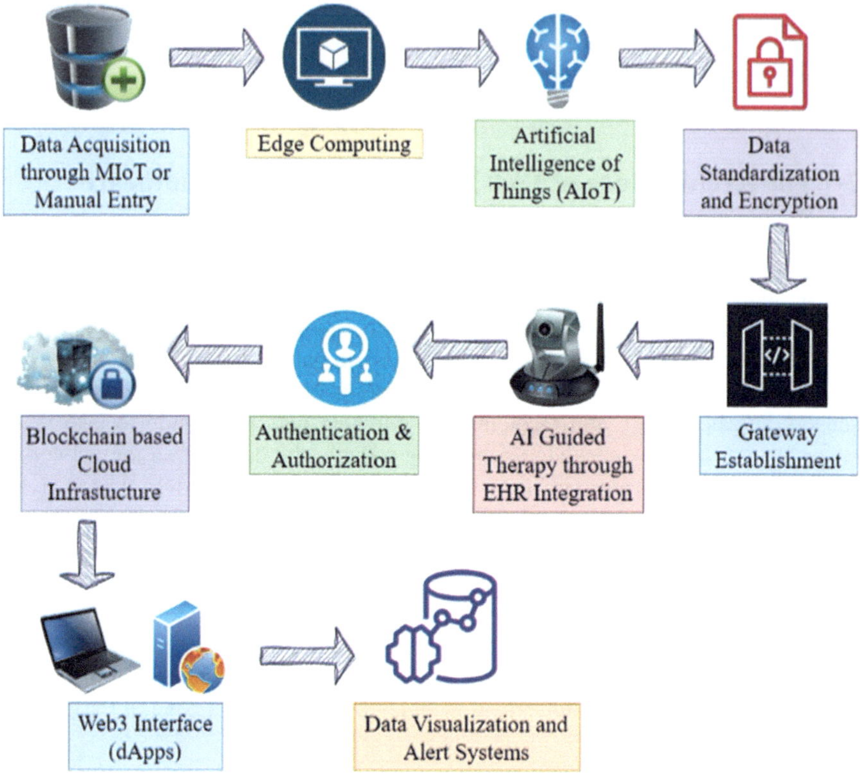

Fig. 1 The architecture of the metaverse healthcare system

2. **Edge Computing**

Edge computing places computing resources closer to where data is generated or consumed. Instead of sending IoT data back to a data center or cloud, edge computing, a technique for computing on-site where data is received or used, allows IoT data to be captured and processed at the edge [17]. Edge computing enables data processing to occur on or near the devices or "edges" of the network. Edge computing can alleviate the strain on network bandwidth by processing data locally. This is especially valuable in scenarios where transmitting large amounts of data to a central server is impractical or costly.

3. **Artificial Intelligence of Things (AIoT)**

Artificial intelligence of things (AIoT) [18] is an emerging technological concept that combines artificial intelligence (AI) and the Internet of Things (IoT) to create a more intelligent and autonomous system of connected devices. AIoT leverages the capabilities of AI, such as machine learning, deep learning, and natural language processing, to enhance the data analysis and decision-making capabilities of IoT devices and systems.

4. **Data Standardization and Encryption**

Standardize data formats and protocols to ensure interoperability. Using healthcare data standards like HL7 (Health Level Seven (HL7): Standard for healthcare electronic data transmissions for clinical data exchange). Implement strong encryption mechanisms (e.g., SSL/TLS) to secure data in transit and at rest. Implementation of the lightweight data encryption technology (the Advanced Encryption Standard (AES)) to maintain data confidentiality. Using lightweight encryption techniques, the healthcare data are stored in the cloud. The Advanced Encryption Standard (AES) is one of the ultralightweight cryptographic techniques with a verified track record.

5. **Establishing a Gateway**

Implementing a gateway for sending and receiving bidirectional cloud-based healthcare data involves setting up a secure, reliable, and compliant infrastructure to facilitate the exchange of health-related information between healthcare providers, patients, and cloud-based systems.

6. **EHR Integration**

Electronic health records [19] are digital representations of a patient's medical history. A health record is assembled, created, and stored electronically using an EHR. If your gateway interacts with electronic health record (EHR) systems, ensure seamless integration with various EHR vendors and platforms commonly used in the healthcare industry.

7. **Authentication and Authorization**

Authentication and authorization [20] are two critical aspects of information security that are fundamental to controlling access to computer systems, networks, applications, and data. They work together to ensure that only authorized users can access resources while maintaining the confidentiality, integrity, and availability of those resources. Multifactor authentication (MFA) [21] is a security mechanism that requires users to provide two or more different authentication factors to verify their identity before granting access to a system, application, or data. MFA enhances security by adding additional layers of verification beyond just a username and password.

8. **Blockchain-Based Data Security and Cloud Infrastructure**

Data security in healthcare is of paramount importance due to the sensitive and personal nature of medical information. Technologies like Blockchain, smart contracts, and non-fungible tokens (NFTs) enable data security and data privacy [22]. Blockchain technology [23] offers a promising solution to enhance data security and integrity within the healthcare system. Any data-driven firm recognizes the need to manage data security, storage, transactions, and integration securely. Blockchain technology can effectively address these pressing problems. This includes blockchain-based applications for data management, data storage on cloud-

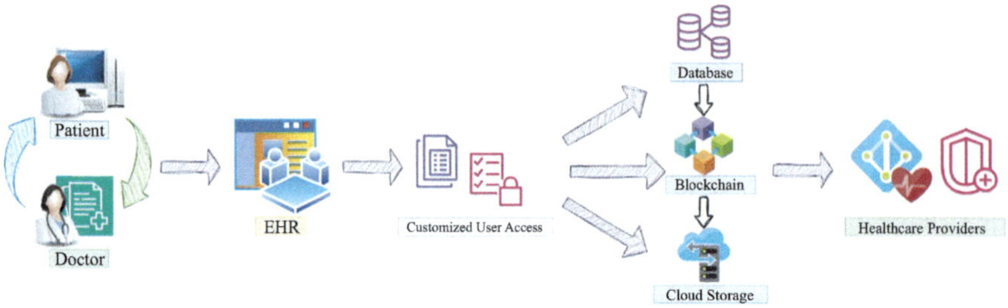

Fig. 2 Blockchain based data security and cloud storage

based services, and electronic health records (EHRs). Patients' interactions with their doctors and specialists generate primary data. This information includes a person's medical background, current health issues, and other physiological details. Each patient's EHR is constructed utilizing the primary information gathered in the first phase. The EHR also contains additional medical data, such as that obtained via nursing care, medical imaging, and drug usage history. Only the owner of this property is granted personalized access control for each patient who owns a sensitive EHR. The EHR owner will select who will be given access after receiving requests for access from parties who wish to view such priceless data. Distributed records are stored in databases and cloud storage, while a blockchain offers exceptional privacy to guarantee tailored, legitimate user access. Ad hoc clinics, community care centers, and hospitals are examples of healthcare providers who are the final users who seek to gain access to a secure delivery of service that will be approved by the owner. For instance, any health record will be visible and accessible on your phone and verified through a distributed ledger like blockchain, to which healthcare professionals will continue to add over time, regardless of where you are treated in the world. The figure depicts the blockchain-based data security and cloud storage system for the healthcare system (Fig. 2).

Identifying a cloud service provider (e.g., AWS, Azure, Google Cloud, and Oracle) that complies with healthcare data security, federated learning, and privacy regulations [24]. Ensure the selected cloud platform supports the necessary services for data storage, processing, and transmission.

9. **Web3 Interface**

A Web3 interface refers to the interaction and communication layer between web applications (front end) and blockchain networks (typically Ethereum) or decentralized applications (dApps) [25]. Web3 interfaces enable web applications to connect to blockchain networks, read data from them, and send transactions or smart contract interactions. This is a fundamental component for building and interacting with blockchain-based decentralized applications.

10. **Data Visualization, Alert System, and Stakeholder Interactions**

The graphical depiction of information and data pictorially or graphically is known as data visualization. Incorporating data visualization, a healthcare alert system [26], and managing stakeholder interactions within the metaverse can significantly enhance the healthcare experience, improve patient outcomes, and ensure the safety and security of virtual healthcare environments. A healthcare alert system in the metaverse plays a critical role in patient safety, emergency response, and healthcare communication. Effective stakeholder interactions within the metaverse healthcare are essential for patient care, safety, and collaborative work with patient caregivers, healthcare providers, healthcare administrators, regulatory bodies, and technology providers.

3 The Metaverse in Healthcare: Use Cases

A metaverse dedicated to "Medical Technology and AI" (MeTAI) can optimize the workflows within AI-driven medical practices, specifically in areas like medical imaging-based diagnosis and therapy. It does so by facilitating the development, testing, evaluation, regulation, adaptation, and enhancement of these technologies. Wang et al. [27] presented a MeTAI ecosystem, focusing on its four primary healthcare applications: virtual comparative scanning, raw data sharing, augmented regulatory science, and the metaverse medical intervention. The subsequent section presents a detailed case study within this metaverse. The metaverse holds a central position within the digital healthcare ecosystem across various domains, including senior care, vascular health, extended and chronic illness management, dentistry, gynecology, oncology, ophthalmology, mental health, physical health, emergency care, as well as medical education and training. In the forthcoming section, we present a few use cases where the metaverse is applied in the realm of digital healthcare.

3.1 Digital Therapeutics for Urology

In the field of urology, there is a significant focus on the development and research of digital therapeutics, which encompass various technologies such as mobile applications, bladder devices, pelvic floor muscle trainers, intelligent toilet systems, mixed reality-assisted training, and surgical procedures, as well as telemedicine for urological consultations. This chapter aims to offer a comprehensive summary of the current influence of the metaverse on digital therapeutics and to outline its existing trends, uses, and prospects within the realm of urology [28].

3.2 The Metaverse in Cancer Care

Moztarzadeh et al. [29] proposed a framework based on digital twins using a machine-learning approach for cancer care. The study examined how a virtual psychological support group in the metaverse impacts the emotional well-being of breast cancer survivors. Six survivors participated, discussing their experiences under the guidance of psycho-oncologists. Before and after the sessions, emotional dimensions and intensity were assessed. The study found that participants gained better emotional control and reduced negative emotions like fear and sadness. The experience in the metaverse was engaging, and the findings suggest potential emotional benefits in using immersive environments for psychological support in this context [30].

3.3 The Metaverse in Fetal Medicine and Gynecology

The metaverse presents significant potential for fostering collaboration among multidisciplinary teams in comprehending fetal malformations through the analysis of ultrasound and magnetic resonance imaging (MRI) files. The identification of fetal abnormalities can be a laborious task. Still, with the utilization of the metaverse as a digital tool, this can be accomplished without the hindrance of geographical limitations [31]. The metaverse represents a non-pharmacological approach aimed at assisting expectant mothers in managing anxiety during pregnancy and pain during labor. Through the provision of education on medical procedures for expectant mothers, facilitating virtual connections between the mother and her unborn child, and redirecting patients' focus away from pain signals during pregnancy [32].

3.4 The Metaverse Medical Education and Training

Orthopedics, which is dedicated to preserving and enhancing the functionality of the skeletal system, including joints, muscles, and the spine, can benefit from the integration of the metaverse. This technology can find applications in medical education, training, patient care, and clinical practice, with a specific focus on orthopedics and rehabilitation, fields closely linked to musculoskeletal health issues. The study also underscores the diverse elements of the metaverse, including virtual and augmented reality, and their potential applications across various medical contexts. These applications encompass training students in clinical skills for rare scenarios, enhancing the safety of clinicians during invasive procedures, and enabling remote teaching [33].

4 The Metaverse in Healthcare: Use Cases

4.1 *Ethical Challenges*

Although the metaverse offers several advantages for healthcare, it also gives rise to ethical considerations. These ethical concerns encompass matters concerning patient confidentiality and data security during virtual consultations. The privacy and security of patient information within the metaverse is a substantial barrier because healthcare data is extremely sensitive. It is crucial to protect against data breaches, unauthorized access, and cyberattacks.

The possibility of biased algorithms in AI-powered healthcare solutions raises another concern. The possibility for depersonalization, loss of the human element in healthcare interactions, and the danger of technology dependence too much in virtual healthcare present ethical concerns. Additionally, not all patients have access to the necessary technology or high-speed Internet required for a seamless metaverse healthcare experience. This can lead to disparities in healthcare access [34]. Thus, it is imperative to guarantee equitable access to these technologies for all patients.

Another and one of the major challenges in visible sight is that people need to be more confident in the healthcare metaverse because it is a new field that is just starting. People tend to trust doctors more than they do AI-based holograms and avatars. By raising the standard of the metaverse healthcare offerings, procedures, and diagnostic tools, the trust gap between patients and the metaverse should be bridged.

4.2 *Benefits*

1. **Telemedicine and Remote Consultation**

A better way to access specialists, remote monitoring, medical education, and assistance for mental health are all made possible by the integration of the metaverse into the healthcare industry. It can improve data visualization, cross geographical boundaries, and promote teamwork. To fully realize the potential of the metaverse-based healthcare solutions, technical needs, ethical issues, and the necessity for seamless electronic health record integration must also be taken into account.

2. **Immersive Medical Training and Simulation**

Healthcare workers can practice difficult procedures, surgeries, and diagnostics in highly realistic, interactive environments thanks to immersive medical training and simulation in the metaverse. It promotes skill development, encourages experience learning, and permits safe experimentation, ultimately raising the standard of healthcare education and training.

3. **Connectivity for People**

   A patient's ability to interact with medical professionals, support groups, and other patients virtually is referred to as a people connection in the metaverse. Patients can join online support groups, go to telehealth consultations with medical specialists, and interact with people who have had or have health concerns comparable to their own. Compared to typical online communication methods, patients can engage in more immersive and engaging dialogue, share information, and seek emotional support. This could improve their healthcare experience and sense of community, particularly when physical proximity is not practical or convenient.

4. **Transparency**

   Increased transparency in the healthcare industry is one of the metaverse's main advantages. Patients are better able to access their medical information, available treatments, and healthcare expenses thanks to this, leading to a more educated and empowered patient experience. Additionally, it can promote data sharing and transparency in medical research, which will ultimately improve patient outcomes and foster greater collaboration in healthcare decision-making.

5. **Effective Collaboration Among the Stakeholders and Healthcare Professionals**

   It is an essential benefit of using the metaverse in healthcare. Breaking down geographic barriers enables immersive, real-time, multidisciplinary communication and cooperation. To improve patient care, research outcomes, and the effectiveness of the healthcare system, healthcare practitioners, researchers, and administrators can work together seamlessly, share insights, and make informed decisions. With improved connectivity and collaboration, healthcare delivery and treatment modalities progress and innovate.

6. **Reduced Travel Costs and Efforts**

   Both patient and healthcare provider travel expenses and time can be considerably decreased with the help of the metaverse in healthcare. Without having to travel to healthcare institutions, patients can get virtual medical consultations and services, saving time and money on transportation. Similar to this, healthcare providers can hold online conferences, meetings, and training sessions without the need for actual travel, increasing accessibility and decreasing costs for all parties. When in-person visits are not required for routine care or consultations, this decrease in travel-related burdens is especially beneficial.

4.3 Limitations

Although the metaverse brings several benefits, it poses several limitations as well. Careful consideration and addressing of these limitations are crucial for realizing the full potential of the metaverse while mitigating its drawbacks. Some of the limitations are mentioned below.

1. **Network and Internet Connectivity**

The seamless delivery of services in the metaverse may be hampered by network and Internet connectivity issues, particularly in areas with weak infrastructure. To guarantee equal access to virtual healthcare, problems including latency, bandwidth needs, and accessibility difficulties in remote places must be solved [35]. Investments in infrastructure and technology are critical for maximizing the potential of the metaverse in healthcare.

2. **Human–Computer Interface**

The depth of communication and diagnosis can be hampered by constraints in haptic feedback, facial expressions, and body language recognition, even when virtual environments try to mimic real-world interactions [36]. For a more thorough and productive healthcare experience in the metaverse, it is crucial to bridge this divide between virtual and real-life interactions.

3. **Interactive Sensors**

While virtual environments can emulate many parts of the physical world, there are limitations to how well they can imitate the tactile input and sensory data collected by actual medical instruments. The precision and realism of medical simulations and diagnoses within the metaverse may be impacted by this [37]. To improve the authenticity of healthcare experiences in virtual worlds, advancements in sensor technology and haptic feedback integration are required.

4. **Necessary Training and Education for the Healthcare Professionals**

To ensure their proficiency and efficacy in virtual healthcare settings, healthcare practitioners in the metaverse must have the necessary training and education. Healthcare professionals require training in utilizing immersive technology, navigating virtual environments, and adjusting to new user interfaces for patient interactions and medical procedures. This includes mastering communication techniques for virtual consultations, comprehending data security and privacy regulations particular to the metaverse, and learning how to use virtual reality (VR) and augmented reality (AR) equipment [38]. The need for ongoing education and skill development will become increasingly important as technology develops to suit the needs of the metaverse's healthcare sector.

5. **Regulatory Policies and Procedures**

There may be a lack of clarity regarding compliance, data security, and patient privacy because of how rapidly virtual healthcare is developing in the metaverse and possibly outpacing the creation of full rules. It is an issue that calls for continual adaptation and cooperation between regulatory and healthcare organizations to strike the correct balance between promoting innovation and protecting patient safety within the limits of current regulatory frameworks [39].

6. **Privacy and Data Security**

There is a higher danger of data breaches and privacy violations as sensitive patient information is shared and maintained in virtual environments. It is crucial to ensure strong encryption, authentication, and adherence to legal requirements for the safety of medical data [40]. The metaverse still faces a significant issue in balancing the advantages of immersive healthcare encounters with the requirement for strict data security measures.

7. **Content Accuracy and Quality of the Transmission**

For patient safety, it is essential to make sure that medical information, diagnoses, and treatment suggestions are appropriately communicated in virtual settings [34]. Technical problems like slowness or malfunctions could prevent the transfer of crucial medical information and reduce the effectiveness of online healthcare exchanges. To get over these restrictions and establish trust in the metaverse-based healthcare services, we must strive for high standards of content accuracy and smooth transmission.

8. **Interoperability Issues**

To handle the metaverse healthcare system, high-end technical infrastructure is required for the content accuracy and the quality of data transmission. The metaverse's immersive healthcare applications demand robust hardware and networks to ensure that medical simulations and educational content are not only accurate but also delivered seamlessly to healthcare professionals and patients alike. This infrastructure is essential to support the immersive nature of healthcare experiences within the metaverse, but it also presents a considerable investment and logistical challenge for healthcare institutions and technology providers. Addressing these technical demands will be pivotal in realizing the full potential of the metaverse in healthcare [35].

5 Result, Discussion, and Future Scope

The metaverse can provide a more cost-effective and efficient way to train healthcare professionals. For example, medical students can use the metaverse to practice complex procedures in a virtual environment without putting patients at risk. Additionally, the metaverse can be used to train healthcare professionals on new equipment and therapeutics without having to purchase or transport expensive equipment. The metaverse can also transform clinical trials by making them more accessible and convenient for patients. Patients can participate in clinical trials from the comfort of their own homes, which can save them time and money on travel. Additionally, the metaverse can be used to monitor patients' health remotely during clinical trials, which can help to improve patient safety and data collection. NFTs can be used to tokenize medical records, prescriptions, and medical bills. This can help to improve the security and portability of medical data. For example, patients could use NFTs to share their medical records with different healthcare providers without having to worry about the data being lost or stolen.

In the future, regulatory policies and procedures [41] must evolve to keep pace with the rapid evolution of virtual healthcare in the metaverse. Privacy and data security issues should be addressed through strong encryption and compliance with legal requirements. Content accuracy and quality of delivery are critical to patient safety and trust. Fundamentally, the role of the metaverse in healthcare is poised to usher in a new era of patient-centered, collaborative, and technologically advanced healthcare. Digital twins can be used to create personalized treatment plans for patients based on their individual genetic makeup and medical history. Doctors could use the metaverse to visualize a patient's digital twin [42] in 3D, which would allow them to better understand the patient's anatomy and physiology. Finally, interoperability issues represent the logistical challenges that need to be overcome to realize the full potential of the medical metaverse.

P4 medicine, a conceptual framework within the healthcare field, is steadily gaining traction for its real-world application. The four "P"s represent participatory, personalized, predictive, and preventive medicine, as elucidated [43]. Of these four "P"s, participatory medicine can seamlessly integrate with the metaverse solutions. Participatory medicine signifies a movement in which patients and healthcare professionals actively cooperate and mutually support each other as equal partners in healthcare. The metaverse has the potential to provide a solution for advancing participatory medicine.

The integration of the metaverse into the healthcare industry represents a transformative leap towards a more accessible, efficient, and patient-centered healthcare system. This digital evolution, driven by cutting-edge technologies such as the medical Internet of Things (MIoT), artificial intelligence of things (AIoT), blockchain, and Web3 interfaces, is poised to revolutionize healthcare across multiple sectors [44]. The metaverse has the potential to revolutionize healthcare in several ways. The metaverse could help to improve access to care, enhance medical training and simulation [45], increase transparency, promote data sharing and collaboration, provide personalized and proactive care, improve patient engagement, and reduce healthcare costs. Through various chapters, effective collaboration among stakeholders improves patient care, research outcomes, and health system efficiency. Additionally, reduced transportation costs and labor benefit both patients and healthcare professionals. The potential for biased algorithms and depersonalization in AI-powered healthcare [46] solutions must be closely monitored. However, the medical metaverse also has ethical challenges and limitations that must be addressed. Health data is highly sensitive, so maintaining patient confidentiality and data security during virtual visits is paramount. Despite the challenges, the potential benefits in terms of improved access, education, and patient outcomes are significant. The healthcare industry, along with technology providers, regulators, and healthcare professionals, must work together to overcome these challenges and harness the full potential of the metaverse to transform healthcare for the better.

6 Conclusion

The early stages of the metaverse-driven healthcare solutions present numerous hurdles, including the need for substantial investments, advanced technological infrastructure, a range of technical experts, adherence to regulatory standards, the development of policies and procedures, ethical frameworks, professional training, engagement with stakeholders, security concerns, and ensuring patient access to the metaverse. The metaverse-based supervisory control system can operate with a central data storage and control system. As a result, multiple specialists will be able to collaborate to make critical decisions together. The system creates an expert-monitored competent care environment with real-time monitoring across the globe. In addition, the system reduces the risk of infection among healthcare workers. The design of a blockchain-based Web3, AI-enabled, digital twin-based, Web3-based supervisory control system utilizing biomedical sensors and wearable medical devices accessible over the local network and the public cloud is essential for the metaverse-based sustainable solutions.

References

1. Kapoor, A., Guha, S., Kanti Das, M., Goswami, K. C., & Yadav, R. (2020). Digital healthcare: The only solution for better healthcare during COVID-19 pandemic? *Indian Heart Journal, 72*(2), 61–64. Author, F., Author, S.: Title of a proceedings paper. In: Editor, F., Editor, S. (eds.) Conference 2016, LNCS, vol. 9999, pp. 1–13. Springer (2016).
2. Alshamrani, M. (2022). IoT and artificial intelligence implementations for remote healthcare monitoring systems: A survey. *Journal of King Saud University – Computer and Information Sciences, 34*(8), 4687–4701.
3. Chen D., & Zhang R. (2022). *Exploring research trends of emerging technologies in health metaverse: A bibliometric analysis*. Available at SSRN3998068. https://doi.org/10.2139/ssrn.3998068.
4. Yang, Y., Siau, K., Xie, W., & Sun, Y. (2022). Smart health: Intelligent healthcare systems in the metaverse, artificial intelligence, and data science era. *Journal of Organizational and End User Computing (JOEUC), 34*(1), 1–14. https://doi.org/10.4018/JOEUC.308814
5. Stephenson, N. (2003). *Snow crash: A novel*. Spectra.
6. Mystakidis, S. (2022). Metaverse. *Metaverse Encyclopedia, 2*(1), 486–497.
7. Dionisio, J. D. N., Iii, W. G. B., & Gilbert, R. (2013). 3D virtual worlds and the metaverse: Current status and future possibilities. *ACM Computing Surveys (CSUR), 45*(3), 1–38.
8. Kapp, K. M., & O'Driscoll, T. (2010). *Learning in 3D: Adding a new dimension to enterprise learning and collaboration*. Pfeiffer & Company.
9. Aapro, M., Bossi, P., Dasari, A., Fallowfield, L., Gascón, P., Geller, M., et al. (2020). Digital health for optimal supportive care in oncology: Benefits, limits, and future perspectives. *Supportive Care in Cancer, 28*, 4589–4612.
10. Khirasaria, R., Singh, V., & Batta, A. (2020). Exploring digital therapeutics: The next paradigm of modern health-care industry. *Perspectives in Clinical Research, 11*(2), 54.
11. Lutz, J., Offidani, E., Taraboanta, L., Lakhan, S. E., & Campellone, T. R. (2022). Appropriate controls for digital therapeutic clinical trials: A narrative review of control conditions in clinical trials of digital therapeutics (DTx) deploying psychosocial, cognitive, or behavioral content. *Frontiers in Digital Health, 4*, 823977.

12. Phan, P., Mitragotri, S., & Zhao, Z. (2023). Digital therapeutics in the clinic. *Bioengineering & Translational Medicine*, e10536.
13. Metaverse Healthcare Platforms. (2023). https://metaverseofthing.com/metaverse/metaverse-web3-healthcare-startups/
14. Turab, M., & Jamil, S. (2023). A comprehensive survey of digital twins in healthcare in the era of metaverse. *BioMedInformatics, 3*(3), 563–584.
15. Akhtar, N. (2021, April 16). *A holistic analysis of Medical Internet of Things (MIoT)*. https://hal.science/hal-03226578
16. Dimitrov, D. (2016). Medical internet of things and big data in healthcare. *Healthcare Informatics Research, 22*(3), 156. https://doi.org/10.4258/hir.2016.22.3.156
17. Hassan, N., Gillani, S., Ahmed, E., Yaqoob, I., & Imran, M. (2018). The role of edge computing in internet of things. *IEEE Communications Magazine, 56*(11), 110–115. https://doi.org/10.1109/mcom.2018.1700906
18. Baker, S., & Wang, X. (2023). Artificial intelligence of things for smarter healthcare: A survey of advancements, challenges, and opportunities. *IEEE Communications Surveys and Tutorials, 25*(2), 1261–1293. https://doi.org/10.1109/comst.2023.3256323
19. Seymour, T., Frantsvog, D., & Graeber, T. (2012). Electronic health records (EHR). *American Journal of Health Sciences, 3*(3), 201–210. https://doi.org/10.19030/ajhs.v3i3.7139
20. Kim, H., & Lee, E. A. (2017). Authentication and authorization for the internet of things. *IT Professional, 19*(5), 27–33. https://doi.org/10.1109/mitp.2017.3680960
21. Ibrokhimov, S., Hui, K. L., Al-Absi, A. A., Lee, H. J., & Sain, M. (2019). Multi-factor authentication in cyber physical system: A state of art survey 2019. In *21st International Conference on Advanced Communication Technology (ICACT)*. https://doi.org/10.23919/icact.2019.8701960
22. Ullah, H., Manickam, S., Obaidat, M., Laghari, S. U. A., & Uddin, M. (2023). *Exploring the potential of metaverse technology in healthcare: Applications, challenges, and future directions*. IEEE Access.
23. Nofer, M., Gomber, P., Hinz, O., & Schiereck, D. (2017). Blockchain. *Business & Information Systems Engineering, 59*(3), 183–187. https://doi.org/10.1007/s12599-017-0467-3
24. Casola, V., Castiglione, A., Choo, K. R., & Esposito, C. (2016). Healthcare-related data in the cloud: Challenges and opportunities. *IEEE Cloud Computing, 3*(6), 10–14. https://doi.org/10.1109/mcc.2016.139
25. Zheng, G., Gao, L., Huang, L., & Guan, J. (2020). Decentralized application (DAPP). In *Springer eBooks* (pp. 253–280). https://doi.org/10.1007/978-981-15-6218-1_9
26. Gotz, D., & Borland, D. (2016). Data-driven healthcare: Challenges and opportunities for interactive visualization. *IEEE Computer Graphics and Applications, 36*(3), 90–96. https://doi.org/10.1109/mcg.2016.59
27. Wang, G., Badal, A., Jia, X., et al. (2022). Development of metaverse for intelligent healthcare. *Nature Machine Intelligence, 4*, 922–929. https://doi.org/10.1038/s42256-022-00549-6
28. Kim, E. J., & Kim, J. Y. (2023). The metaverse for healthcare: Trends, applications, and future directions of digital therapeutics for urology. *International Neurourology Journal, 27*(Suppl 1), S3.
29. Moztarzadeh, O., Jamshidi, M., Sargolzaei, S., Jamshidi, A., Baghalipour, N., Malekzadeh Moghani, M., & Hauer, L. (2023). Metaverse and healthcare: Machine learning-enabled digital twins of cancer. *Bioengineering, 10*(4), 455.
30. Durosini, I., Strika, M., Pizzoli, S. F. M., & Pravettoni, G. (2023, September). Emotions and "sense of presence" in the psycho-verse: Psychological support for breast cancer survivors in the metaverse. In *International conference on extended reality* (pp. 417–426). Springer Nature.
31. Werner, H., Tonni, G., & Lopes, J. (2023). Metaverse in fetal medicine. In *In: 3D physical and virtual models in fetal medicine*. Springer. https://doi.org/10.1007/978-3-031-14855-2_7
32. Hajesmaeel-Gohari, S., Sarpourian, F., & Shafiei, E. (2021). Virtual reality applications to assist pregnant women: A scoping review. *BMC Pregnancy and Childbirth, 21*(1), 1–8.
33. Román-Belmonte, J. M., Rodríguez-Merchán, E. C., & la Corte-Rodríguez, H. D. (2023). Metaverse applied to musculoskeletal pathology: Orthoverse and rehabverse. *Postgraduate Medicine, 135*(5), 440–448.

34. Akyildiz, I. F., Guo, H., Dai, R., & Gerstacker, W. H. (2023). MulseMedia communication research challenges for metaverse in 6G wireless systems. *arXiv (Cornell University)*. https://doi.org/10.48550/arxiv.2306.16359
35. Chengoden, R., Victor, N., Huynh-The, T., Yenduri, G., Jhaveri, R. H., Alazab, M., et al. (2023). *Metaverse for healthcare: A survey on potential applications, challenges and future directions*. IEEE Access.
36. Ali, S., Abdullah, N., Armand, T. P. T., Athar, A., Hussain, A., Ali, M., Muhammad, Y., Joo, M., & Kim, H. C. (2023). Metaverse in healthcare integrated with explainable AI and blockchain: Enabling immersiveness, ensuring trust, and providing patient data security. *Sensors, 23*(2), 565. https://doi.org/10.3390/s2302056
37. Rawat, D. B., & Alami, H. E. (2023). Metaverse: Requirements, architecture, standards, status, challenges, and perspectives. *IEEE Internet of Things Magazine, 6*(1), 14–18. https://doi.org/10.1109/iotm.001.2200258
38. Lee, C. W. (2022). Application of metaverse service to healthcare industry: A strategic perspective. *International Journal of Environmental Research and Public Health, 19*(20), 13038. https://doi.org/10.3390/ijerph192013038
39. Koohang, A., Nord, J. H., Ooi, K., Tan, G. W., Al-Emran, M., Aw, E. C., Baabdullah, A. M., Buhalis, D., Cham, T., Dennis, C., Dutot, V., Dwivedi, Y. K., Hughes, L., Mogaji, E., Pandey, N., Phau, I., Raman, R., Sharma, A., Sigala, M., et al. (2023). Shaping the metaverse into reality: A holistic multidisciplinary understanding of opportunities, challenges, and avenues for future investigation. *Journal of Computer Information Systems, 63*(3), 735–765. https://doi.org/10.1080/08874417.2023.2165197
40. Letafati, M., & Otoum, S. (2023). On the privacy and security for e-health services in the metaverse: An overview. *Ad Hoc Networks*, 103262. https://doi.org/10.1016/j.adhoc.2023.103262
41. Rosenberg, L. Regulation of the metaverse: A roadmap: The risks and regulatory solutions for largescale consumer platforms. In *Proceedings of the 6th ICVARS'22* (pp. 21–26). Association for Computing Machinery. https://doi.org/10.1145/3546607.3546611
42. Pregowska, A., Osial, M., Dolega-Dolegowski, D., Kolecki, R., & Proniewska, K. (2022). Information and communication technologies combined with mixed reality as supporting tools in medical education. *Electronics, 11*, 3778. https://doi.org/10.3390/electronics11223778
43. Delpierre, C., & Lefèvre, T. (2023). Precision and personalized medicine: What their current definition says and silences about the model of health they promote. Implication for the development of personalized health. *Frontiers in Sociology, 8*, 1112159.
44. Petrigna, L., & Musumeci, G. (2022). The Metaverse: A new challenge for the healthcare system: A scoping review. *Journal of Functional Morphology and Kinesiology, 7*(3), 63. https://doi.org/10.3390/jfmk7030063. PMID: 36135421; PMCID: PMC9501644.
45. Onu, P., Pradhan, A., & Mbohwa, C. (2023). Potential to use metaverse for future teaching and learning. *Education and Information Technologies*. https://doi.org/10.1007/s10639-023-12167-9
46. Scherz, P. (2022). Data ethics, AI, and accompaniment: The dangers of depersonalization in catholic health care. *Theological Studies, 83*(2), 271–292. https://doi.org/10.1177/00405639221096770

The Metaverse in Healthcare: The Emerging Future of the Next Generation

Nidhi Malik, Nisha Arya, and Siddhant Gupta

1 Introduction

"Snow Crash," in 1992, Neal Stephenson released this science fiction book, which essentially explores the idea of the "metaverse," wherein millions of users can interact and participate in a digital environment created by computers in a variety of ways. The term "metaverse" is defined as a digital world that allows participants to participate in activities like gaming, socializing, and shopping using real-time immersive technologies. The metaverse is considerably more than just a "virtual world," despite the term being used frequently. It actually consists of a network of virtual environments connected by a common protocol or platform. The primary goal of this technology is to provide users with an immersive and seamless experience by making it simple for users to move between different virtual settings and integrate their real-world identities and things into the virtual world. By enabling us to experience new and previously impractical things in the physical world, such as work, education, and social relationships, the metaverse has the ability to push the limits of human expression and creativity.

As the metaverse becomes more well-known, tech firms, investors, and entrepreneurs are making large investments in it. There is a lot of potential for the metaverse to expand into a big industry and economic force, opening up new possibilities for employment, innovation, and development.

The structure of this chapter is as follows: Section 1 includes an introduction to the metaverse, the history of the metaverse, and an understanding of mixed, virtual, and augmented reality, along with the potential advantages of this in healthcare. Section 2 presents the literature work. Section 3 deals with applications

N. Malik (✉) · N. Arya · S. Gupta
The NorthCap University, Gurugram, Haryana, India
e-mail: nidhimalik@ncuindia.edu

C. L. Chowdhary (ed.), *The Metaverse for the Healthcare Industry*,
https://doi.org/10.1007/978-3-031-60073-9_3

of the metaverse, with a main focus on usage in the healthcare sector. In Section 4, we talked about market research, the metaverse's evolution, and the rise of the healthcare sector in relation to the metaverse market. Section 5 presents the metaverse's tools and technologies, as well as the companies developing them, their products, and the metaverse's tools and technologies that are currently used by the companies in the healthcare sector. Case study has also been included in this section. Section 6 concludes the chapter.

1.1 History

The metaverse concept came into light in 1992, which describes a fully immersive virtual world, initially announced in a novel titled "Snow Crash," published by an author named Neal Stephenson. He basically illustrates that there is a digital space where people can collaborate with each other in an imaginary world in a fully immersive way.

In the years following the publication of Snow Crash, this metaverse concept has gained so much popularity in the tech world. In 1995, an inventor named Mark Pesce, who is also a cocreator of the VRML, also known as virtual reality modeling language, gave a presentation in which he talked about the "3D Web" as a metaverse-like environment. He observes a network of interconnected virtual worlds where people can travel and explore alongside one another. Online multiplayer games like World of Warcraft and Second Life, where players may create their own avatars and interact with one another, are where the idea of the metaverse first started to take shape in the early 2000s.

The development of virtual reality and blockchain technologies has increased interest in the metaverse recently. But still, the concept of the metaverse is evolving due to many changes and developments. Figure 1 displays the emergence of the metaverse from previous years [4].

1.2 Mixed, Virtual, and Augmented Reality

1.2.1 Mixed Reality

This technology is a cutting-edge technology that merges AR and VR to provide users with a unique and interactive experience. In this technology, digital objects are projected onto the real world, which enables the users to engage with both digital as well as real objects at the same time in the real world. It was first introduced in 1994 by Fumio Kishino and Paul Milgram.

This technology primarily relies on a device called a head-mounted display (HMD), which helps in tracking the user's position and movement using numerous sensors that are installed on the gadget. The user can interact with a variety of

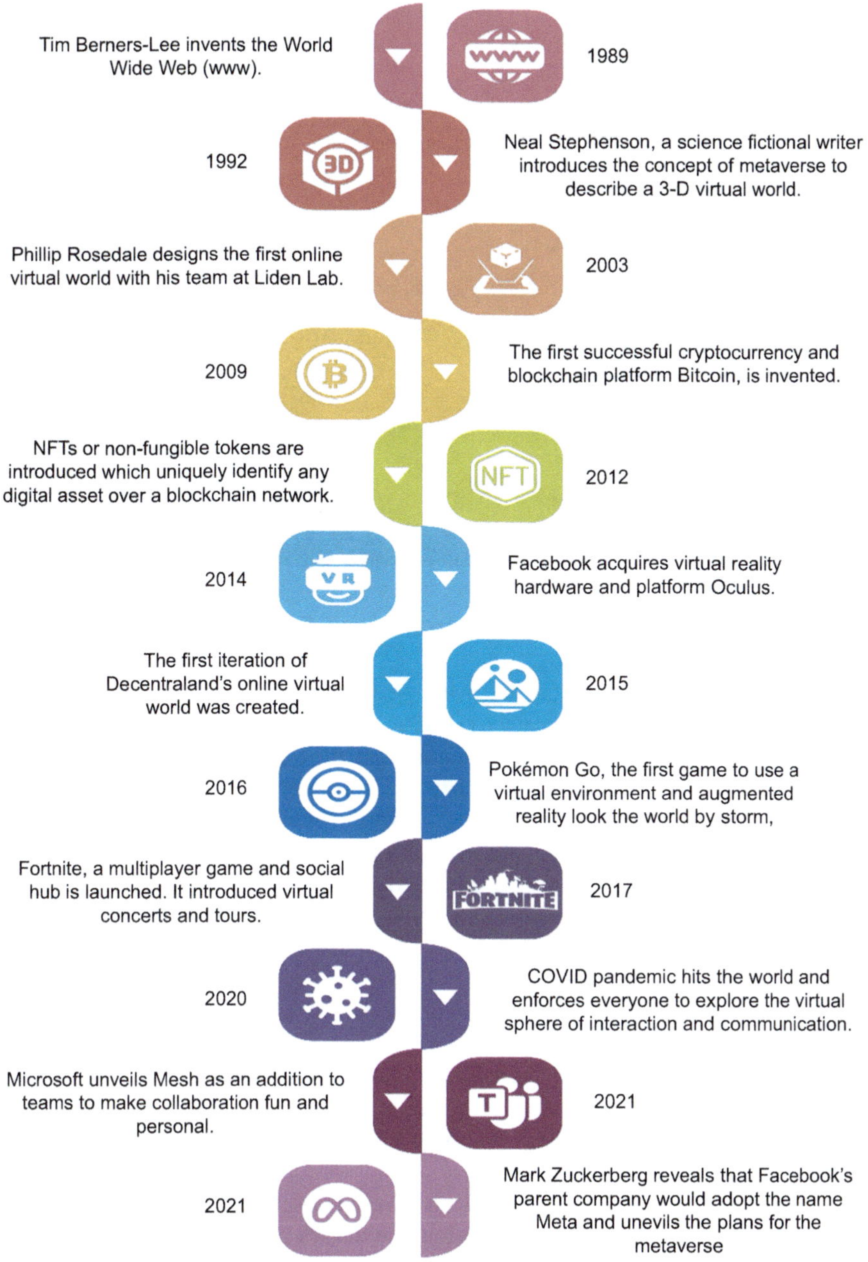

Fig. 1 The metaverse emerged due to a series of historical events

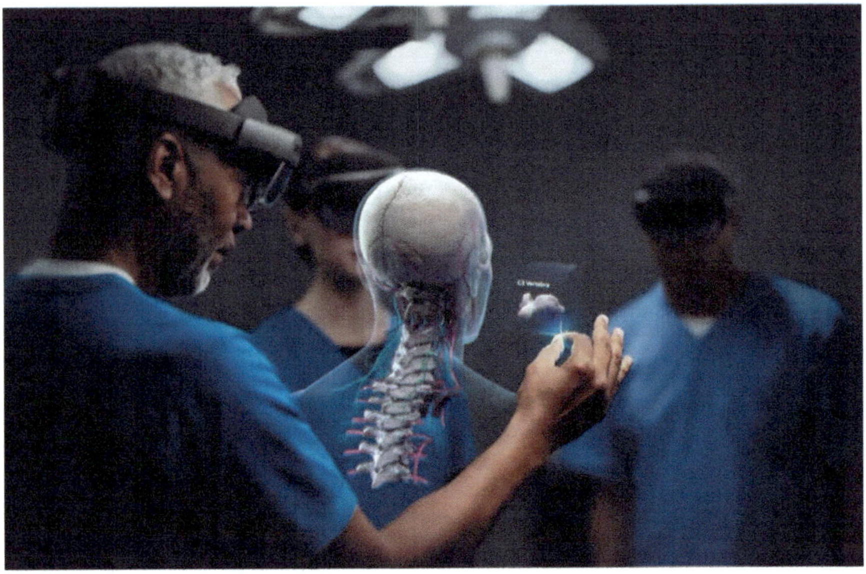

Fig. 2 Mixed reality in the healthcare sector

virtual objects more effectively by using gestures, verbal commands, and other techniques with the use of this device (HMDs). This technology offers more smooth and intuitive methods to interact with digital content, which is a huge benefit.

It offers several benefits in a variety of industries, including the healthcare industry where it enables doctors to interact with digital items in the real world. In order to better understand the patient's condition and available treatments, clinicians can use mixed reality to visualize patient data or medical imaging in 3D. The utilization of mixed reality in the healthcare sector can be observed in Fig. 2 [4].

1.2.2 Virtual Reality

A three-dimensional image or digitally simulated environment that the viewer can interact with is produced by this technical innovation. Through a head-mounted display, or HMD, or any other immersive technology, the user can explore and engage.

The user is immersed in the virtual space or three-dimensional image in such a way as to create a sensation of immersion that causes them to feel as though they have been transported there. The user's movements are used to update the virtual world in real time, creating an immersive experience. Users of this technology can interact with the virtual environment by using a variety of input tools, such as virtual reality headsets and motion controllers.

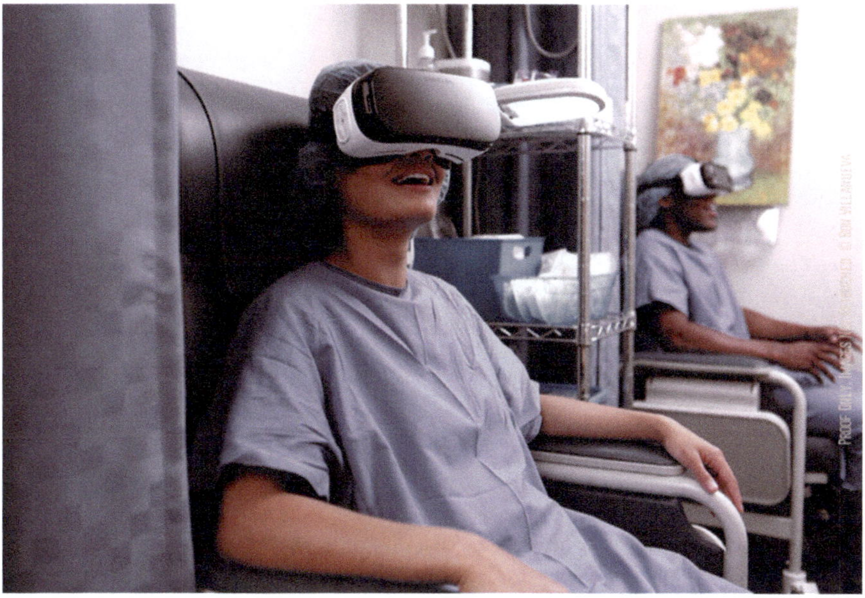

Fig. 3 Virtual reality in the healthcare sector

In 1968, computer scientist Ivan Sutherland created the first virtual reality headset, termed "The Sword of Damocles," which is still in use today. It also has a lot of benefits in a variety of industries, including the healthcare industry, where it enables surgical training for medical students. It also helps doctors to simulate patient treatment plans. It can also help patients to manage pain and anxiety during and after any medical procedures or post-surgery by providing a calming and distracting environment. Figure 3 describes how virtual reality is used in the healthcare sector.

1.2.3 Augmented Reality

It is an experience that can be experienced through technology that combines digital objects with the user's physical world environment, creating interactive and immersive experiences through the use of images, animations, etc. It basically combines the physical world with digital information, which can be experienced through a specialized headset or glasses, smartphone, tablet, etc.

Also, Ivan Sutherland, who was a computer scientist, invented the first augmented reality system along with the first virtual headset, which was called "The Sword of Damocles," in 1968. It also has a number of advantages in various sectors, including the healthcare sector, where it enables medical students to simulate

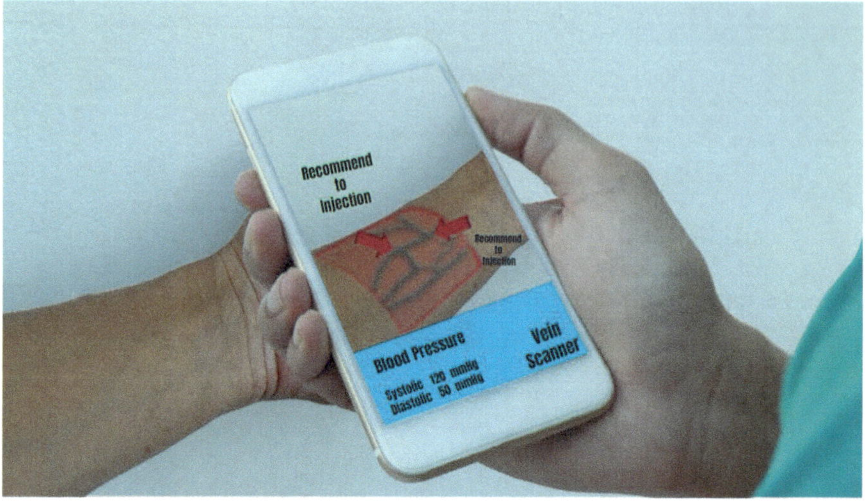

Fig. 4 Augmented reality in the healthcare sector

anatomy and learn complex procedures during medical training. Additionally, this technology also allows doctors to view patient data or medical images in real time with respect to the patient's body.

It is further divided into two parts:

- Marker-Based Technology: Basically, it uses the sensors to track the markers to produce a virtual projection in the actual world, such as a QR code, etc.
- Markerless Technology: It basically uses computer vision and other technologies to track the user's surroundings without the need for any markers that are needed in marker-based technology.

The utilization of AR in the healthcare industry can be observed in Fig. 4.

2 Literature Review

In the past few years, the terminology of the metaverse has become very popular. Many researchers and developers had started to explore the capabilities of virtual worlds as a new kind of social and economic system. In this section of the research chapter, we will provide an overview of some of the existing research that is happening in the metaverse, including research on many related topics like augmented, virtual reality, etc.

Artificial intelligence, blockchain, digital twins, MR, AR, and VR are just a few of the established and emerging technologies that have been combined to create the metaverse [14]. In recent years, researchers and businesses have invested more money on the technology [15]. As a new computing platform, the metaverse has enormous financial potential and is attracting the interest of industry giants like Apple and Google (Huang et al., 2022; Lee et al., 2021). Additionally, this technology will advance more in the upcoming years due to the development of sensor technology, blockchain technology, the launch of Web 3.0, the expansion of AR and VR technologies, and the most recent interest shown in the metaverse by CEO Mark Zuckerberg [15]. Also, the metaverse can alter employment opportunities and present new lifestyle and production options [16]. The metaverse is anticipated to have an impact on our daily life and the economy in addition to a variety of businesses [37]. By 2027, 30% of individuals are predicted to spend up to 2 h each day in the metaverse, which is expected to have a substantial impact on our daily lives and economy [11].

In terms of education, the metaverse has the potential to be used in the teaching and learning process [31]. It is also expected to revolutionize the healthcare and medical fields, transforming patient care and medical training. People who have utilized virtual reality (VR) or augmented reality (AR) educational programs or the metaverse goods and services are more inclined to feel that the fourth industrialization or the digital transformation will have more positive consequences on our lives than negative ones, according to a survey conducted in Korea [35].

Furthermore, the metaverse is not just about gaming and entertainment. It has been used in exergames to speed up the healing process for patients undergoing rehabilitation [36]. Here, exergame is a term that refers to a virtual reality game that allows many players to exercise simultaneously and is intended to speed up the healing process for patients undergoing rehabilitation, according to a study by Park et al. [35]. Using AR and VR together has been shown to reduce physical demand when compared to using either technology alone [34]. The metaverse has great potential and may alter how we interact with one another and the world at large.

The metaverse has the ability to encourage collaboration between medical professionals, students, and patients by utilizing virtual environments and technology like digital whiteboards, digital twins, and 3D avatars as well as by offering rewards through tokenization [24]. Healthcare professionals and patients can communicate from the comfort of their homes and take part in procedures, training sessions, and other healthcare-related metaverse-based activities thanks to the construction of digital avatars [1]. Dental therapies can be delivered more effectively when 3D digital images are used, and oral health can be taught to dental professionals and students [22]. The BRM all-in-one machine, which serves as an example of the metaverse in medicine, can offer technical support for the best possible use of the Meta-Internet of Things (MIoT), which blends IoT with the metaverse [23]. The management of obesity and NCDs can now be seen as relevant from the viewpoints of social prescribing, patient education, and clinical care in the field of healthcare [17]. VR therapy is advantageous for those with eating disorders and autism since research has shown that it reduces pain, anxiety, and stress symptoms while improving cognitive and social skills [25, 33]. In emergency care, studies linked to VR are more numerous than those related to AR, yet AR has more promise for classification of diagnoses and application of treatments. The metaverse's principal application technologies, AR and VR, are most frequently applied in the sector of education [26]. The healthcare industry relies heavily on eye and physical contact, as well as gestures and facial expressions, and the metaverse cannot take its place [27]. A promising way to improve healthcare outcomes is the suggested use of digital twin technology for the assessment and management of human health. However, there are many barriers that need to be removed before digital twin technology can be fully used in the healthcare industry, including assuring data security, privacy, and quality. Medical twin technology, which may be used to build a virtual world that is equal to reality, forecast treatment outcomes, and recommend the best drug, is one of the key areas to consider. A concept known as a "medical twin" creates identical twins in digital space utilizing digital twin service technology and verifies them using various tests in the healthcare sector [12]. Technology like Accuvein's, which projects the map and locates the patient's own veins on their skin, can be used for intravenous injections [29]. For people with social anxiety, a VR social abilities workshop was highly helpful since it allowed them to interact and learn communication skills, which raised their self-esteem [30]. The effectiveness of telehealth in its most basic form can be on par with or even better than traditional physical clinic delivery, but it depends on the medical indication and particular type of patient interaction, and it might not be appropriate for all patients [32]. The metaverse can be used in the treatment of cancer as well [40]. For instance, a tumor that was cancerous from a patient's spine was removed using Augmedics headsets by Johns Hopkins neurosurgeons. The four stages of the evolution of the medical metaverse (meta-medicine) are virtual-real linkage, the fusion of virtual and real, holographic simulation, and holographic construction [20]. It is crucial for the advancement of meta-medicine that trustworthy technological systems and cutting-edge technologies like Web3.0, 5G networks, the blockchain technology, and Internet of Things are used [20]. While it was shown that digital personality had a beneficial moderating effect in the association between mental health and digital healthcare centered in the metaverse, mental health was also found to play a substantial intermediary role in the connection between eSport performance and the metaverse-based digital healthcare (Cai et al., 2023).

Also, apart from healthcare, there are more advantages in the field of industry. According to Tlili et al. [38], the three major values of Industry 5.0 – resilience, human-centeredness, and sustainability – have the potential to be fulfilled by the metaverse in a variety of ways. It can also be used in marketing, as it helps brands boost their originality and appeal to their target audience as customers are able to see the brand's product live and may use it in the virtual world [42].

The metaverse is a fast-growing virtual world, and as its data volume, value, and volume rise, so does the demand for security and dependability [42]. By enabling interoperability between different systems and assuring secure and decentralized data storage and management, blockchain technology offers a potential remedy [18]. Moreover, by examining technical aspects like consensus mechanisms, network administration, and blockchain interoperability, the blockchain has the potential to revolutionize the immersive experience [19]. DAOs, cross-chain interoperability, and hybrid innovative consensus algorithms are some recommendations for technical developments to further improve the blockchain's technical capabilities in the metaverse. The metaverse can be protected from possible threats by utilizing technology like blockchain and artificial intelligence, according to research.

To secure the metaverse's incorporation into our daily lives as it develops, there are several problems that need to be solved. Numerous concerns need to be resolved for the metaverse to be properly integrated [28]. Although the integration of the physical, social, cognitive, and cyber environments in the metaverse has advantages [21], there are also considerable worries regarding security, behavior, appropriateness, safety, privacy, ethics, and governance [13]. According to Ning et al. [3], the metaverse is also having some moral and ethical issues, like violations of intellectual property rights, an unfavorable environment, and false information being published and spread. Companies must convince both business and private users that the applications of the metaverse are not only appropriate but also beneficial in order to increase user confidence in the metaverse [39].

Also, there are many websites that have worked on the metaverse, and we can take their help in related work. Some of those are:

- High Fidelity: This virtual world platform intends to offer a completely decentralized and open digital world where users may purchase, own, and govern their virtual goods and engage in impressively immersive social interactions. Researchers have explored the potential of this virtual platform for virtual real estate development, with some arguing that it represents a new kind of real estate market (e.g., Pilkington, 2019).
- Second Life: It is a digital realm where individuals can communicate with each other by designing their own avatars and take part in various activities, such as socializing, gaming, and e-commerce. IBM and Linden Labs estimated that the conference enhanced productivity and prevented $320,000 in venue and travel expenses by allowing delegates to return to their occupations immediately after the event (News, 2009). Additionally, QTLabs hosts gatherings in Second Life to facilitate and visualize discussions.

Marketing, education, and healthcare are just a few of the fields that the metaverse has an impact on and have been discussed in this portion of the chapter. Also, we discussed the opportunities and potential issues the metaverse may provide. We also take a look at some well-known metaverse systems, like Second Life and High Fidelity, which have received extensive research from academics across a variety of disciplines.

3 Applications of the Metaverse

The establishment of several industries, including gaming, social media, education, healthcare, real estate, fashion, sports, tourism, and many more, has been facilitated by the metaverse's rapid growth throughout all sectors of the economy. It is crucial to remember that the metaverse can be used to a number of different scenarios, including:

- Gaming: Players can enter a virtual world, play games from the comfort of their homes, and have the same experience as if they were playing in the real world thanks to the metaverse technology used in this industry.
- Education: This industry's use of technology offers students fantastic chances to communicate with and learn from their peers in a collaborative and interactive environment that can help them better understand difficult ideas (Kye et al.). From the comfort of their homes, students can experience what it would be like to be physically seated in the classroom with the teachers and their other classmates. Students can use this technology to explore virtual worlds such as historical sites from antiquity, the solar system from geography, and other topics addressed in those subjects [41].
- Virtual Interviews: This technology may be highly beneficial in virtual interviews since it gives both the job seeker and the interviewer a decent platform, which is important because the job seeker frequently has to go to another city or state for the interview. With the use of this technology, job candidates may do interviews while relaxing in their homes rather than spending the majority of their time traveling. Additionally, it benefits the interviewer since it creates an atmosphere in which both the job applicant and the interviewer feel as though they are physically there and therefore less likely to cheat during the interview.
- Virtual Events: In virtual events, this technology is really useful. Most of the time, many people are not able to attend various events like conferences, seminars, celebrations, sports events, etc., due to some restrictions like travel, health problems, etc. So, this technology allows these people to participate in events with other people and feel as if they are physically present at the event. This can make it possible for individuals all over the world to take part in events that they otherwise might not be able to.

3.1 Various Applications in Healthcare Sector

One sector where the virtual world known as the metaverse is growing in popularity is healthcare. The metaverse can be used in a variety of ways in the healthcare industry that benefit both patients and professionals.

Table 1 lists some of the key ways that the metaverse technology is being used in the healthcare sector.

Table 1 Main applications of the metaverse in healthcare

Topic	Description
Virtual consultations	The use of the metaverse technology in the medical industry has made it feasible for patients to consult with their healthcare providers virtually while relaxing in the comfort of their homes
Medical training	Healthcare workers have received medical instruction using the metaverse technology. Without endangering actual patients, medical students can practice surgical techniques and medicinal treatments using digital simulations
Medical research	The use of the metaverse technology could revolutionize medical research. Instead of performing trials on real patients, researchers can utilize virtual reality simulations to evaluate the effects of drugs and treatments. Clinical trial development for drugs could be accelerated and made more efficient as a result
Patient education	The metaverse technology can also be used to educate patients about their health conditions and treatment options. Patients can interact with virtual simulations of the human body to better understand how their condition is affecting their health, and learn about the treatments that are available to them
Mental health	The metaverse technology has been used to develop virtual reality therapy for mental health conditions such as anxiety, depression, etc. without leaving their homes, patients can engage with virtual surroundings and receive medical care from a healthcare professional

We may now delve more into one of the metaverse's most exciting applications after looking at its established uses in healthcare:

- Medical education is a promising area for the metaverse in healthcare. A career in healthcare calls for a great deal of care and consideration. The patient's life could be at jeopardy from any error. However, getting trained in the medical area can be expensive, time-consuming, and costly mistakes made in practice. Therefore, the metaverse in the healthcare sector allows medical experts a secure and controlled setting to hone their talents. By using realistic simulations of complex medical operations, the metaverse enables healthcare professionals to practice their skills without running the danger of making mistakes that would have occurred with more conventional training techniques. Medical students can utilize the metaverse to practically practice operations and develop their diagnostic abilities, such as diagnosing patients in a virtual hospital.
- The metaverse can do more than just provide medical training. It can be used for virtual medical consultations too. This can improve telehealth and virtual consultations, providing an interactive and personalized experience for both healthcare providers and patients, leading to better outcomes. It can particularly benefit patients with chronic conditions or disabilities who face challenges accessing traditional healthcare services.
- The metaverse can also offer a virtual tour of a patient's anatomy, which can improve their understanding of their condition and treatment options and reduce the anxiety and fear associated with medical procedures as they can experience it

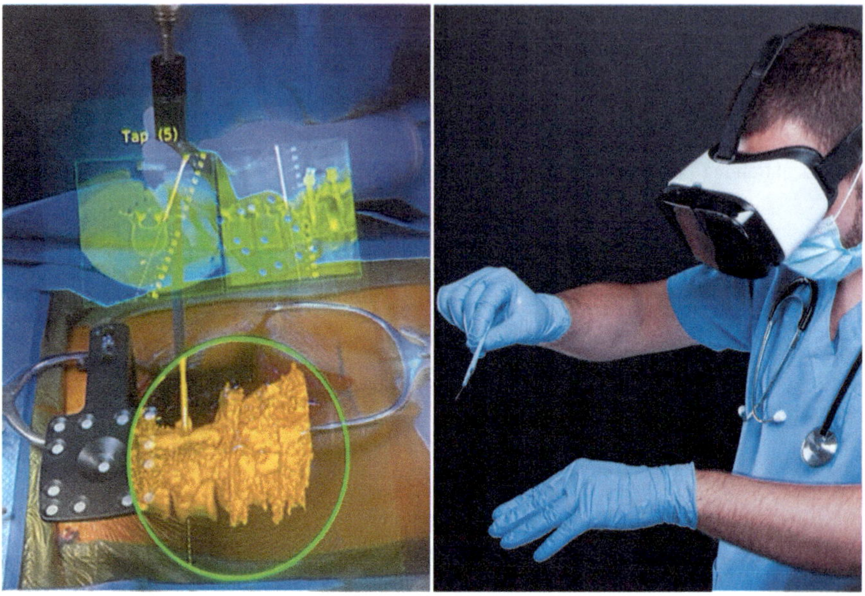

Fig. 5 The metaverse in the healthcare sector

prior to the real medical procedures and know whether any risk is associated with them or not. It can also provide a relaxing virtual environment for the patients so that they get engaged in those environments and forget about the anxiety and fear they had before the medical procedures.

The metaverse can transform healthcare by offering a secure and engaging space for medical training, consultations, and procedures, ultimately leading to better patient outcomes, cost savings, and improved quality of care. The metaverse is crucial to the future of healthcare.

Figure 5 displays how the metaverse is used in the healthcare sector (Yanko Design, 2022).

4 Market Analysis

The metaverse has been around for several years, and the concept has been popularized in science fiction and popular culture. However, the actual development of the metaverse as a functional and accessible digital world has only recently gained momentum. Many companies are recognizing the potential of AR and VR technologies and, as a result, are investing heavily in the development of a fully realized metaverse. Market analysis in the metaverse shows that it is a rapidly growing industry with tremendous potential for innovation and expansion.

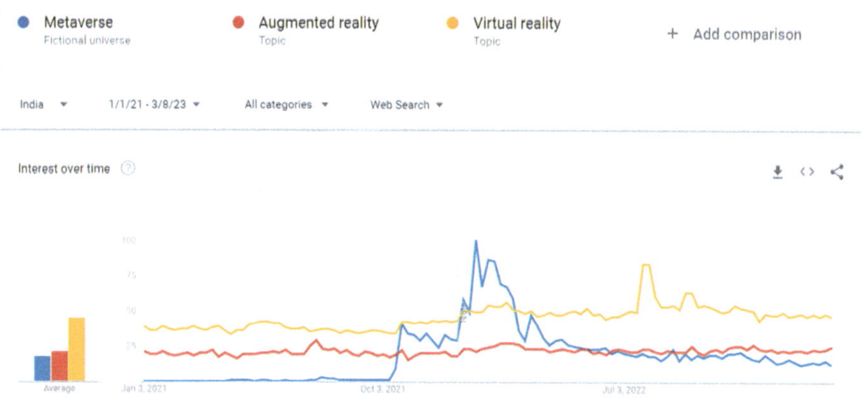

Fig. 6 Trends in the metaverse from the previous year [10]

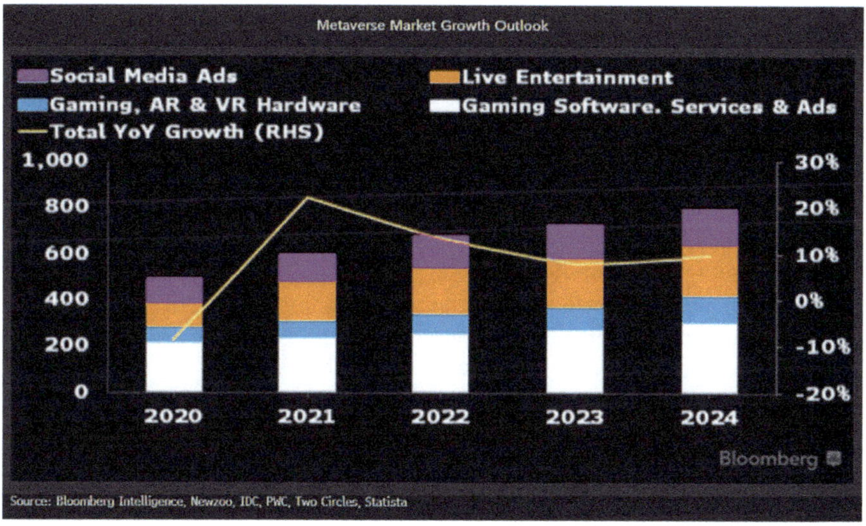

Fig. 7 The metaverse market growth in different industries

If we talk about trends, then in Fig. 6, which describes a graph [7], it basically highlights trends in the metaverse from the previous year, including the adoption of augmented and virtual reality technologies.

Also, the metaverse market in different industries is growing rapidly compared to past years, according to Bloomberg Intelligence; see Fig. 7, which basically depicts a graph displaying the metaverse market growth outlook from 2020 to 2024 (Bloomberg, 2021).

The metaverse market is hoping to experience rapid growth in the coming years. According to a report published by MarketsandMarkets, the market for the metaverse is anticipated to experience a significant increase in growth in the next few years. It is to see a substantial increase in value over the next several years, with estimates indicating a growth from $61.8 billion in 2022 to $426.9 billion by 2027, with a 47.2% CAGR, which is the compound annual growth rate. This growth is being driven by factors such as increasing investment in VR and AR technologies, growing demand for immersive gaming experiences, and the increasing adoption of the metaverse platforms in industries such as healthcare, education, and retail.

Companies like Microsoft, Facebook, HTC, Google, and Unity Technologies are just a few of the key players in this field. These companies' significant investments in the metaverse technology are anticipated to accelerate market growth in the near future.

In terms of popularity, the metaverse is still not particularly well known to the general public, but as more companies and developers engage in the technology, knowledge of it is expanding. As the metaverse becomes more accessible and user-friendly, it is expected to become a mainstream platform for entertainment, social networking, and other applications.

In the near future, it is expected that the healthcare market's use of the metaverse will increase significantly. According to a report by InsightAce Analytic, the global metaverse market in the healthcare sector is assumed to rise to $71.6 billion by 2030 from $6.57 billion in 2022, with a 35.4% CAGR, which is the compound annual growth rate throughout the projected timeline 2023–2031.

Also, according to Globe NewsWire's published Precedence Research Report on August 24, 2022, the metaverse market in the healthcare sector is assumed to rise to $72.10 billion by 2030 from $6.85 billion in 2021, with a 29.89% CAGR, which is the compound annual growth rate over the projected timeline of 2022–2030.

Take the reference to Fig. 8, which describes the growth of the metaverse market size in the healthcare industry (Precedence Research, 2022).

Overall, the metaverse market is a promising industry that is experiencing significant growth and has the ability to transform various sectors and create new opportunities for innovation and growth, whether in the healthcare industry or any other industry.

5 Tools and Technologies Used in the Metaverse

The metaverse is a digital universe where many users can feel like they communicate with each other like in physical form. There are number of tools and technologies that are used to create, access, and interact with the metaverse, some of which include.

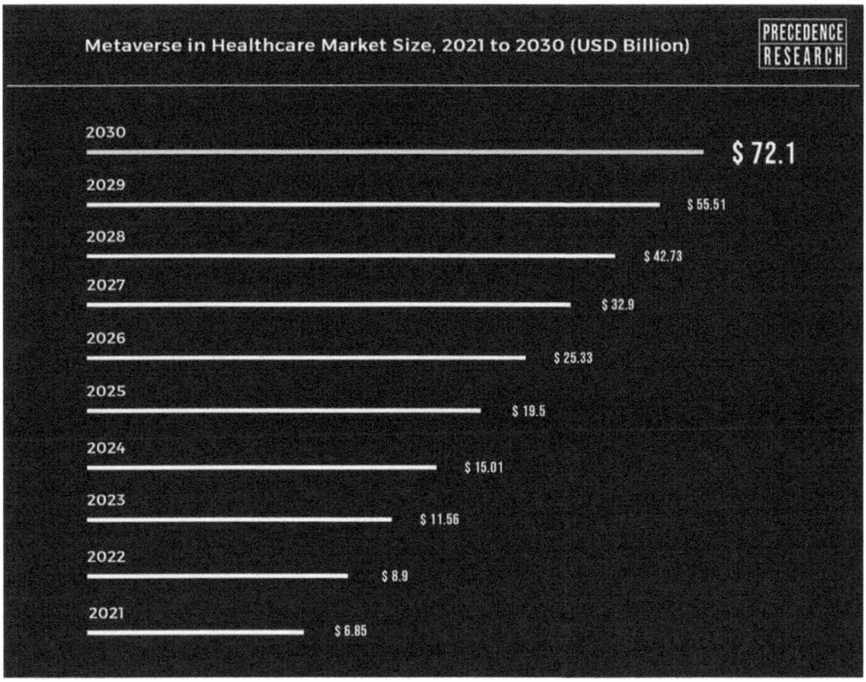

Fig. 8 The metaverse market size in healthcare

- VR headsets: These are the devices that allow the users to get into the metaverse and experience it as if they were physically present in it. Some examples of these devices include the HTC Vive and the Oculus Quest.
- AR devices: With the help of gadgets like the Microsoft HoloLens, people may interact with the digital world while still being aware of their actual surroundings.
- 3D modeling software: The 3D elements that are utilized to fill the metaverse are made using programs like Blender and Maya.
- Game engines: Unity and Unreal Engine are two well-known examples of how game engines can be used to develop interactive and immersive experiences for the metaverse.
- Blockchain technology: Inside the metaverse, blockchain technology is utilized to build decentralized, secure virtual economies and digital assets that users may trade and own.
- Artificial intelligence (AI): The use of AI technology is necessary for the creation of intelligent virtual assistants in the metaverse.
- Motion capture: This technology is used to record real-world actors' movements and convert them into believable motions for virtual avatars in the metaverse. Systems for motion capture like Vicon and OptiTrack are well-liked.

Table 2 Big giants active in the metaverse

Company	Products	Programming languages
Facebook	Spark AR, horizon workrooms, and oculus VR headsets	Java, C++, and python
Unity Technologies	Unity game engine	C# and C++
Epic games	Unreal engine game engine	C++ and blueprint
Microsoft	Azure cloud services, HoloLens AR headsets, and Minecraft	C#, C++, and python
Apple	ARKit	Swift and objective-C
Roblox	Roblox platform	Lua and C++

Lists of some big giants active in the metaverse, along with examples of their offerings and programming languages, are presented in Table 2.

5.1 *In Healthcare Sector*

The usage of the metaverse in healthcare is a new field with a lot of potential. The following are some of the tools and technologies being researched in this area:

- Virtual reality (VR): It has the ability to provide patients with intensely immersive experiences, such as virtual worlds that can be used for cognitive therapy, pain management, or anxiety reduction. Virtual reality can also be used to mimic operations or emergency situations for medical staff training.
- Augmented reality (AR): By enabling students and experts to interact with 3D models of medical equipment and the human body, AR technology can be used in medical education and training. In order to help patients visualize and comprehend their conditions and therapies, augmented reality (AR) can also be used in patient education.
- Wearable technology: Remote patient monitoring and individualized care are now possible thanks to wearable technology like smartwatches and fitness trackers that gather health metrics like activity levels, blood pressure, and heart rate in real time.

These are only a few examples of the tools and technology under consideration for the use of the metaverse in the healthcare industry. The companies, along with the tools or technologies used in the healthcare metaverse, are presented in Table 3.

Table 3 Healthcare companies that are using the metaverse

Company name	Definition	Tools/technologies used	Programming languages
Teladoc health	It is a telemedicine company that provides virtual medical consultations and monitoring	Telemedicine	Not disclosed
XRHealth	It is a company that provides VR and AR therapy and rehabilitation for patients	Wearable technology and virtual reality (VR)	Unity (game engine)
HoloPatient	It is a company that uses augmented reality to create simulations for medical education and training	Augmented reality (AR)	Unity (game engine)
Osso VR	It is a company that provides VR training for medical and surgical professionals	Virtual reality (VR)	Unity (game engine)
Surgical Theater	It is a company that uses virtual reality to help surgeons plan and practice complex procedures before they actually perform them	Virtual reality (VR)	Unity (game engine)

5.2 *Case Study: Brain Hack – Exploring the Brain Hippocampus*

Objective Develop an immersive markerless AR application to educate and train users on the anatomy and functions of the hippocampus, catering to healthcare professionals, students, and individuals interested in neuroscience.

Key Features

Virtual Exploration: Users can explore a detailed 360-degree 3D model of the hippocampus in their scanned physical environment using markerless AR technology. Pinch-to-zoom and rotate gestures allow users to examine the structure from different angles.

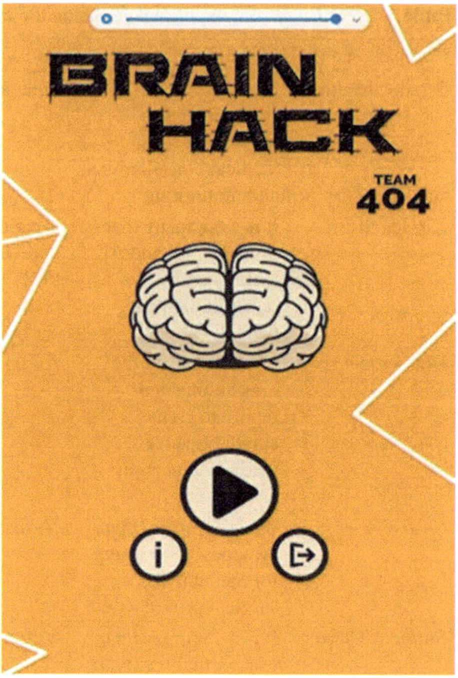

Fig. 9 Home screen

- Brain blood flow: Animating the brain's blood flow system.
- Interactive learning modules: Divided into modules covering anatomy, functions, and related functions. Users interact with virtual elements to understand the role.
- Implementation: Developed for AR-enabled application for Android, smartphones, and tablets.
- Technology used: Utilizes advanced computer vision for accurate markerless tracking with AR Core and SDK, 3D studio max for brain asset (Figs. 9, 10, 11, 12, 13, 14, 15 and 16).

Outcomes

- Increased engagement and retention of information due to the immersive and interactive nature of AR.
- Positive feedback from users regarding the effectiveness of gamification and simulations.

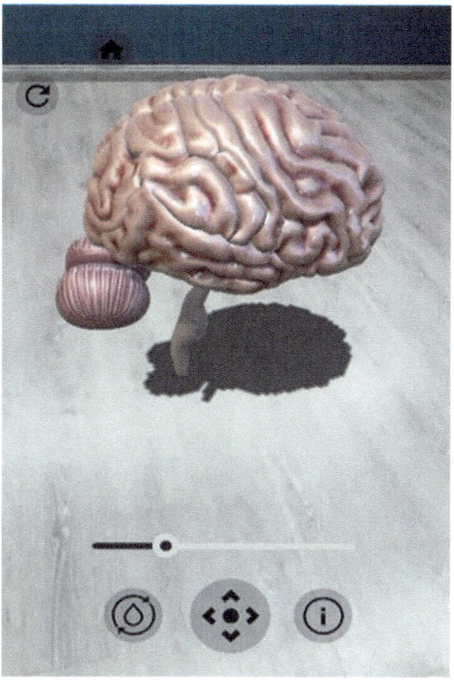

Fig. 10 Augmenting 3D 360-degree brain model

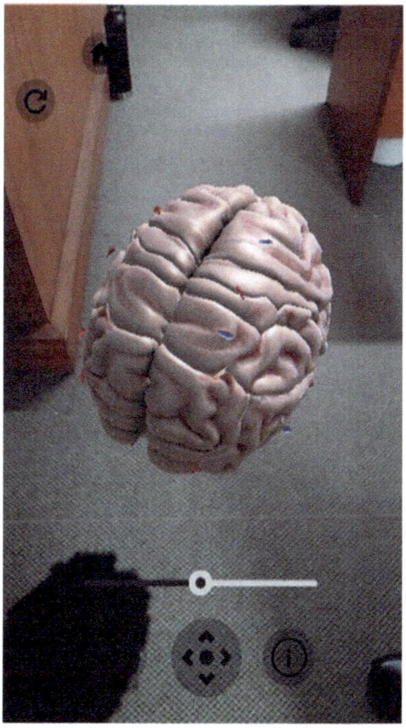

Fig. 11 Blood flow

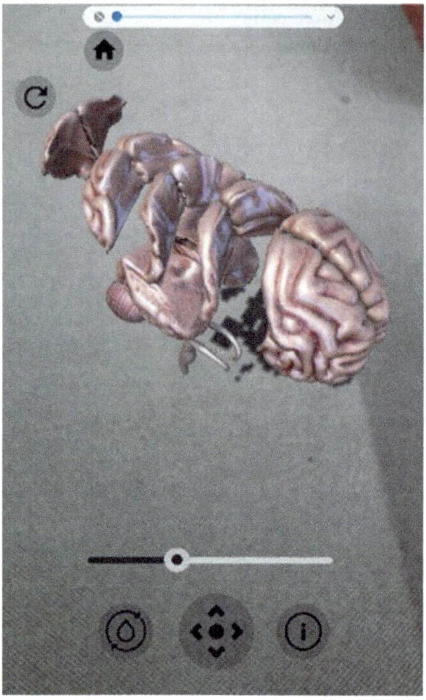

Fig. 12 Dissection

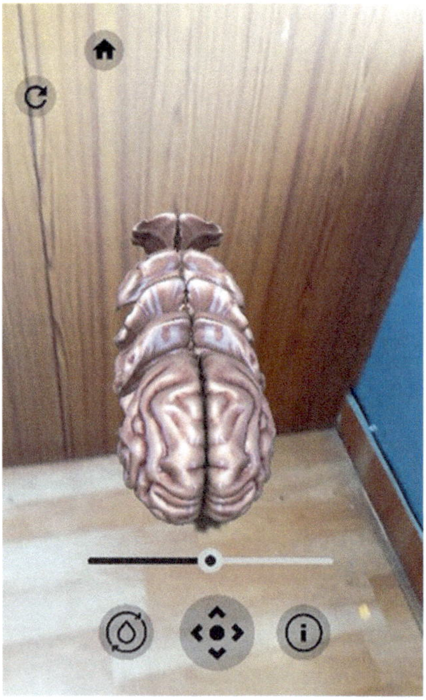

Fig. 13 View in 360 by rotating through UI slider

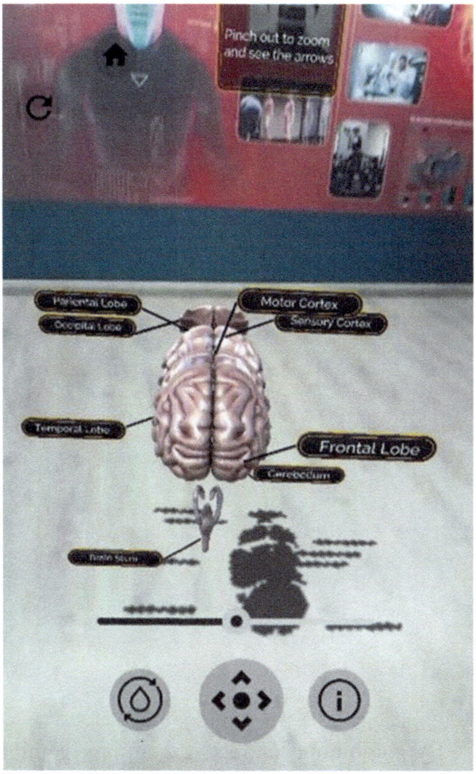

Fig. 14 Labeling of all parts of brain

Additional Features

- Gamified Challenges: Memory challenges and quizzes where users match functions with specific regions of the hippocampus. Points, badges, or levels to gamify the learning process and encourage continued engagement.
- Real-Time Feedback: Immediate feedback on quiz performance, providing explanations for correct and incorrect answers. Performance metrics are displayed in a user-friendly interface.
- Simulated Scenarios: Simulations of real-life scenarios demonstrating the impact of hippocampal damage on spatial navigation or memory recall. Users make decisions based on their understanding of hippocampal functions.
- Collaborative Learning: Multiuser support, allowing collaborative exploration and problem-solving in AR. Virtual classrooms or study groups facilitated by shared AR environments.
- Accessibility Features: Voice-activated commands for navigation and interaction. Customizable text size, color contrast, and other accessibility features.
- Progress Tracking: Personalized dashboards displaying completed modules, achievements, and areas for improvement. Recommendations for additional learning based on user performance.

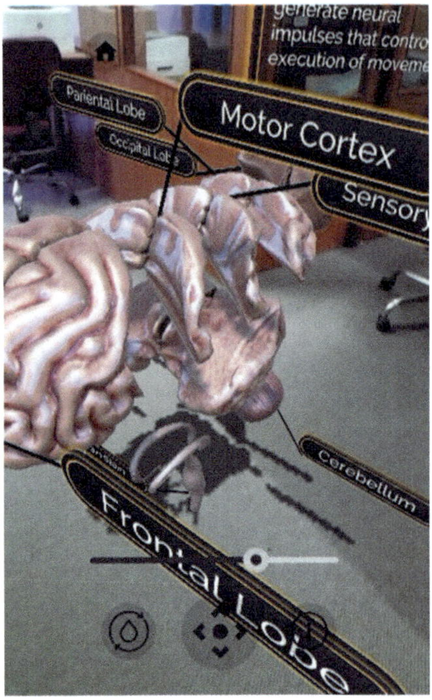

Fig. 15 Zoom in and zoom out the 3D brain

By combining interactive learning, gamification, and simulated scenarios, this application provides an engaging and effective platform for understanding the complexities of the hippocampus and its functions. As AR technology continues to evolve, such applications contribute to a new era of experiential and accessible learning in the field of neuroscience. A hypothetical case study for an educational and training markerless AR application focused on a specific part of the brain – let us say, the hippocampus, which plays a crucial role in memory and spatial navigation.

6 Conclusion

The idea of the metaverse is swiftly developing and has the potential to have both positive and negative effects on society. Many surveys and research chapters that have been published previously indicate that the development and popularity of the metaverse will increase in the coming years. Moreover, many people are now taking an interest in the metaverse, and many big giants have started investing in it, which ultimately helps in its growth. The metaverse can be an emerging future for the next generation as they can interact with each other from the comfort of their homes. The metaverse has vast transformative potential across multiple industries, spanning from healthcare and education to entertainment and gaming. Specifically, the development of the metaverse in healthcare presents a unique opportunity to

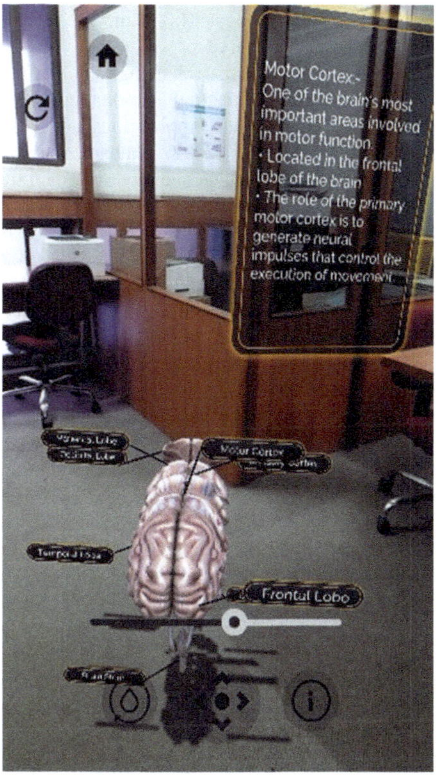

Fig. 16 Further displaying the functionality of the part of brain

transform the way we approach medical training, patient care, and access to health services. However, with a good thing comes a bad thing also, as with the metaverse, some disadvantages will also come along with advantages like security, addiction, and negative social impacts. In conclusion, the metaverse is a fast-changing concept with significant possibility for both beneficial and harmful impacts on society. To ensure the responsible deployment of the metaverse, it is crucial to thoughtfully assess its potential impacts and take measures to minimize any adverse effects.

References

1. Chengoden, R., Victor, N., Huynh-The, T., Yenduri, G., Jhaveri, R. H., Alazab, M., Bhattacharya, S., Hegde, P., Maddikunta, P. K. R., & Gadekallu, T. R. (2022). Metaverse for healthcare: A survey on potential applications, challenges and future directions. *arXiv (Cornell University)*. https://doi.org/10.48550/arXiv.2209.04160
2. Ali, S., Sikandar, A., Abdullah, T. P. T. A., Athar, A., Hussain, A., Ali, M., Yaseen, M., Joo, M.-I., & Kim, H.-C. (2023). Metaverse in healthcare integrated with explainable AI and blockchain: Enabling immersiveness, ensuring trust, and providing patient data security. *Sensors, 23*(2), 565. https://doi.org/10.3390/s23020565

3. Ning, H., Wang, H., Lin, Y., Wang, W., Dhelim, S., Farha, F., et al. (2023). A survey on the metaverse: The state-of-the-art, technologies, applications, and challenges. *IEEE Internet of Things Journal*. https://www.researchgate.net/publication/356375388_A_Survey_on_Metaverse_the_State-of-the-art_Technologies_Applications_and_Challenges
4. CNBCTV18.com. (2022, January 4). *Explained: The history of metaverse*. https://www.cnbctv18.com/technology/explained-the-history-of-Metaverse-12015212.htm
5. Softweb Solutions. (2022, February 14). *How mixed reality applications are empowering the healthcare sector?*https://www.softwebsolutions.com/resources/mixed-reality-application-in-healthcare-industry.html
6. Pennic, J. (2016, June 30). How virtual reality can improve patient experience in healthcare. *Hit Consultant*. https://hitconsultant.net/2016/06/30/virtual-reality patient-experience/
7. HPN Online. (2022, September 21). *AR in healthcare: From medical training to patient education*. https://www.hpnonline.com/blog/blog/21281564/ar-in-healthcare-from-medical-training-to-patient-education
8. Torres, J. (2022, May 15). The Metaverse has the power to improve healthcare, and it has already begun – Yanko Design. *Yanko Design – Modern Industrial Design News*. https://www.yankodesign.com/2022/05/15/the-Metaverse-has-the-power-to-improve-healthcare-and-it-has-already-begun/
9. Google Trends. (2023). *Explore what the world is searching: /m/054_cb, /m/0lqtr, /m/07_ny*. Retrieved March 8, 2023, from https://trends.google.com/trends/explore?date=2021-01-01%202023-03-08&geo=IN&q=%2Fm%2F054_cb,%2Fm%2F0lqtr,%2Fm%2F07_ny
10. Bloomberg. (2021, September 13). *Metaverse may be $800 nillion market, next tech platform*. Retrieved March 8, 2023, from https://www.bloomberg.com/professional/blog/Metaverse-may-be-800-billion-market-next-tech-platform/
11. InsightAce Analytic. *Metaverse in healthcare market size, growth, scope and future trends analysis report to 2031*. https://www.insightaceanalytic.com/report/global-Metaverse-in-healthcare-market-/1226
12. Research, P. (2022, August 24). Metaverse in healthcare market size to hit USD 72.10 Bn by 2030. *GlobeNewswire News Room*. https://www.globenewswire.com/en/news-release/2022/08/24/2503869/0/en/Metaverse-in-Healthcare-Market-Size-to-Hit-USD-72-10-Bn-by-2030.html
13. Huang, J., Sun, P., & Zhang, W. (2022, March 26). *Analysis of the future prospects for the metaverse*. Atlantis Press. https://doi.org/10.2991/aebmr.k.220307.312
14. Lee, L.-H., Braud, T., Zhou, P., Wang, L., Xu, D., Lin, Z., Kumar, A., Bermejo, C., & Hui, P. (2021). All one needs to know about Metaverse: A complete survey on technological singularity, virtual ecosystem, and research agenda. https://doi.org/10.13140/RG.2.2.11200.05124/8
15. Dwivedi, Y. K., Hughes, L., Baabdullah, A. M., Ribeiro-Navarrete, S., Giannakis, M., Al-Debei, M. M., Dennehy, D., Metri, B. A., Buhalis, D., Cheung, C. M. K., Conboy, K., Doyle, R., Dubey, R., Dutot, V., Felix, R., Goyal, D., Gustafsson, A., Hinsch, C., Jebabli, I., et al. (2022). Metaverse beyond the hype: Multidisciplinary perspectives on emerging challenges, opportunities, and agenda for research, practice and policy. *International Journal of Information Management, 66*, 102542. https://doi.org/10.1016/j.ijinfomgt.2022.102542
16. Trunfio, M., & Rossi, S. (2022). Advances in metaverse investigation: Streams of research and future agenda. *Virtual Worlds, 1*(2), 103–129. https://doi.org/10.3390/virtualworlds1020007
17. Guan, S., Lei, S., Qian, Y., Rong, Y., & Tang, Z. (2022). Review on metaverse's market development. *Highlights in Business, Economics and Management, 1*, 14–17. https://doi.org/10.54097/hbem.v1i.2311
18. Zhang, X., Chen, Y., Hu, L., & Wang, Y. (2022, September 8). The Metaverse in education: Definition, framework, features, potential applications, challenges, and future research topics. *Frontiers*. https://doi.org/10.3389/fpsyg.2022.1016300

19. Thomason, J. (2021, December 31). *MetaHealth – How will the metaverse change health care?*https://dergipark.org.tr/en/download/article-file/2167692
20. Song, Y., & Qin, J. (2022). Metaverse and personal healthcare. *Procedia Computer Science, 210*, 189–197. https://doi.org/10.1016/j.procs.2022.10.136
21. Huynh-The, T., Gadekallu, T. R., Wang, W., Yenduri, G., Ranaweera, P., Pham, Q., Da Costa, D. B., & Liyanage, M. (2023). Blockchain for the metaverse: A review. *Future Generation Computer Systems, 143*, 401–419. https://doi.org/10.1016/j.future.2023.02.008
22. Mengting, S., Xie, L., Liu, Y., Kecheng, L., Jiang, B., Lu, Y., Yang, Y., Yu, H., Song, Y., Bai, C., & Yang, D. (2022). The Metaverse in current digital medicine. *Clinical eHealth, 5*, 52–57. https://doi.org/10.1016/j.ceh.2022.07.002
23. Shi, F., Ning, H., Zhang, X., Li, R., Tian, Q., Zhang, S., Zheng, Y., Guo, Y., & Daneshmand, M. (2023). A new technology perspective of the metaverse: Its essence, framework and challenges. *Digital Communications and Networks*. https://doi.org/10.1016/j.dcan.2023.02.017
24. Garavand, A., & Aslani, N. (2022). Metaverse phenomenon and its impact on health: A scoping review. *Informatics in Medicine Unlocked, 32*, 101029. https://doi.org/10.1016/j.imu.2022.101029
25. Yang, D., Zhou, J., Chen, R., Song, Y., Song, Z., Zhang, X., Wang, Q., Wang, K., Zhou, C., Zhang, L., Bai, L., Wang, Y., Lu, Y., Xin, H., Powell, C. A., Thüemmler, C., Chavannes, N. H., Chen, W., Wu, L., & Bai, C. (2022). Expert consensus on the metaverse in medicine. *Clinical eHealth, 5*, 1–9. https://doi.org/10.1016/j.ceh.2022.02.001
26. Thomason, J. (2022). Metaverse, token economies, and non-communicable diseases. *Global Health Journal, 6*(3), 164–167. https://doi.org/10.1016/j.glohj.2022.07.001
27. Cerasa, A., Gaggioli, A., Marino, F., Riva, G., & Pioggia, G. (2022). The promise of the metaverse in mental health: The new era of MEDverse. *Heliyon, 8*(11), e11762. https://doi.org/10.1016/j.heliyon.2022.e11762
28. Wu, T., & Ho, C. B. (2022). A scoping review of metaverse in emergency medicine. *Australasian Emergency Care, 26*(1), 75–83. https://doi.org/10.1016/j.auec.2022.08.002
29. Petrigna, L., & Musumeci, G. (2022). The metaverse: A new challenge for the healthcare system: A scoping review. *Journal of Functional Morphology and Kinesiology, 7*(3), 63. https://doi.org/10.3390/jfmk7030063
30. Lee, C. W. (2022). Application of metaverse service to healthcare industry: A strategic perspective. *International Journal of Environmental Research and Public Health, 19*(20), 13038. https://doi.org/10.3390/ijerph192013038
31. Bhugaonkar, K., Bhugaonkar, R., & Masne, N. S. (2022). The trend of metaverse and augmented & virtual reality extending to the healthcare system. *Cureus*. https://doi.org/10.7759/cureus.29071
32. Usmani, S. S., Sharath, M., & Mehendale, M. (2022). Future of mental health in the metaverse. *General Psychiatry, 35*, e100825. https://doi.org/10.1136/gpsych-2022-100825
33. Zhou, H., Gao, J., & Chen, Y. (2022). The paradigm and future value of the metaverse for the intervention of cognitive decline. *Frontiers in Public Health, 10*. https://doi.org/10.3389/fpubh.2022.1016680
34. Qiu, C. S., Majeed, A., Khan, S., & Watson, M. (2022). Transforming health through the metaverse. *Journal of the Royal Society of Medicine, 115*(12), 484–486. https://doi.org/10.1177/01410768221144763
35. Xi, N., Chen, J., Gama, F., Riar, M., & Hamari, J. (2022). The challenges of entering the metaverse: An experiment on the effect of extended reality on workload. *Information Systems Frontiers*. https://doi.org/10.1007/s10796-022-10244-x
36. Cai, L., Huang, Z., Feng, Q., Chang, X., & Yan, K. (2023). Co-transformation of digital health and eSport in metaverse: Moderating effects of digital personality on mental health in Multiplayer Online Battle Arena (MOBA). *International Journal of Environmental Research and Public Health, 20*(1), 760. https://doi.org/10.3390/ijerph20010760

37. Park, J., Lee, K., & Chung, D. R. (2022). Public interest in the digital transformation accelerated by the COVID-19 pandemic and perception of its future impact. *The Korean Journal of Internal Medicine, 37*(6), 1223–1233. https://doi.org/10.3904/kjim.2022.129
38. Shah, S. H. H., Karlsen, A., Solberg, M., & Hameed, I. A. (2022). A social VR-based collaborative exergame for rehabilitation: Codesign, development and user study. *Virtual Reality*. https://doi.org/10.1007/s10055-022-00721-8
39. Kye, B., Han, N., Kim, E., Park, Y., & Jo, S. (2021). Educational applications of metaverse: Possibilities and limitations. *Journal of Educational Evaluation for Health Professions, 18*, 32. https://doi.org/10.3352/jeehp.2021.18.32
40. Tlili, A., Huang, R., & Kinshuk, N. (2023). Metaverse for climbing the ladder toward 'Industry 5.0' and 'Society 5.0'? *Service Industries Journal, 43*(3–4), 260–287. https://doi.org/10.1080/02642069.2023.2178644
41. Zeng, Y., Zeng, L., Zhang, C., & Cheng, A. S. K. (2022). The metaverse in cancer care: Applications and challenges. *Asia-Pacific Journal of Oncology Nursing, 9*(12), 100111. https://doi.org/10.1016/j.apjon.2022.100111
42. Di Pietro, R., & Cresci, S. (2021). Metaverse: Security and privacy issues. In *2021 third IEEE international conference on trust, privacy and security in intelligent systems and applications (TPS-ISA)* (pp. 281–288). IEEE. https://arxiv.org/pdf/2205.07590.pdf

The Social and Ethical Challenges of the Metaverse

Zahra Alidousti Shahraki and Mohsen Aghabozorgi Nafchi

1 Introduction

The metaverse can be considered the next generation of the Internet after web and mobile technology [1]. It can affect the entire life of humanity and provide the possibility of experiencing a virtual universe alongside a real environment. People can interact with each other, play games, and perform economic activities. The most important point in the development of the metaverse environment is the progress made in recent years in technologies such as extended reality (XR), virtual reality (VR), augmented reality (AR), and mixed reality (MR), along with other technologies such as blockchain, non-fungible tokens (NFT) and 6G, wearable devices, brain-computer interface (BCI), decentralization, and artificial intelligence.

The most important aspect of the metaverse is that it cannot be considered an isolated environment for a specific group of people and ignores the challenges faced by individuals that interact with it. In other words, the metaverse is an environment in which people interact with various interests and behaviors without any restrictions. For example, with the increase in the elderly population worldwide, managing the needs of this group of people has attracted the attention of many scientists, especially governments. Research in this field shows that the use of the metaverse capacities and their technologies to help the elderly is welcomed. However, the most important point is whether the elderly use the metaverse's services in an environment free of interactions with other age groups. If this is true, there is no need to worry, but if the elderly want to interact with various people and groups in the same environment, they will definitely witness many problems in the

Z. A. Shahraki (✉)
Department of Computer Engineering, University of Isfahan, Isfahan, Iran

M. A. Nafchi
Department of Computer Science and Engineering, Shiraz University, Shiraz, Iran

C. L. Chowdhary (ed.), *The Metaverse for the Healthcare Industry*,
https://doi.org/10.1007/978-3-031-60073-9_4

metaverse environment. And the need to design special tools and pay attention to ethical issues in this field is seen more and more today.

Therefore, according to this chapter, the basic need for detailed research on the side effects of the metaverse environment on different groups of society should be prioritized. Because of the importance of this, in the following chapter, the social and ethical issues and challenges faced by certain individuals and groups are examined.

2 Seven Layers of the Metaverse

Using the topic of the metaverse layering for the analysis of questions related to the metaverse can be considered an important step for a specific pattern related to the social and ethical challenges of the metaverse. The author of this chapter divides the metaverse environment into seven layers [2]:

2.1 Experience

One of the important layers of the metaverse is the user experience, in which users perform activities such as social life, shopping, and others based on it. In a metaverse environment, by using VR, users can understand experiences that were not possible before, such as 3D games; therefore, the metaverse provides a new experience for users with its technologies. Consequently, new experiences also present new challenges for users, such as security, privacy, and many ethical issues that have not been addressed in previous systems. For example, the personal information of a user can be used to create an avatar and be used by people in various ways, such as pornography, and he/she may face many mental problems by observing herself in the virtual world.

2.2 Discovery

This layer can be divided into two parts, "push and pull." On the one hand, the issue of push makes users actively seek new information and experiences; on the other hand, pull is an outward process and includes processes that inform users of what events and happenings are expected in the metaverse. One of the characteristics of the metaverse is that the processes and programs are real time. For example, users in this environment can enter a game; on the one hand, they can play in real time, and on the other hand, they can observe the interactions of other users. Platforms apply this feature to increase the appeal of their games.

2.3 Creator Economy

One of the important aspects of the metaverse is its economic aspect, which, with the help of AR tools, VR can create 3D environments that cannot be implemented in previous generations of the Internet, and it creates many potential markets and economies. For example, content production, which is currently being developed with great popularity in social networks, is an important economic aspect of the new world. This matter will continue into the virtual world of the metaverse. They will also attract their followers to the metaverse and interact with them. Among their economic activities, it is possible to sell NFTs and commercial goods, interact with brands, influence users using avatars, and use them in things such as fashion.

Therefore, the metaverse is a win-win environment for everyone, but it is necessary to look more carefully at whether ethical issues such as intellectual property, which already exist on the Internet and social networks, will be in the metaverse environment or a new generation of ethical issues will emerge.

For example, one of the challenges is to encourage more purchases on social networks, which threatens society's health. This matter in the metaverse increases the risk of mental diseases, addiction to social networks, and more purchases with the development of new technologies. By using new methods of social media marketing, companies can easily collect users' information in the metaverse environment and send advertisements based on it. If a company gains access to tools around the user that record user information, it can easily find the user's location, private tools, and behavioral characteristics; even access the user's brain signals with the help of a wearable device; make the most of the targeted advertisements; and easily keep the customer in hand. Based on his/her interests, he/she should create content, publish advertisements, and encourage the user to buy. Now, the basic question here is: If a user does not have the ability to buy, what effect will these colorful advertisements have on their mental health?

2.4 Spatial Computing

Spatial computing is a technology that can simultaneously provide humanity with the experience of virtual and real environments at the same time. Discussions such as AR, VR, and MR have taken a step forward by using this technology. It has been implemented in many services, such as 3D environments, that can be used to display objects in 3D. Therefore, users can enjoy 3D games and witness a new generation of user interfaces that work with the help of gesture recognition.

2.5 Decentralization

The metaverse has provided a decentralization environment using new technologies such as blockchain, in which the user can perform all kinds of activities in the provided virtual space without worrying about the concentration of data in one company and reduce concerns about security and privacy. On the other hand, we will witness a new exchange space in the economic world that is based on people's individual transactions. It also enables people to form virtual communities alongside governments and achieve their goals in various fields. Therefore, this issue raises concerns for governments about controlling people's interactions in the metaverse. The freedom created has many benefits, but we cannot ignore the sinister activities of destructive groups and smuggling in this environment. For example, one of the concerns of governments is the transfer of money with the help of digital currencies, which will challenge the economies of countries in the near future. Governments should familiarize themselves with the challenges of a decentralized environment and keep themselves up to date.

2.6 Human Interface

In recent years, new technologies have been developed for human-machine interfaces. These new tools have allowed people to experience environments such as AR, VR, and MR. Among the examples of tools that have been developed with the aim of communicating with the virtual world, wearable tools can be mentioned. For example, a brain-computer interface (BCI) is a tool that, by analyzing brain signals, provides the necessary commands to various devices to interact with the real or virtual world. In the near future, the development of wearable devices and their use in the metaverse environments will provide many attractions for user interaction in this environment. However, the challenges of sharing user information through wearable devices and privacy threats should not be ignored. Moreover, in relation to the development of these tools, we should not forget to make tools according to the needs of the disabled and elderly.

2.7 Infrastructure

A metaverse environment with a complex structure requires strong infrastructure to implement and simulate a virtual environment. Infrastructure that can perform high-volume calculations using artificial intelligence and blockchain technology tools. But on the other hand, complex tools with high computing power produce a lot of heat, which can bring the challenge of global warming and energy production into a new phase. In addition, the production of materials needed to build hardware components for the metaverse could increase concerns about the contamination of the Earth with hazardous materials.

3 Ethical Issues on the Metaverse and People with Disabilities

One of the important issues that must be considered when designing a new technology is the challenge of using it for people with different physical and movement limitations. For example, with the spread of the disease and widespread acceptance of online education systems, one of the topics that attracted the attention of experts was the ability of people with disabilities, especially blind people, to benefit from online education environments. Using the online education environment was very convenient for a normal person, but the facilities intended for blind people were very few, and these people could not easily use the features of this technology with shortcut keys. In terms of accessibility, blind people should be able to understand the concept of videos, deaf people should be able to view caption videos, physically disabled people should be able to enter commands in voice, and people with cognitive impairments should be able to easily work with applications and learn the work steps without engaging their minds [3].

These issues also apply to the metaverse environment, and the question that occupies the minds of disabled people is the extent to which they can easily use this environment. Are there special facilities for blind people and people with various disabilities? The VR headsets had controls for the right and left hands. Many controls have keys that are difficult to press owing to their small size. In addition, they have joysticks that are difficult to hold, which is very difficult for disabled people who need special facilities. Here, the role of gesture devices can be considered in helping these people. In this type of device, users can perform the required movements in a virtual environment by moving their hands to the left and right. In addition, disabled people also have problems with accessibility to the metaverse environment and interacting with it. For example, a person with mobility problems can pick the desired product from one row of a virtual store.

Despite this, blind people can still perform the required movements in a metaverse environment. For example, Ara is the name of a smart device that can detect objects and transmit them to a blind person in the form of vibration [4]. One application of this device in the field of the metaverse is to create a feeling of being close to an object in a virtual journey between two cities.

Figure 1 shows the group of disabled people related to the metaverse, which will be examined in the following, and the problems related to them in this environment.

Fig. 1 Metaverse and people with disabilities

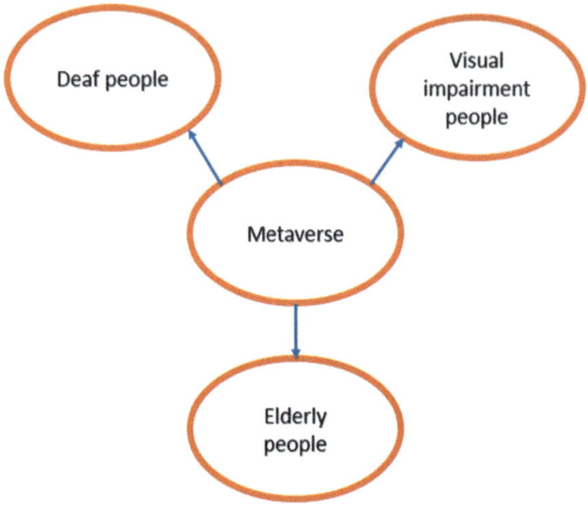

3.1 *People with Visual Impairment*

3.1.1 Accessibility

An important topic in the field of using the metaverse technology is the number of facilities considered for blind people during the use of this new technology. For example, for this group of people, a screen-reading tool should be considered that can provide the necessary explanations to users through audio descriptions [5].

3.1.2 Privacy

Camera-based assistive technologies can be considered tools that provide information about the blind to this group of people. For example, more advanced smart glasses, in addition to analyzing data in front of people, also provide the possibility of analyzing data collected from behind [6]. The combination of this technology with the metaverse increases the concerns of blind people in the field of privacy, and great care should be taken when using these types of tools to prevent compromising privacy.

Among other tools, we can mention smart voice assistants, which have embedded cameras and microphones, which have expanded the concerns in the field of privacy, especially for blind people, because here a new concept is created in the field of privacy, and that is "tangible privacy." It is important to turn the microphone and camera on and off. When the user can feel whether these expressions are on or off, their confidence about whether they are off or on also increases [7], so installing installable controls so that the user can check whether the device is on or off increases the user's trust, increases reliability, and decreases privacy concerns.

3.2 *Deaf People*

One of the tools that can be considered for deaf people in a metaverse environment is sign language interpretation for communication and interaction with the metaverse environment. Thus, an individual can interact using sign language in a virtual environment. In addition, the use of text-to-speech conversion tools can play an important role in the participation of deaf people in a metaverse environment, so that their avatar can speak easily.

3.3 *Elderly People*

The elderly are a group of people in society who are considered more vulnerable, and special care must be taken into account in the design of technology for them, for example, in the field of security, the participation of an elderly person in the metaverse environment and the use of tools related to it, such as wearable devices, despite the many benefits in terms of the possibility of diagnosing diseases and communicating with health centers in emergency situations, abusing from this situation is possibility. It provides that it is easy to get the information of the elderly person, and in addition to obtaining the virtual information of the elderly person, it is also dangerous for the physical life of the person, and the living environment of the elderly person can be threatened by thieves. To better understand the issue of paying attention to the elderly in a metaverse environment, effective factors in motivating the participation of the elderly and creating risks for them have been investigated. The factors that cause the presence of more elderly people in the Internet environment are [8]:

3.3.1 Security and Behavioral Skills

Limited Information/Skills on Security Risks

Lack of skills and knowledge about the dangers of the Internet environment and unwillingness to learn about the risks that threaten them in the Internet environment can cause serious harm to the elderly. Therefore, the presence of the elderly in a metaverse environment can cause many problems for them in the near future. It is possible that some people are of the opinion that the current elderly generation is less familiar with the Internet environment and because of this, it causes more harm to them than the generation that is getting old, but this fact should not be forgotten that in old age, the ability of the individual's skills is reduced; for this reason, in each period, the elderly are less familiar with technology than young people in the same period.

The Desire to Receive Services in the Simplest Way

Evidence shows that the elderly are looking for the easiest way to access their banking services, such as by asking friends and neighbors for help [9]. This situation has also affected the reluctance of the elderly to accept advanced methods of determining the identity of users in the Internet environment, and the reluctance of the elderly to use new security methods, such as the use of antiviruses or storing passwords. In the near future, with the development of the metaverse environment on the one hand and the rapid progress of various technologies, new methods of information and identity thcft cannot be compared to new technologies. Therefore, with the unwillingness of the elderly to learn methods of determining identity, serious problems are created for them. However, it should not be overlooked that the design of programs and services for the elderly, especially now that the world is facing an aging crisis, has conditions that must be carefully considered in future metaverse environments. For example, when designing an application for the elderly, special attention should be paid to their ability to use the services provided, because the elderly face factors such as reduced vision, hearing, and thinking; for this reason, it is not possible to use complex methods.

Perhaps some people believe that the development of new technologies such as wearable devices will solve their problems, but on the other hand, the elderly face new problems due to a lack of familiarity with the dangers of new technologies. More attention should be paid to designers in the metaverse environments.

Vulnerability to Certain Fraud

Research [9] shows that the elderly are easily trapped by fraudsters who send posts similar to bank, police, and government messages. This is because of their trust in these centers. By sending messages and claiming problems with payment, account security, or refunds, fraudsters try to collect valuable information about the elderly to achieve their goals. Precious information that can easily remove the entire wealth of an elderly person, wealth that is impossible to renew for the elderly, or is replaced by difficult conditions, should therefore be kept private.

The vulnerability of the elderly is not limited to sending messages, and the most important issue is finding the behavioral alcoves of people, especially the elderly, to find new methods of Internet fraud, which can cause many problems for the elderly in the metaverse environment.

3.3.2 Issues Related to Health and Society

Figure 2 shows the health and society concerns related to the metaverse, which will be examined in the following.

Reduction of Health and Strength of Movement

One of the important topics that increase the desire of the elderly to use online services, especially in the fields of finance, social services, and health, is the decrease in the health and strength of the elderly to perform physical work. For this reason, they share all the details of their information in interactions on the Internet, which exposes their lives to serious risks, such as theft of personal information.

Memory Problems and Cognitive Deficits

Short-term memory impairment and forgetfulness can make it difficult for elderly people to understand the occurrence of fraud, remember its details, and report fraud to the authorities. Cognitive deficits (reduction in the power of cruelty) or the speed of perception (reduction in the processing of images and sounds) can cause irreparable risks in the Internet environment because they are unable to understand and evaluate the risks. For example, in topics such as phishing, these types of messages cannot be distinguished from original messages. Moreover, they cannot use the desired commands to increase the security of their personal information. This study can affect the activities of the elderly in the metaverse environment and in

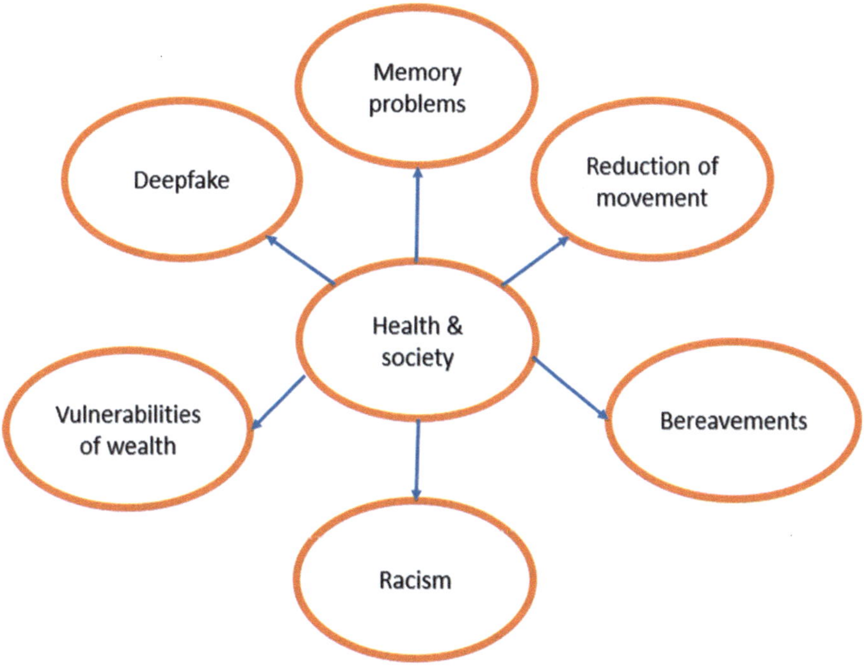

Fig. 2 Health and society concerns related to the metaverse

the complex environments provided by different companies. Despite this weakness, the personal information of the elderly can be easily threatened.

Separation from Society and Loneliness

A large number of elderly people live alone and are members of small communities. For this reason, with the expansion of social networks, there is a great desire to participate in interactions created on the Internet, which causes many challenges and the presence of fraudsters who abuse the trust of the elderly. Therefore, fraudsters engage in activities to achieve their goals by establishing communication and increasing their sense of trust. This type of fraud is called grooming, and people are prone to it due to loneliness and the desire to participate in social groups.

Bereavements

Bereavement scams are a type of fraud in which a person uses the opportunity created by the death of a person to contact the family of the deceased with a trick, for example, an insurance agent that tries to deceive them [10].

One of the most important and vulnerable cases among the elderly is financial management after stress or bereavement; therefore, in these cases, the elderly face a problem in identifying a fraudulent person and becoming a victim. This issue is seen more in the case of people whose financial matters are managed by their spouses, who have died now [8].

Wealth

After years of hard work, the elderly have wealth in their old age, which attracts the attention of fraudsters owing to their lack of familiarity with security issues in cyberspace and the absence of checking their bank accounts. According to the points mentioned, the elderly population is a large, vulnerable group that easily faces all kinds of scams in the internet environment. Because of their physical condition and reduced physical abilities, they are unable to defend themselves against scammers. Despite this fact, the many advantages of a metaverse environment for the elderly can be dangerous for their security and create many social consequences for governments, which require strict measures in the field of creating security surveys according to the temperament of the elderly. It is worth mentioning that issues such as people who are victims of Internet fraud with the title of greedy or naïve can play an important role in reporting fraud cases among the elderly because they are afraid and embarrassed to label themselves with these titles. Moreover, the elderly fear that reporting fraud will make them known as someone who is unable to cope with their work and will limit their lifestyle [8].

Of course, it goes without saying that the aforementioned vulnerabilities are related to a generation that has not fully used Internet services, and the next generation will be more alert in this field; however, new technologies will also create new methods of defrauding the elderly. Therefore, by examining the challenges faced by the elderly in the Internet environment, it is necessary to educate the elderly in relation to the harm of cyberspace and the metaverse environment in the near future.

Racism

In 2016, ProPublica reporters reported that Facebook classified people based on race and sent ads to them based on this classification [11]. This happened when Facebook did not ask users about their race. However, Facebook recognizes its race by using the activity of users (liking posts and web pages) on this platform and collecting and analyzing it. In addition, the issue of selling avatars in virtual environments before the metaverse was faced with racist and sexist harassment, so avatars, which are graphic images representing people in the virtual environment, are priced at different prices based on race. Another issue is the frequently removed comments of black women on Facebook regarding racism and sexism [12]. These are small examples that consider the issue of race and ethnicity in the virtual environment before the development of the metaverse virtual environment.

Deepfake

"Deepfake" is a word that is derived from joining two words "Deep learning" and "fake," which was initially started by a Reddit user in 2017 by publishing videos on social networks in "that mapped the faces of stars like Scarlett Johansson onto sexual performers" [13]. Most of the uses of deepfakes can be considered in pornographic topics [14]. However, its use in politics has also been considered [15]. In the near future, with the development of new technologies in the field of artificial intelligence, a new generation of Deepfake images and videos will be designed in the metaverse, which will affect people's private and social lives.

4 Government

The metaverse infrastructure is developing at a very fast pace, and we will witness the emergence of new technologies and applications in this field using artificial intelligence tools. However, the most important issue is the attention of governments and legislators to the new uses of the metaverse.

For example, how should intellectual property challenges be faced in the future in the metaverse environment, and what are the laws in this field? How are issues, such as taxes and sales, in this environment? How is monitoring of issues such as cyberbullying managed in a metaverse environment? To prevent security challenges, how is the identification operation applied in this environment? Topics, such as user personal data, are supported against various risks. However, the most important challenge in a metaverse environment is the decentralized world, so that user data are widely accessible [16].

Countries can only act to block infrastructure and cannot directly enter and have a comprehensive global law on topics such as how to operate in this environment and sharing and acquiring user data. Any country can monitor its companies and startups and impose restrictions. However, implementing a general rule that can be used worldwide is challenging. The mentioned materials, in connection with topics such as cyberbullying, deepfakes, security, and privacy, show the importance and role of governments in dealing with and preventing such incidents. To achieve a secure online environment for everyone, the most important issue is matching the real information of users with the virtual information of users [17]. In these cases, there is a need to approve new laws.

5 Intellectual Property

In the metaverse, the things that are made, such as buildings, marketplaces, or avatars, cannot be considered programs, but they can be considered in the artistic works group; therefore, they are included in copyright law, and the intellectual rights of their creators must be protected.

In the continuation of this discussion, two situations are created:

1. In this case, a company provides the necessary infrastructure, and the user has the ability to create new elements. In this situation, terms and conditions can delegate intellectual property to the service provider company.
2. In this case, the user does not have the ability to create a new element and can use only the facilities provided by the company. Therefore, the spiritual owner of the element is the same provider company.

6 NFTs

Non-Fungible Tokens (NFTs) are defined as "new digital assets, powered by blockchain technology, in which all the transactions are recorded" [18].

The owner of an NFT is stored in the blockchain, and the owner can sell it and use it in transactions. NFTs can contain artwork, video, film, or real estate and can be created by anyone, even with little programming knowledge. However, the most important issue is the law of copyright and the intellectual property of products. When a person buys an NFT, he/she only buys a digital token and does not own the copyright or license for that product [19]. For example, when buying an NFT, including a signed book, the person buys a copy of that product and is not the original owner of the original copy. In this case, the smart contracts stored in the blockchain can be considered an agreement and a contract between the seller and the buyer. Therefore, with a little investigation, it can be concluded that there are no specific rules in the field of NFTs [18].

If a seller wants to transfer the intellectual rights of his/her work, he/she must act in accordance with the rules that are related to the real world. For example, in England, copyright transfer operations under the Copyright Designs and Patents Act 1988 (CDPA) require a copyright assignment that is "in writing signed by or on behalf of the assignor." Because of the extent and virtual nature of NFTs, they will face new challenges.

7 Education in the Metaverse

One aspect that should be given special attention in the field of the metaverse is the issue of training users for better and healthier interaction with this environment without many borders. The metaverse environments, with many advances in artificial intelligence technologies, are very advanced environments prone to many risks in areas such as security, privacy, cyberbullying, and deepfakes. An environment that competes among different companies and creates many fields in the interactions between the user and the virtual world is a double-edged sword that can affect the life of humanity. The metaverse is more than just a social networking environment. Currently, social networks by themselves have affected most aspects of people's lives, and there is not a day that we do not witness various crimes in cyberspace. However, the crimes committed in the current social network environments are not comparable to Internet crimes in the metaverse environment. For example, think that with the help of artificial intelligence, the information collected from a user is used to make a game, and this character is used in future interactive environments, such as porn interactive environments.

With little precision, many psychologically damaging effects can be considered by the user. A user who does not have the ability to stop the harassment and spread of the desired content because of the absence of rules or the presence of rules without limits and boundaries of interactions in the metaverse environment must only watch the destruction of his personality in the virtual world. Therefore, governments and organizations related to education should pay special attention to the issue of prevention before treatment, i.e., education of their users. Users should be aware of the consequences of their actions and activities on the Internet. For example, every day, we see many pictures of children broadcast in the virtual environment by parents. Parents who do not know without enough awareness of the results of this act—that is, sharing their children's data on the Internet—broadcast them. However, the most important point is that in the current Internet environment, the problem of sharing users' data, especially children, ends with viewing photos or videos, whereas in the metaverse environment, the same data can be used to create different characters in games and movies, which has irreparable effects on human interaction. However, with little precision and increased awareness of humanity, it is possible to reduce the heavy burden of the various metaverse effects in different fields. A highly complex environment with many attractions attracts users, willingly or unwillingly. However, teaching users about the risks can clarify the sense of the dangerousness of the metaverse environment for them, and as a result, users interact more carefully and obsessively in a metaverse environment.

Education of children, elderly people, and disabled people in relation to the risks and challenges of the metaverse environment should be considered because they are exposed to many risks in the Internet environment, and they should be familiar with the challenges of this environment and how to interact with it.

But the issue of education is not only for users, and government decision-makers in countries around the world should not be forgotten in the field of education. Large amounts of data are stored by the government. For example, different user data exist in the field of health. Therefore, one of the most important concerns for governments is training employees to address the challenges of the metaverse environment. Another example found in the field of government challenges and the need to train employees in relation to this environment is the field of politics and the political propaganda of representatives. An example of this type of action is Trump's advertising and the use of social network services to change users' opinions about an election rival. This issue reveals the necessity of training government employees in the field of the challenges of the metaverse environment.

Companies should also pay special attention to their employees and provide them with the necessary training related to the metaverse threats. To prevent the margins that the metaverse environment will cause in the future due to the unfamiliarity of the employees with this environment. Topics such as endangering the security and privacy of the company.

8 Physical and Mental Health

One of the most important issues in the field of technologies used in the metaverse environment is the physical and mental health of users. The previous experience of using the Internet shows that users easily become addicted to new technologies, endangering their physical and mental health.

In an online survey conducted among 1050 users regarding the dangers of the metaverse, 47 percent cited addiction to simulated reality and 41 percent cited privacy and mental health issues as major threats to this environment [20].

Celine Merkx and Jeroen Nawijn's research on the use of VR in the field of tourism experience shows that users have become addicted to using the simulated environment and have no desire to leave the environment. Some users even considered selling their devices to finance the launch of virtual reality. Behavior seen among addicts. In addition, other users claimed that they did not want to use this technology initially, but after the first experience, their senses were aroused for further use. Users have also stated that while using the VR headset, they felt isolation and loneliness, similar to visiting the moon [21].

9 Security and Privacy

One of the important challenges in the field of user privacy in a metaverse environment is the collection and analysis of user behavior using data collected by sensors and their activities in the program environment.

One of the advantages of the metaverse is that each user is shown as a three-dimensional avatar [22, 23]. However, this issue also creates challenges for the users. On the one hand, it collects a large amount of user data [24]. On the other hand, the collection of this volume of data provides the conditions for big data analytics and user behavior analysis, and therefore concerns about the improper use of data, for example, their analysis and sale, increase ethical concern in this field. This is increasingly appearing [25]. For example, Facebook and Cornell University researchers in their research analyzed user feedback in front of the same information but from negative and positive aspects. The results of this research show that negative and positive posts affect users' feelings about news [26]. After the publication of the results of this research, there was a wave of concern among users regarding the unauthorized use of their data. However, Facebook believed that when users signed up for an account, they accepted the company's slogans, and the company could use their data. Moreover, the posts analyzed were visible to other users [23].

10 Case Study

The study of Nick Munn and his colleagues on the concerns related to the development of the metaverse states that although topics such as user privacy can be threatened in this environment, but with the development of new security methods, the necessary ground for the expansion of the metaverse and the use of its facilities can be provided [27].

11 Conclusion

Recent developments in the field of information technology have affected all aspects of humanity. One of these aspects is extensive development in the field of virtual environments. The virtual environment, called the metaverse, creates many changes in the social, economic, and cultural interactions of humans along with the real environment. Changes will not be without challenges. Whenever new technologies are discussed, new challenges remain open in that field. The metaverse will also not be without challenges, owing to its many attractions. For example, there are many concerns regarding the security, privacy, and interactions of people with disabilities and the elderly in this environment. In this chapter, an attempt is made to deal with issues that are rarely addressed in other scientific writings related to the metaverse.

References

1. Grider, D., & Maximo, M. (2021). *THE METAVERSE: Web 3.0 Virtual Cloud Economies.* https://grayscale.com/wp-content/uploads/2021/11/Grayscale_Metaverse_Report_Nov2021.pdf. Accessed 30 Aug 2023.
2. Gupta, R., & Pal, S. K. (2023). Seven layers of Metaverse. In *Introduction to Metaverse: Technology landscape, applications, and challenges* (pp. 45–66). Springer.
3. Caldwell, B., et al. (2008). Web content accessibility guidelines (WCAG) 2.0. *WWW Consort, 290*, 1–34.
4. Dickstein, L. (2022). *A wearable cane strap technologies Ara.* https://time.com/collection/best-inventions-2022/6230641/strap-technologies-ara/. Accessed 08 May 2023.
5. Alexiou, G. (2022). *What type of accessibility features need to be present in the Metaverse?*https://www.forbes.com/sites/gusalexiou/2022/03/31/is-the-Metaverse-likely-to-be-accessible-and-inclusive-of-people-with-disabilities/. Accessed 08 May 2023.
6. Akter, T., Ahmed, T., Kapadia, A., & Swaminathan, M. (2022). Shared privacy concerns of the visually impaired and sighted bystanders with camera-based assistive technologies. *ACM Transactions on Accessible Computing, 15*(2), 1–33.
7. Ahmad, I., Akter, T., Buher, Z., Farzan, R., Kapadia, A., & Lee, A. J. (2022). Tangible privacy for smart voice assistants: Bystanders' perceptions of physical device controls. *Proceedings of the ACM on Human-Computer Interaction, 6*(CSCW2), 1–31.
8. Tripathi, K., Cooper, C., & Burton, A. (2020). *Older adults as victims of online financial crime.* UCL. https://www.ucl.ac.uk/future-crime/sites/future_crime/files/ucl_policy_briefing_-_older_people_and_financial_crime_december21.pdf. Accessed 02 Sep 2023.
9. A. UK. (2015). Only the tip of the iceberg: Fraud against older people. *Evidence Review.* [Online]. Available: https://www.ageuk.org.uk/globalassets/age-uk/documents/reports-and-publications/reports-and-briefings/safe-at-home/rb_april15_only_the_tip_of_the_iceberg.pdf
10. Barclays. (2023). *Bereavement Scams.* https://www.barclays.co.uk/fraud-and-scams/bereavement-scams/. Accessed 02 Sep 2023.
11. Angwin, J., & Jr, T. P. (2016). Facebook lets advertisers exclude users by race. *ProPublica.* https://www.propublica.org/article/facebook-lets-advertisers-exclude-users-by-race. Accessed 06 Aug 2023.
12. Adeyemo, B. (2021). *I'm a Black woman and the Metaverse scares me—Here's how to make the next iteration of the internet inclusive.* https://theconversation.com/im-a-black-woman-and-the-Metaverse-scares-me-heres-how-to-make-the-next-iteration-of-the-internet-inclusive-173310. Accessed 07 Aug 2023.
13. Wu, H., Hui, P., & Zhou, P. (2023). Deepfake in the Metaverse: An outlook survey. arXiv Prepr. arXiv2306.07011.
14. Ajder, H., Patrini, G., Cavalli, F., & Cullen, L. (2019). *The state of Deepfakes: Landscape, threats, and impact.* [Online]. Available: https://regmedia.co.uk/2019/10/08/deepfake_report.pdf
15. Maddocks, S. (2020). 'A Deepfake porn plot intended to silence me': Exploring continuities between pornographic and 'political' deep fakes. *Porn Studies, 7*(4), 415–423.

16. Caserta, R. (2023). *The Metaverse: Why governments should care*. https://kpmg.com/xx/en/blogs/home/posts/2023/01/the-Metaverse-why-governments-should-care.html. Accessed 12 Aug 2023.
17. Wu, H., & Zhang, W. (2023). Digital identity, privacy security, and their legal safeguards in the Metaverse. *Security and Safety, 2*, 2023011.
18. CE. (2022). *Intellectual property in the Metaverse*. Episode IV: Copyright. https://intellectual-property-helpdesk.ec.europa.eu/news-events/news/intellectual-property-Metaverse-episode-iv-copyright-2022-06-30_en. Accessed 12 Aug 2023.
19. Macura, A. (2023). *NFTs & Copyright: What do you own?*https://www.searchenginejournal.com/nft-copyright/481280/#close. Accessed 15 Aug 2023.
20. Statista. (2021). *Dangers of the Metaverse according to internet users worldwide in 2021*.
21. Merkx, C., & Nawijn, J. (2021). Virtual reality tourism experiences: Addiction and isolation. *Tourism Management, 87*, 104394. https://doi.org/10.1016/j.tourman.2021.104394
22. Narin, N. G. (2021). A content analysis of the Metaverse articles. *Journal of Metaverse, 1*(1), 17–24.
23. Anshari, M., Syafrudin, M., Fitriyani, N. L., & Razzaq, A. (2022). Ethical responsibility and sustainability (ERS) development in a Metaverse business model. *Sustainability, 14*(23). https://doi.org/10.3390/su142315805
24. Kato, R., Kikuchi, Y., Yem, V., & Ikei, Y. (2022). Reality Avatar for customer conversation in the Metaverse. In *Human interface and the management of information: Applications in complex technological environments: Thematic area*, HIMI 2022, Held as Part of the 24th HCI International Conference, HCII 2022, Virtual Event, June 26 July 1, 2022, Proceedings, Part II, 2022, pp. 131–145.
25. Fernandez, C. B., & Hui, P. (2022). Life, the Metaverse and everything: An overview of privacy, ethics, and governance in Metaverse. In *2022 IEEE 42nd international conference on distributed computing systems workshops (ICDCSW)* (pp. 272–277).
26. Chambers, C. (2014). *Facebook fiasco: Was Cornell's study of 'emotional contagion' an ethics breach?*https://www.theguardian.com/science/head-quarters/2014/jul/01/facebook-cornell-study-emotional-contagion-ethics-breach. Accessed 01 May 2024.
27. Munn, N., & Weijers, D. (2023). The real ethical problem with metaverses. *Frontiers in Human Dynamics, 5*. https://doi.org/10.3389/fhumd.2023.1226848

Harnessing the Potential of the Metaverse in Medical Education and Training

Aiesha Kuna and D. Lakshmi

1 Introduction

The term "metaverse" was first used in the novel "Snow Crash" written by N. Stephenson (2003) [1], based in a dystopian fantasy describing the escapades of the protagonist, Hiro, within a virtual world wherein he could make purchases, explore, and even defeat real-world enemies within this "metaverse," explain Rabindra Ratan et al. (2021) [2]. Bringing this concept to life, standing at the pinnacle of the evolution of computer systems is the metaverse—an extension of extended reality (XR), virtual reality (VR), augmented reality (AR), and mixed reality (MR). The metaverse is, essentially, a virtual world that may compose of elements from the real world, which allows us to traverse within itself using an avatar to represent ourselves. We may make financial transactions, actions, indulge in entertainment, sports, or perform any activity that we do in the real world within the metaverse. This opens up a wide spectrum of possibilities for human–computer, human–human, or even human–object interaction on a whole new level. While immersive technologies are believed to have been around since the 1960s, they have begun to catch the public eye upwards of 2016, which was when head-mounted displays (HMDs) were popularized according to Foxman (2018) [8]. With its rapid development, immersive technologies began to take over most industries.

The next step in the path that technology has paved for the world to follow its footsteps in is undoubtedly the metaverse. Figure 1 details the major categories of the metaverse technology, while Fig. 2 shows the various steps being undertaken in the development of the metaverse so far, with reference to the analysis of Lee (2022) [11], Gelernter (1993) [12], Evans et al. (2017) [13], and Orchard et al. (2022) [14]. With major companies now eyeing its growth and Huang et al. (2022) [15]

A. Kuna · D. Lakshmi (✉)
School of Computing Science Engineering and Artificial Intelligence (SCAI), VIT Bhopal University, Bhopal, Madhya Pradesh, India

C. L. Chowdhary (ed.), *The Metaverse for the Healthcare Industry*,
https://doi.org/10.1007/978-3-031-60073-9_5

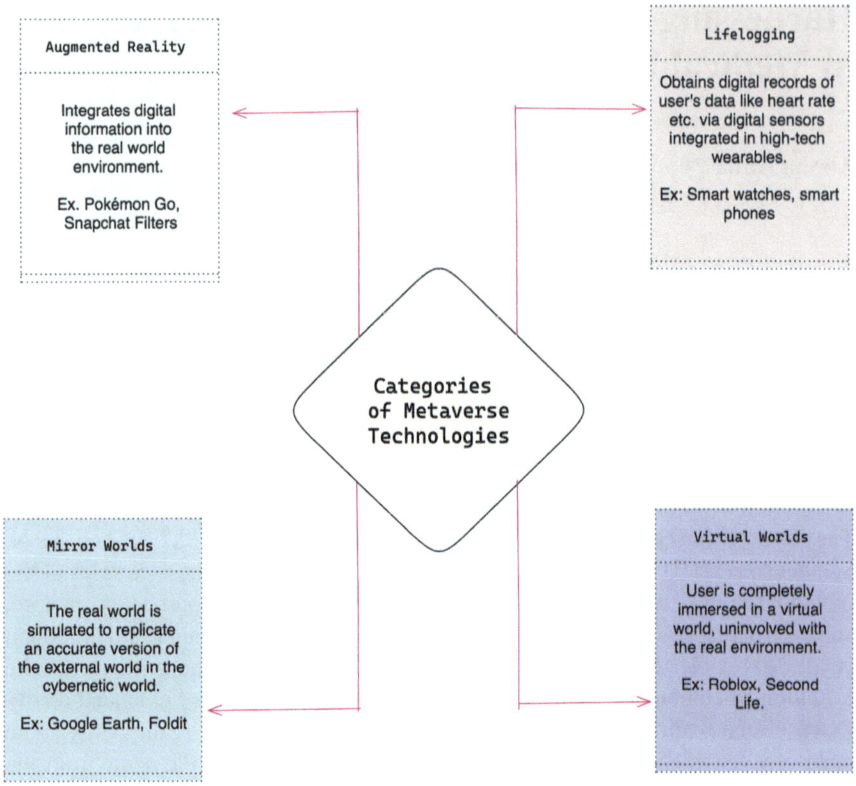

Fig. 1 Categories of the metaverse technologies

estimating them to be investing over $50 billion in the creation and development of the metaverse, all heads turn to the next important question: *How would the metaverse be implemented in general healthcare?*

Healthcare is an essential industry for human survival which has been present as far as time can tell. Maintaining good physical, mental, general, and social health of an individual and largely the entire human population is integral for the progression of society as stressed by R. Chengoden et al. (2023) [9]. Illness and disease have always plagued the earth, threatening life; however, development and progress in medical sciences have allowed us to flourish and get to where our society stands today. With developments in technology leading to improvement in various fields, the healthcare industry finds various applications of VR, AR, MR, and XR in its functions. For example, Z. Qu et al. (2022) [10] detail the immersive technologies being used in the "Remote GP Consultation" project, which is run by the Silver Chain Group. This project allows a nurse to check the patients' health data and consult with a remote holographic doctor enabled with AR technology. The purpose of this project is to help a nurse who needs to speak to a doctor who may be busy helping patients—so he or she can look through Microsoft HoloLens to see patients'

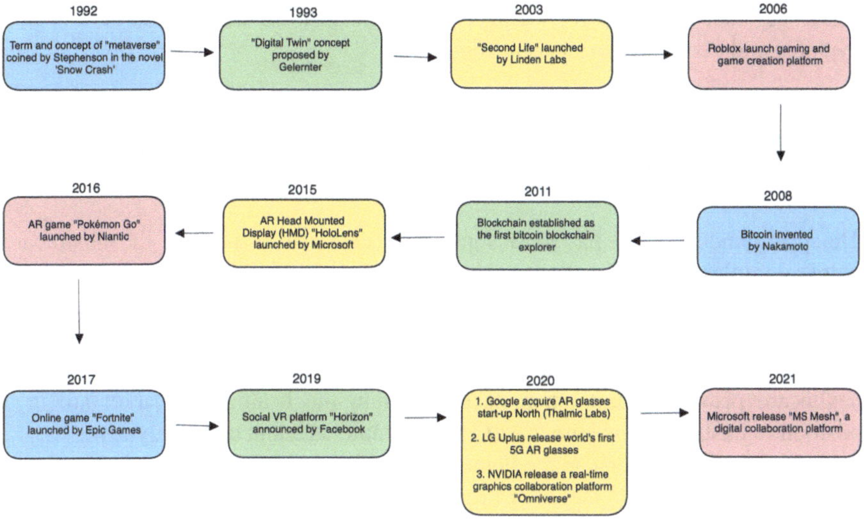

Fig. 2 Timeline of the metaverse

data and speak to a holographic doctor. The HoloLens VR/AR/MR technology allows for the doctors to stay in their current location while still helping out and finishing their job. Further down the line, this project could accommodate patients receiving similar care in the comfort of their own homes. This is a good example of how much easier immersive technologies make healthcare professionals' work as well as making the recovery process more convenient for the patient. Naturally, this commands urgency to draw our attention to the future prospects of the metaverse in the realm of healthcare.

2 Key Study Parameters

Harnessing the minds of young or aspiring professionals in the medical field, who are more willing to utilize newer technologies as compared to existing health professionals, may be made possible by understanding and taking advantage of the valuable resource we call the metaverse. Delving into the multifaceted ways in which the metaverse, a virtual and immersive digital environment, is being harnessed to enhance medical learning, skills acquisition, and professional development, this chapter explores the transformative potential of the metaverse in the realm of medicine—more specifically in medical education and training. Through an examination of innovative applications, technologies, and emerging trends, this study aims to provide insights into the evolving landscape of medical education within the metaverse. By analyzing its impact on accessibility, collaboration, simulation, and experiential learning, we seek to elucidate the possibilities and challenges that lie ahead for medical educators, institutions, and learners in this dynamic and evolving educational frontier.

3 Significance of the Metaverse in the Healthcare Industry

The post-pandemic era has seen some very clear shifts in how the healthcare industry implements technology or simply operates at all. Chengoden et al. (2023) [9] observe that at present, consumers lean more towards using virtual healthcare systems and related digital innovations as compared to the pre-pandemic conditions and on average choose to make much healthier lifestyle choices. Governments, healthcare providers, and other stakeholders in the healthcare market are in a position to hastily endorse the use of interoperable data and data analytics.

Although the metaverse in medicine has not been implemented yet, the predicted size of this market is too large to be ignored. By 2032, the expected market growth of the global medical metaverse is predicted to reach about USD 98.34 billion, estimating a compound annual growth rate (CAGR) of 29.4% from 2023 to 2032, computes Velleriya Ivanova (2023) [16]. A major factor in the popularization of the usage of the metaverse in the healthcare industry is the COVID-19 pandemic. During the pandemic, telemedicine (or teleconsultation) was heavily relied upon as people were unable to move out of their homes. Pre-pandemic, only 43% of healthcare facilities could offer remote services to their patients. Due to the effects of the pandemic, healthcare facilities were pushed to find ways to provide therapy without patients having to physically be present at the facility. Owing to this rapid digitalization, now about 95% of health facilities provide remote services, according to Kala et al. (2022) [6]. With the metaverse, teleconsultations can be furthered by 3D clinical visits between patients and doctors in a virtual office or any other location virtually. This would give a more "realistic" feel as compared to a website or video consultation.

The metaverse could also be instrumental in helping healthcare professionals diagnose diseases and planning the subsequent required treatment. The doctors at the Johns Hopkins Hospital have gone so far as to use AR glasses "Augmed" to help perform surgery in 2020, Chengoden et al. (2023) [9]. The metaverse may also be used for reconstruction and performance of plastic surgeries, which require immense precision, also giving the patient an opportunity to tentatively view what the results may look like, Wilson (2022) [17]. In general medicine, integrating the data of the patient's vitals, CT scans, health records, and genetic test results to create a digital simulation of the patient's anatomy and physiology, the use of digital twins solutions in the metaverse will keep the patients well-informed and engaged in their treatment, as hypothesized by Hassani et al. (2022) [18].

The implementation of the metaverse in healthcare is not limited solely to patient–doctor interactions. Largely, we can find broad areas of interest for its application as highlighted in Fig. 3. While all aspects of this transformation are

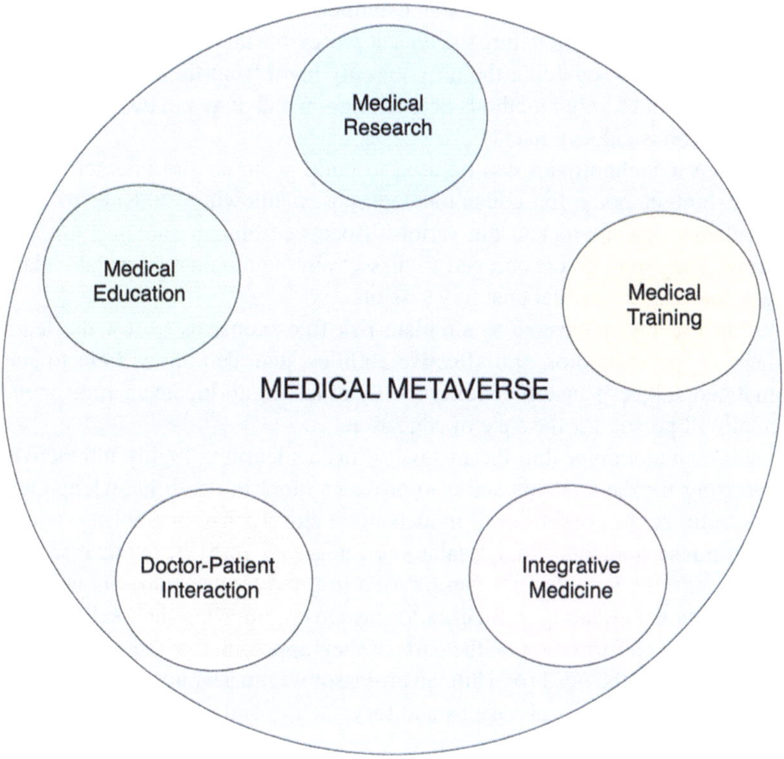

Fig. 3 Broad areas of application of the metaverse in medicine

important, in this chapter, we aim to further expand the advantages of implementing the metaverse in medical education, training, and research.

3.1 The Metaverse in Medical Education

"Medical education" can be used to refer to the knowledge imparted to a patient by health professionals to better understand their ailments or to the education undertaken by students that aspire to work in the healthcare industry—basically, students of any doctorate or nursing school. Extended reality and its expansion via the metaverse can take the understandability of complex medical concepts to an unprecedented level in multiple ways including:

- Tetra Signum developed a virtual medical education platform centered around surgical education. This platform was also used by a university to conduct remote lectures and discussions, and also allowed students to observe remote operating rooms with doctors of various countries including Japan, Singapore, and the UK,

S. Han et al. (2020) [19]. This is an example of how we could make use of the metaverse's open world nature to connect professors and doctors from around the world to students, enabling them to not only learn from the best of the best but also understand foreign methods of teaching—which may not have been possible in strictly physical seminars.

- AR and VR technologies can be used to build accurate and interactive models of the human body for educational purposes, allowing students to explore, understand, and appreciate the various aspects of human anatomy much more deeply. They may be encouraged to dissect and manipulate a virtual cadaver to make full use of a virtual anatomy session.
- We can use the metaverse to simulate risk-free scenarios to test the learners' cognitive, psychomotor, and affective abilities, and also allow them to study a simulated subject's health condition without having to inconvenience or risk an actually ill person for the sake of education.
- Using a simulation within the metaverse makes learning highly interactive and interesting for the students and also provides more in-depth knowledge as they can scrutinize the conditions or models more closely than in real life.
- Detecting sensors and analytical tools integrated into the metaverse and its supporting hardware devices can be used to provide instantaneous feedback to the practitioners relating to their motor responses, boosting their self-confidence and providing information on the parts of their approach that they must still work on. Eliminating the need for a human professor within a simulation would require mandatory installation of various auditory, tactile, and visual sensors providing continuous feedback.
- Post the COVID-19 pandemic, medical professors observed that the students' hands-on experiences and interactions with patients were severely impeded, which are crucial to foster good practice and understanding in a learner. As a solution, Chen et al. (2022) [20] suggested that adopting an immersive, blended pedagogy combining traditional classroom instruction alongside immersive sessions in the metaverse would provide the most rounded curriculum and see an enhancement in student engagement as well as outcomes—especially within the fields of patient care and scientific enquiry.
- Yang et al. (2022) [5] made use of the BRM all-in-one machine to make use of holographic emulation to demonstrate the mechanism of lung cancer induced by smoking cigarettes. Students were provided an immersive experience allowing them to observe closely the alveolar damage caused by the cigarette smoke and take note of its relationship with the onset of lung cancer. Figure 4 highlights the network architecture of the AR vision glasses that incorporate the BRM all-in-one machine.
- Suh et al. (2023) [3] proposed that the development of full-scale scenario-based simulator training can aid in the development of interpersonal communication skills, teamwork, leadership, decision-making, the capacity to prioritize tasks under time constraints, and stress management. Medical students can practice their clinical skills, such as analyzing medical histories, doing physical exams,

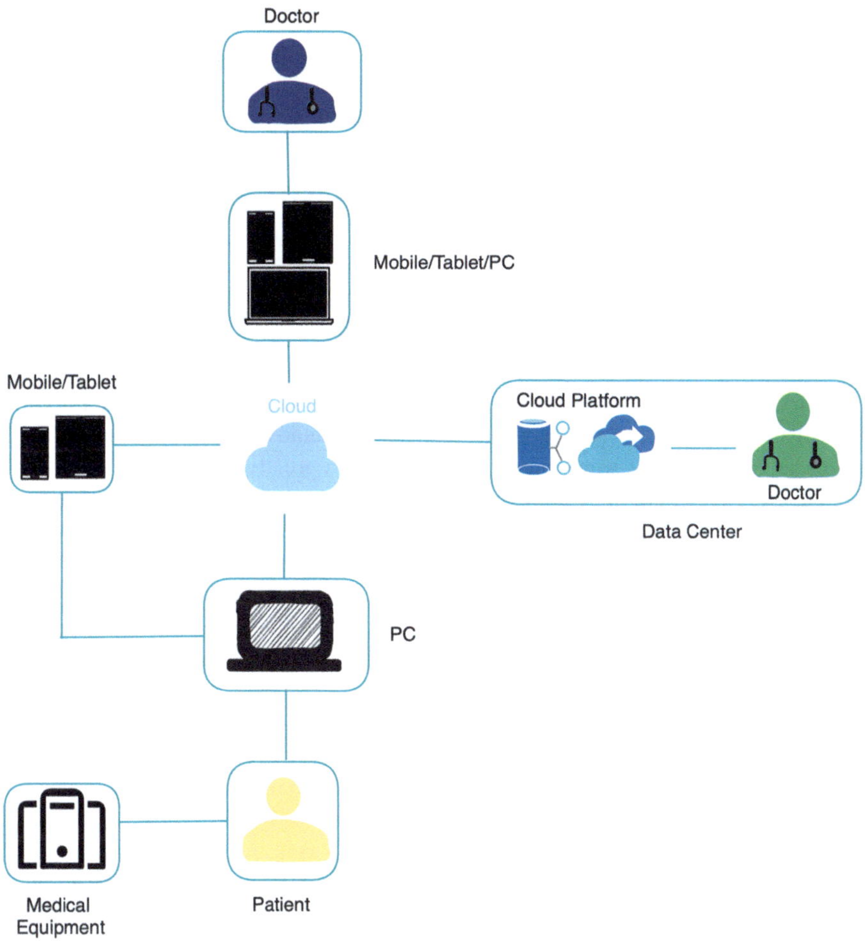

Fig. 4 Network architecture of Qian-AR glasses implementing the BRM all-in-one machine

and conversing with patients in virtual patient interactions using the full-scale scenario-based simulator.

- A study conducted by Kidd et al. (2012) [26] measured the effectiveness of a Second Life simulation as a teaching strategy for undergraduate mental health nursing students. The use of Second Life in baccalaureate, accelerated baccalaureate, and master's nursing programs "enables role playing, collaboration, real-time interactions between students and faculty, and experimentation," as observed by Skiba D.J. (2009) [27]. Students' part of the study attested that the usage of Second Life as part of their program was moderately effective, although slightly difficult on the technical aspect.
- Patients or even people not belonging to the medical field who may want to educate themselves on various health conditions or understand better ways to

improve their health. General medical education can be made more accessible and laid out in layman terms for the greater part of the population to access by dispatching the use of the metaverse. Immersive learning would allow easy absorption of this knowledge for those interested and increase the power to retain what is learned. This would revolutionize medical literacy among people or help a patient more clearly understand their condition rather than just go by what their doctor explains to them.

3.2 The Metaverse in Medical Research

The metaverse is a transformative concept, still having vague and varied definitions. Due to its immersive and global nature, it opens up a relatively new and exciting field of research which, if it were to bear fruition, would greatly enhance the quality of human life. In the field of health information, the metaverse can facilitate immersive research in controlled virtual environments. Suh et al. (2023) [3] highlight that the advantage of the metaverse over traditional research methodologies is that it promotes accessible collaboration between the team(s) involved, even remotely, and that it allows us to create an ideal environment for running tests without putting anybody at risk; further, it reduces chances of error in maintaining a controlled environment.

Among all medical fields, the psychology domain seems to find the most use cases for research within the metaverse. Bhugaonkar et al. (2022) [21] hypothesized that the metaverse stands to aid psychologists in studying social interactions and communication. This is confirmed by a study conducted by Krijn et al. (2004) [22] and their team of psychologists who made use of virtual reality exposure therapy (VRET) as an alternative to traditional exposure therapy to treat patients struggling with anxiety disorders. VRET is a type of therapy that simulates an anxiety-inducing scenario virtually in a safe and controlled environment to guide the patient to get over their anxiety. The result of their research was that VRET was much more effective in treating social anxiety, phobias, and post-traumatic stress disorders as compared to traditional exposure therapy.

Spiers and Maguire (2007) [23] conducted a neuroscience study using VR to investigate the neural mechanisms that underlie spatial memory. The researchers were able to monitor the parts of the brain that were selectively activated while performing tasks requiring spatial memory. During the conduction of this experiment, the researchers noted that having the subjects navigate through a virtual environment triggered more activity in the hippocampus (the region of the brain widely associated with memory) in comparison to having them view static images. From this study, we can derive the vast potential of VR or the metaverse in real-world applications for studying brain functions thoroughly.

Zhao et al. (2022) [24] also drew attention to the appeal of using the metaverse to present data from research in an easy-to-understand form or broadcast the findings to a wider audience using powerful interactive 3D visualizations of the data. In this way, we can take complicated calculations, derivations, and findings and compile them into a form that makes it quick to grasp and understand the final result of the research conducted, making it fun and exciting.

3.3 The Metaverse in Medical Training

Seeing as the growth of the metaverse in the medical edutech sector is on an upward curve, its implications on medical training must also be looked out for, as indicated by Ahuja et al. (2023) [4]. By taking advantage of the low-risk nature of the metaverse as a platform, students can be effectively trained in the necessary physical skills, complex clinical cases, or important ethical issues. As previously discussed, VR finds many applications in preclinical and clinical practice. Similarly, it may facilitate precision training for nursing students in clinical skills competency.

In a study conducted by Dyer et al. (2018) [25], an application was created to simulate immersive experiences to train students at the University of New England for aging services. The students were put in generated scenarios to observe and deal with age-related conditions like macular degeneration and high-frequency hearing loss by being put in the patients' shoes, allowing them to get a taste of what a real person suffering from the same may experience. As a result, the researchers observed that students from medical, physician assistant, physical therapy, and nursing schools into whose curriculum this method of training was integrated fostered much greater empathy for multiple age-related degenerative diseases.

Using extended reality, surgical skills can be trained in a risk-free environment. As the risk factor is potentially eliminated, even students in the first year who are just starting out may also gain hands-on experience in an immersive and informative virtual scenario. Research in this field hints that including remote observation and assistance during surgery is a viable possibility with the evolution of the metaverse and extended reality systems.

On May 29, 2021, under the supervision of the Asian Thoracic Surgery Education Group at the 29th Online Conference of the Asian Heart and Thoracic Surgery Society, an outreach program was held using XR technology. This program was aimed at providing training in lung cancer surgery to more than 200 thoracic surgeons from multiple Asian countries and also from Manchester University, UK. The participants were instructed to set up their avatar and use a head-mounted display or a computer of their choice to enter a skillfully crafted virtual 360° environment broadcasted from the smart operating room in the Seoul National University Bundang Hospital. Koo (2021) [7] further expanded that those that received this training greatly appreciated how it was as if they were in the operating theater with the instructors, thanks to the high-definition surgical cameras and sound quality broadcasted and hosted in an interactive environment where they may switch angles or position to observe the techniques demonstrated as they feel comfortable.

4 Building a Bridge Between Nursing School and Effective Patient Care

Incorporating virtual reality into the curriculum of nursing school better prepares students for their looming exposure to the real-life patient care scene. Through the metaverse, the methodologies of providing proper care to patients may be indoctrinated into the nursing students so they may be well-built to handle people with various requirements from the get-go. The metaverse can simulate patients with different diseases, symptoms, and needs for their care, thereby allowing a student to grasp the best possible ways to provide comfort and treatment to the patient hands-on. Further, familiarizing the youth with technological advances pertaining to their application in the field of medicine would encourage them to use them to their benefit even as practitioners, potentially facilitating the popularization of accessing healthcare through virtual systems. Shorey et al. [30] conducted an analysis of multiple studies on nursing students (mostly conducted in developing countries) which determined that using virtual reality for training had a higher rate of time–cost-effectiveness as compared to mannequin-based simulations and face-to-face lectures.

In practice, doctors would be able to open virtual clinics for consultation and even use digital twins of their patients to conduct detailed examinations virtually. A patient's scan or test data can also be uploaded onto their digital profile to allow the doctor to diagnose them on the basis of these online, even if they are in a remote location. Table 1 highlights some of the various fields of applications of virtual reality in nursing education and patient care. Figure 5 summarizes the possible areas of applying the metaverse in medicine, which is a more in-depth expansion of Fig. 3.

Table 1 Applications of virtual reality in nursing education and patient care

Application	Description
Clinical skills practice	Students can practice their clinical skills using hyperrealistic, high-fidelity virtual simulations
Critical thinking	The enhancement of critical thinking and decision-making skills in nursing students is facilitated through the utilization of scenario-based simulations
Interprofessional learning	Interprofessional learning and teamwork among healthcare providers are promoted through the use of collaborative virtual simulations
Pain management	Virtual reality interventions are set up to alleviate discomfort and improve the comfort of patients when they may be experiencing some sort of pain that medicines or other numbing elements are unable to suppress
Anxiety and stress relief	In tune with the previous point, virtual reality simulations aid in diminishing anxiety and stress levels among patients undergoing medical procedures
Patient education	Virtual reality is employed for interactive patient education, aiming to empower and engage patients in their healthcare

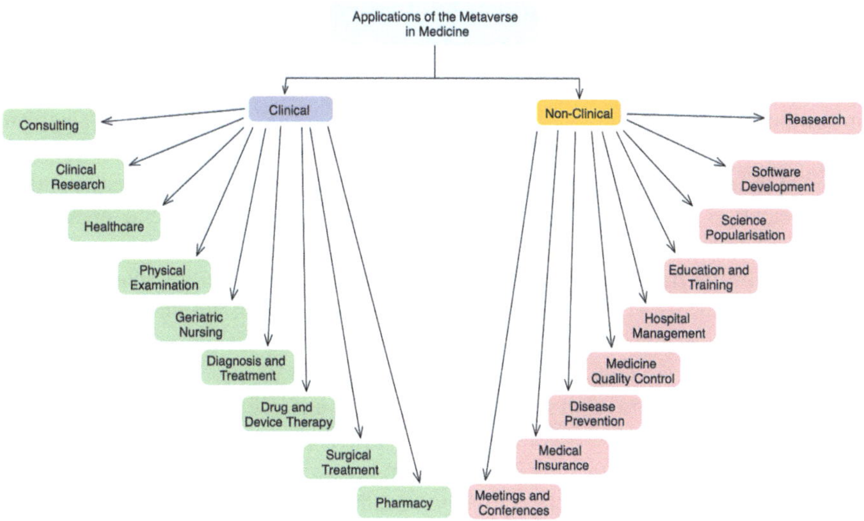

Fig. 5 Major clinical and nonclinical application scenarios for the metaverse in medicine

5 The Metaverse in Integrative Medicine

According to Gannotta et al. (2018) [31], integrative medicine is the treatment of patients through spiritual, emotional, mental, and environmental in addition to the physical means. Dyer et al. (2022) [32] concluded through their analysis that there are many studies that point to the fact that utilizing integrative medicine as a mode of treatment helps to promote the value of a better quality of life. The metaverse broadens the horizons of integrative medicine by allowing users to channel their energy into various activities like virtual yoga, guided meditation, nutritional advice, and similar mind-body therapies. Roblox, a sort of the metaverse platform, has a certain section dedicated to allow users to dive into a world of virtual mindfulness and practice guided yoga and meditation. This space was an initiative by Alo Yoga and has had a collective count of 55 million visits so far from all across the globe. The research of Gonçalves et al. (2012) [33] shows that this form of therapy applying to both the mind and body is also believed to be useful in helping patients suffering from PTSD, anxiety, or other illnesses onset by mental distress as well. There is also the possibility of allowing patients to be introduced to integrative medicine through the metaverse in order to allow them to test the waters and perhaps be less resistive towards the possibility of person-to-person sessions of integrative therapy.

6 Limitations of the Medical Metaverse

Despite the countless advantages and possibilities that deployment of the metaverse in the healthcare industry brings, there are certain limitations to how far we can go with its implementation and things to consider before we push for its large-scale usage in the field of medicine. Among the most concerning of these is the regulation and protection of data and privacy. The security, management, and privacy of patients' information is considered to be of top priority for health institutions, as explained by Petrigna et al. (2022) [28]. Therefore, unless we are able to impose strict regulations for ethical data collection and management within the metaverse, its usage in the healthcare industry may not be feasible. Further, Suh et al. (2023) [3] point out that medical professionals would have to go beyond their domain to study cybersecurity and similar courses in order to preserve patient privacy.

Another issue to consider is the varying Internet strength and bandwidth among professionals. People with slow Wi-Fi or low bandwidth, especially those in rural areas, may suffer from heavy lag in image streaming while attempting to access the metaverse. Also, students as well as professors would require the proper equipment supporting the requirements to enable usage of the metaverse; these devices are still worth quite a hefty price and may be inaccessible to a good many of those in the field of medical education.

Also, Suh et al. (2023) [3] observe that prolonged usage of VR and AR devices can induce discomfort, dizziness, headaches, or even nausea. Studies have also depicted that incessant usage of AR or VR technologies can lead to a "post-VR sadness," contributing to a transient depressive mood or a sort of ill feeling on extended use. Peckmann et al. (2022) [29] noted that people that spent a large amount of time playing a VR game displayed higher rates of depersonalization-derealization (DPDR) disorder than those accustomed to PC gaming, which causes an individual to feel disconnected from their physical body. However, Ahuja et al. (2022) [4] muse that although this may be true for VR gaming, it is still unknown whether usage of VR in the medical field would trigger a similar response.

Considering all these factors, it is clear that the true and widespread implementation of the metaverse in the medical field can be actively pursued and taken advantage of after addressing its negative implications and finding optimal solutions for them.

7 Conclusion

The metaverse undoubtedly represents a groundbreaking concept that holds the potential to revolutionize various aspects of healthcare, including medical education, research, and training. Via its flexibility, interoperability, feedback system, and engagement, the metaverse offers a new dimension for immersive learning, skill development, and innovative research in the field of medicine.

The significance of the metaverse in healthcare is underscored by its rapid growth, with substantial investments being made by major companies and a projected market size exceeding USD 98 billion by 2032. The post-pandemic shift towards virtual healthcare systems and digital innovations has further highlighted the relevance and timeliness of integrating the metaverse into healthcare practices.

In the realm of medical education, the metaverse offers opportunities for global collaboration, interactive learning experiences, and risk-free simulation scenarios. It enables students to gain hands-on experience, understand complex medical concepts, and develop critical skills in a dynamic and engaging virtual environment. Medical professionals can utilize the metaverse not only to educate their patients but also to enhance their own training and professional development.

In medical research, the metaverse provides a safe and controlled platform for immersive studies, particularly in psychology and neuroscience. Researchers can explore social interactions, study brain functions, and present data in interactive 3D visualizations, making complex research findings more accessible to a wider audience.

Medical training in the metaverse offers low-risk, immersive scenarios for students to hone their skills, from clinical practice to surgical procedures. It has the potential to bridge the gap between theory and practice, ensuring that future healthcare professionals are well-prepared and empathetic in their approach.

It is clear that the metaverse holds great promise for reshaping the landscape of medical education, research, and training. As we continue to navigate the evolving metaverse, it is imperative that healthcare professionals, institutions, and policymakers collaborate to ensure its responsible and ethical integration into the field of medicine for active use in clinical settings, patient treatment and care, smart diagnosis, medical education, or any other application which engineers the useful integration of modern technology into increasing the quality of both work and education within the healthcare industry. Embracing this transformative technology has the potential to enhance patient care, advance medical knowledge, and prepare the next generation of healthcare professionals for the challenges and opportunities of the future.

References

1. Stephenson, N. (2003). *Snow crash: A novel*. Spectra.
2. Ratan, R., & Lei, Y. (2021, November 1). Down to earth. *What is the metaverse? 2 media and information experts explain*. Accessed on July 4, 2022.
3. Suh, I., McKinney, T., & Siu, K. C. (2023, April). Current perspective of metaverse application in medical education, research and patient care. In *Virtual worlds* (Vol. 2, pp. 115–128). MDPI.
4. Ahuja, A. S., Polascik, B. W., Doddapaneni, D., Byrnes, E. S., & Sridhar, J. (2023). The digital metaverse: Applications in artificial intelligence, medical education, and integrative health. *Integrative Medicine Research, 12*(1), 100917.
5. Yang, D., Zhou, J., Chen, R., Song, Y., Song, Z., Zhang, X., Wang, Q., Wang, K., Zhou, C., Sun, J., Zhang, L., Bai, L., Yuehong Wang, X., Wang, Y. L., Xin, H., Powell, C. A., Thüemmler,

C., Chavannes, N. H., Chen, W., Wu, L., & Bai, C. (2022). Expert consensus on the metaverse in medicine. *Clinical eHealth, 5*, 1–9. https://doi.org/10.1016/j.ceh.2022.02.001. ISSN 2588-9141, https://www.sciencedirect.com/science/article/pii/S2588914122000016
6. Kala, N. (2022). Revolutionizing medical education with metaverse. *International Journal of Scientific Research in Computer Science, Engineering and Information Technology, 8*, 26–32.
7. Koo, H. (2021). Training in lung cancer surgery through the metaverse, including extended reality, in the smart operating room of Seoul National University Bundang Hospital, Korea. *Journal of Educational Evaluation for Health Professions, 18.*
8. Foxman, M. H. (2018). *Playing with virtual reality: Early adopters of commercial immersive technology*. Doctoral dissertation, Columbia University.
9. Chengoden, R., Victor, N., Huynh-The, T., Yenduri, G., Jhaveri, R. H., Alazab, M., Bhattacharya, S., Hegde, P., Maddikunta, P. K. R., & Gadekallu, T. R. (2023). Metaverse for healthcare: A survey on potential applications, challenges and future directions. *IEEE Access, 11*, 12765–12795. https://doi.org/10.1109/ACCESS.2023.3241628
10. Qu, Z., Lau, C. W., Simoff, S. J., Kennedy, P. J., Nguyen, Q. V., & Catchpoole, D. R. (2022). Review of innovative immersive technologies for healthcare applications. *Innovations in Digital Health, Diagnostics, and Biomarkers, 2*(2022), 27–39.
11. Lee, C. W. (2022). Application of metaverse service to healthcare industry: A strategic perspective. *International Journal of Environmental Research and Public Health, 19*(20), 13038.
12. Gelernter, D. (1993). *Mirror worlds: Or the day software puts the universe in a shoebox ... How it will happen and what it will mean*. Oxford University Press.
13. Evans, G., Miller, J., Pena, M. I., MacAllister, A., & Winer, E. (2017, May). Evaluating the Microsoft HoloLens through an augmented reality assembly application. In *Degraded environments: Sensing, processing, and display 2017* (Vol. 10197, pp. 282–297). SPIE.
14. Orchard, A., O'Gorman, M., La Vecchia, C., & Lajoie, J. (2022, April). Augmented reality smart glasses in focus: A user group report. In *CHI conference on human factors in computing systems extended abstracts* (pp. 1–7).
15. Huang, J., Sun, P., & Zhang, W. (2022, March). Analysis of the future prospects for the Metaverse. In *2022 7th international conference on financial innovation and economic development (ICFIED 2022)* (pp. 1899–1904). Atlantis Press.
16. Ivanova, V. (2023). The metaverse: A new frontier in healthcare. *Brain and Nerves, 75*(10), 1115–1120. https://doi.org/10.11477/mf.1416202485
17. Wilson, T. (2022). *The metaverse and healthcare: Opportunities, challenges, and tips for tech pioneers*.
18. Hassani, H., Huang, X., & MacFeely, S. (2022). Impactful digital twin in the healthcare revolution. *Big Data and Cognitive Computing, 6*(3), 83.
19. Han, S., & Bang, M. Y. (2020). *Domestic XR usage trend in the non-face-to-face era*. Software Policy & Research Institute (SPRI).
20. Chen, Y., Lin, W., Zheng, Y., Xue, T., Chen, C., & Chen, G. (2022). *Application of active learning strategies in metaverse to improve student engagement: An immersive blended pedagogy bridging patient care and scientific inquiry in pandemic*. Available at SSRN 4098179.
21. Bhugaonkar, K., Bhugaonkar, R., & Masne, N. (2022). The trend of metaverse and augmented & virtual reality extending to the healthcare system. *Cureus, 14*(9).
22. Krijn, M., Emmelkamp, P. M., Olafsson, R. P., & Biemond, R. (2004). Virtual reality exposure therapy of anxiety disorders: A review. *Clinical Psychology Review, 24*(3), 259–281.
23. Spiers, H. J., & Maguire, E. A. (2007). Neural substrates of driving behaviour. *NeuroImage, 36*(1), 245–255.
24. Zhao, Y., Jiang, J., Chen, Y., Liu, R., Yang, Y., Xue, X., & Chen, S. (2022). Metaverse: Perspectives from graphics, interactions and visualization. *Visual Informatics, 6*(1), 56–67.
25. Dyer, E., Swartzlander, B. J., & Gugliucci, M. R. (2018). Using virtual reality in medical education to teach empathy. *Journal of the Medical Library Association: JMLA, 106*(4), 498.

26. Kidd, L. I., Knisley, S. J., & Morgan, K. I. (2012). Effectiveness of a Second Life® simulation as a teaching strategy for undergraduate mental health nursing students. *Journal of Psychosocial Nursing and Mental Health Services, 50*(7), 28–37.
27. Skiba, D. J. (2009). Nursing education 2.0: A second look at Second Life. *Nursing Education Perspectives, 30*(2), 129–131.
28. Petrigna, L., & Musumeci, G. (2022). The metaverse: A new challenge for the healthcare system: A scoping review. *Journal of Functional Morphology and Kinesiology, 7*(3), 63.
29. Peckmann, C., Kannen, K., Pensel, M. C., Lux, S., Philipsen, A., & Braun, N. (2022). Virtual reality induces symptoms of depersonalization and derealization: A longitudinal randomised control trial. *Computers in Human Behavior, 131*, 107233.
30. Shorey, S., & Ng, E. D. (2021). The use of virtual reality simulation among nursing students and registered nurses: A systematic review. *Nurse Education Today, 98*, 104662.
31. Gannotta, R., Malik, S., Chan, A. Y., Urgun, K., Hsu, F., & Vadera, S. (2018). Integrative medicine as a vital component of patient care. *Cureus, 10*(8).
32. Dyer, N. L., Surdam, J., Srinivasan, R., Agarwal, A., & Dusek, J. A. (2022). The impact of individualized complementary and integrative health interventions provided in clinical settings on quality of life: A systematic review of practice-based research. *Journal of Integrative and Complementary Medicine, 28*(8), 618–640.
33. Gonçalves, R., Pedrozo, A. L., Coutinho, E. S. F., Figueira, I., & Ventura, P. (2012). Efficacy of virtual reality exposure therapy in the treatment of PTSD: A systematic review. *PLoS One, 7*(12), e48469.

Metaverse in Medicine: Medical Internet of Things (MIoT)

Seyedeh Yasaman Hosseini Mirmahaleh and Amir Masoud Rahmani

1 Introduction

Modern lifestyles and environmental variations increase the probability of individuals contracting background diseases such as diabetes mellitus, cardiovascular and respiratory diseases, brain disorders such as Alzheimer's and Parkinson's, acute depression, and different types of cancers. Timely diagnosis and prediction of diseases have been shown to have a positive impact in preventing patient mortality and restoring their health to normal status. However, traditional medicine-based approaches may not always be effective in achieving these goals. Smart cities are emerging to link various intelligent devices with humans to simplify and improve the quality of modern life, including medical-based applications. Researchers have introduced the Internet of Things (IoT) technology for transferring and processing information to support economic, medical, management, and natural event areas. Artificial intelligence (AI) has also emerged to solve challenges based on the human brain structure by inferring different events and reactions and making decisions in the face of complicated problems. To address the high-risk nature of medical science, AI and machine learning (ML) algorithms have been integrated into medical science to predict and diagnose diseases with high accuracy and minimal delay [1, 2]. With the growing demand for intelligent healthcare, Medical IoT (MIoT) has emerged as a subset of IoT applications that handles medical devices and patients or joins people to monitor their vital signs and receive healthcare services. However, managing communications between different components of Medical IoT

S. Y. H. Mirmahaleh (✉)
Department of Electrical Engineering, Science and Technology, Lille University, Lille, France
e-mail: Yasaman-Hosseini@ieee.org

A. M. Rahmani
Future Technology Research Center, National Yunlin University of Science and Technology, Douliou, Yunlin, Taiwan

C. L. Chowdhary (ed.), *The Metaverse for the Healthcare Industry*,
https://doi.org/10.1007/978-3-031-60073-9_6

and supporting its perception layers have become a challenge due to the increasing information traffic from sensors' outputs [3, 4]. Due to the challenges of raising the nodes of MIoT, ciphertext-policy attribute-based encryption (CP-ABE) algorithms and other cryptography protocols applied to the information transaction between various biosensors, wearable, and other medical sensors as the wireless body area network (WBAN) to improve the security by defining agreement keys between doctors and patients [5, 6]. Some case studies attempted to handle the issue by providing trust-aware approaches to prevent sharing malicious data in the fog level of IoT via managing the detected faults, which covers MIoT [7, 8]. The Q-learning method helped to prepare a secure platform for data transactions between edge nodes in healthcare-based IoT applications by employing the rewarding method and the Markov decision process [9, 10]. The researchers proved the role of blockchain-based approaches to protect the patients' privacy records and recommendations of the doctors or other healthcare service providers (HSPs) to requesters in Medical IoT by guaranteeing its security [11, 12]. Besides security problems, MIoT faced the challenges of timely diagnosing and predicting diseases and decision-making to dedicate a suitable healthcare service to requesters in dangerous conditions to protect human health. To overcome the issues, the case studies usually targeted a specific disease (a type of cancer, background diseases, brain disorders, etc.) to monitor the vital signs and other efficient factors in the patients or susceptible people. In contrast, a generalized method is more efficient than it is for timely decision-making [13–15]. The high sensitivity of medical applications to device accessibility, power resource management, and service availability are two critical characteristics to follow for improving the efficiency of MIoT-based applications, which are almost invisible in satisfying the feature. The reviewed approaches and problems indicate the significance of different methods that can improve energy efficiency and latency of Medical IoT besides overcoming availability, security, and timely decision-making; predicting; and diagnosing concerns.

At first, the metaverse idea was welcomed by gamers via creating a virtual space of the actual and physical life of the people and their environment, where it covers different applications and emerges beyond the game area. The technology provided an appropriate platform to cover chronic diseases (chronic pulmonary, liver disorder, etc.) and other risky maladies (skin disorders, cancers, etc.) by employing various AI-based methods and simulations [16–18]. While there have been some discussions among specialists about the unclarity of fair distribution of medical services in the metaverse, its properties prove that it can improve availability, timely decision-making, diagnosing, and predicting in MIoT with a massive number of nodes.

In this chapter, we aim to analyze the effectiveness of different approaches in improving or hindering the efficiency of Medical IoT regarding availability, diagnosing, predicting, total energy, and delay. We will also explore the role of the metaverse in supporting these objectives. The chapter will investigate efficient solutions to address the challenges faced by the reviewed methods, improve the performance of MIoT, and introduce new methods.

2 Q-Learning-Based Approach

This section of the chapter attends to Q-learning method efficiency in Medical IoT, which also covers reinforcement and other unsupervised algorithms on timely decision-making, availability, prediction, and diagnosis. We first define three MIoT-based applications with different service priorities to analyze the role of different approaches in improving or deteriorating the performance of Medical IoT infrastructure. The applications help to create a realistic view of the operations and processes of the various methods in supporting service providing and estimating their impact on total energy and delay. Figure 1a–c indicate three defined applications inspired by the actual medical devices, services, and requirements. Applications (1)–(3) support providing services to patients or susceptible people with background diseases and Alzheimer's and identify who is infected by COVID-19 and other viruses. The case studies and statistics indicated a rising number of patients with the diseases and their hazardous situations in jeopardizing human life and increasing the probability of dying and losing routine activities, which justifies the reason for following them [19–21].

In MIoT-based applications, any people and devices joined to its infrastructure are identified as its members, which are connected by the network, as shown in Fig. 2.

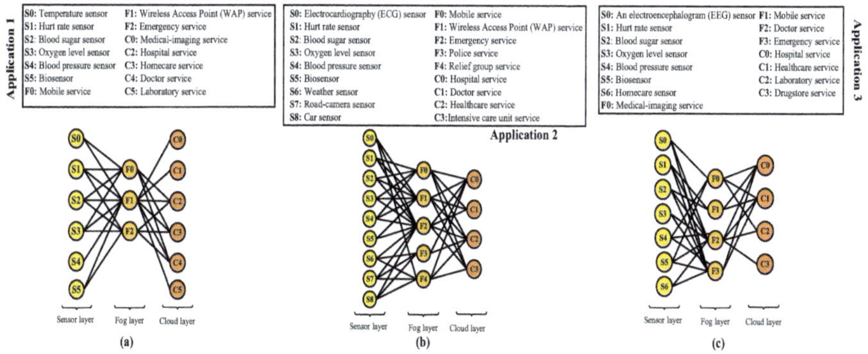

Fig. 1 The three MIoT-based applications: (**a**) Application 1 covers identifying patients with COVID-19 and other dangerous viruses; (**b**) Application 2 covers detecting the patients with background diseases in risky conditions; (**c**) Application 3 covers timely diagnosing and predicting Alzheimer's

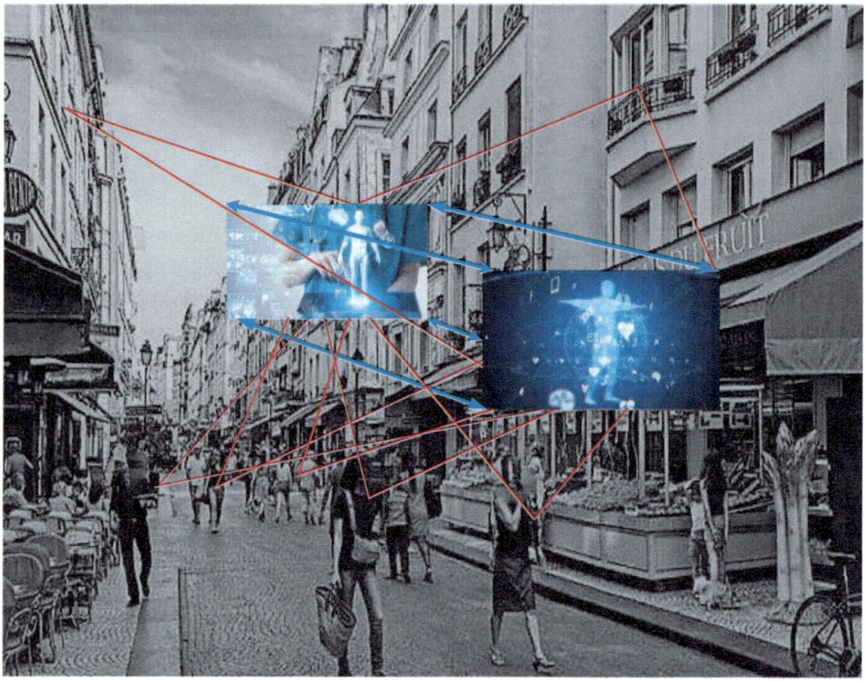

Fig. 2 A schematic of a simple view of MIoT users

In the Q-learning method, we describe an initial lookup table of the states and operations or processes that must be implemented in each state and set or reset an element of the Q matrix. The relationship between the states (as nodes) and their statuses (as links) is indicated by the Q graph with V vertices and E edges when the Q matrix defines the situation of the states. This chapter first tries to explain the operations of Q-learning by utilizing the Markov model process and mapping their nodes onto the vertices of the Q matrix, as shown in Fig. 3a–c. State mapping can clarify the operations of the learning method and its strong points in decentralized applications and supporting vehicle medical devices.

Figure 3a, b illustrate state mapping of the primary nodes of applications 1–3 onto the vertices of $Q1$, $Q2$, and $Q3$ Graphs, where its nodes can be increased by joining new components and users of MIoT, respectively. The figures focus on mapping operations for the states of the applications thought are available and active at t time (such as availability of S0 on application 1 at t time). The following state diagram and its matrix describe the Markov model process for application 1 when sensor node 0 (S0) is active at t time:

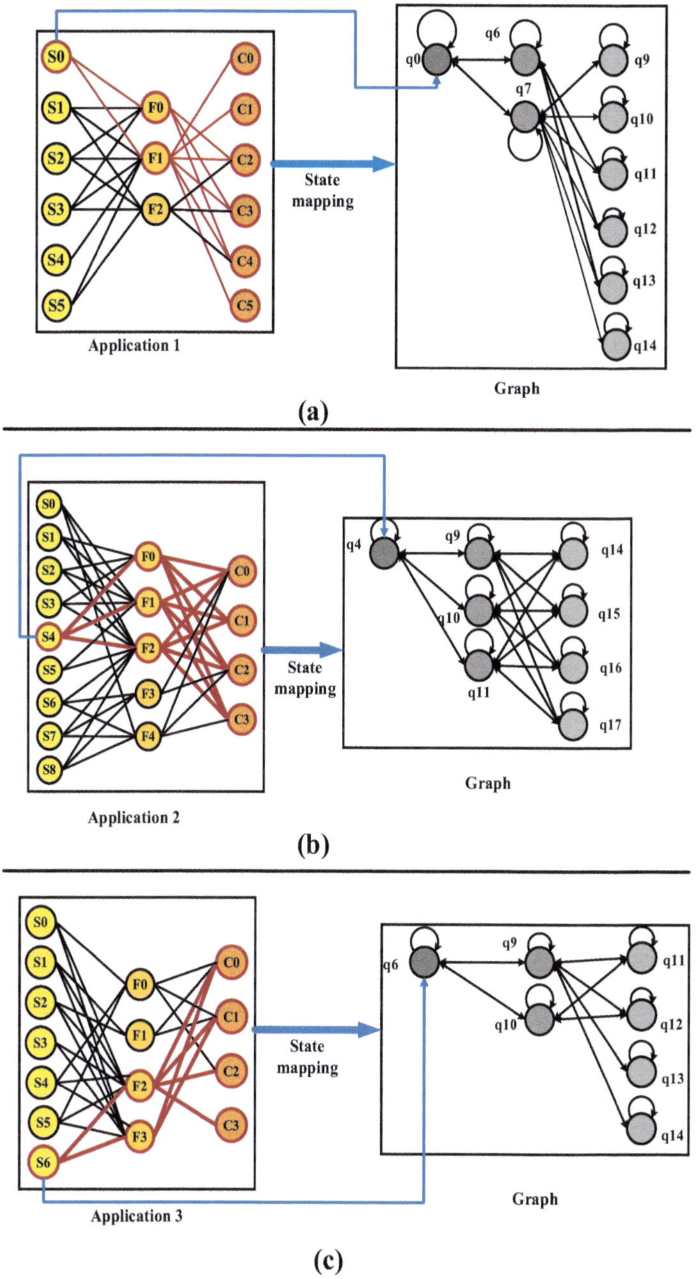

Fig. 3 The state mapping of three applications onto vertices of a graph, along with their active nodes at time *t*. The active nodes and paths are highlighted in red; (**a**) shows the state mapping of application 1, where S0 is an active sensor at time *t*; (**b**) shows the state mapping of application 2, where S4 is an active sensor at time *t*; (**c**) shows the state mapping of application 3, where S6 is an active sensor at time *t*

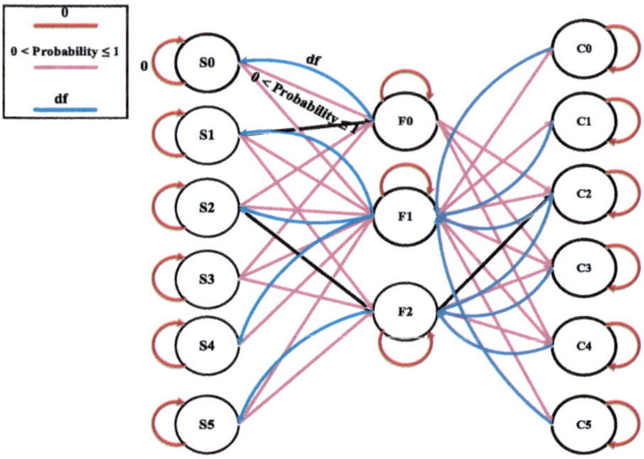

$$G = (V, E)\ G_Q = (m, n)\ Q = \begin{matrix} \\ \text{State}_0 \\ \text{State}_1 \\ \vdots \\ \text{State}_m \end{matrix} \begin{bmatrix} \text{State}_0 & \text{State}_1 & \dots & \text{State}_m \\ q_{0,0} & q_{0,1} & \dots & q_{0,j} \\ q_{1,0} & q_{1,1} & \dots & q_{1,j} \\ \vdots & \vdots & \dots & \vdots \\ q_{i,0} & q_{i,1} & \dots & q_{i,j} \end{bmatrix}$$

$$[Q]_{i\times j} = \begin{cases} i = m \\ j = m \end{cases}$$

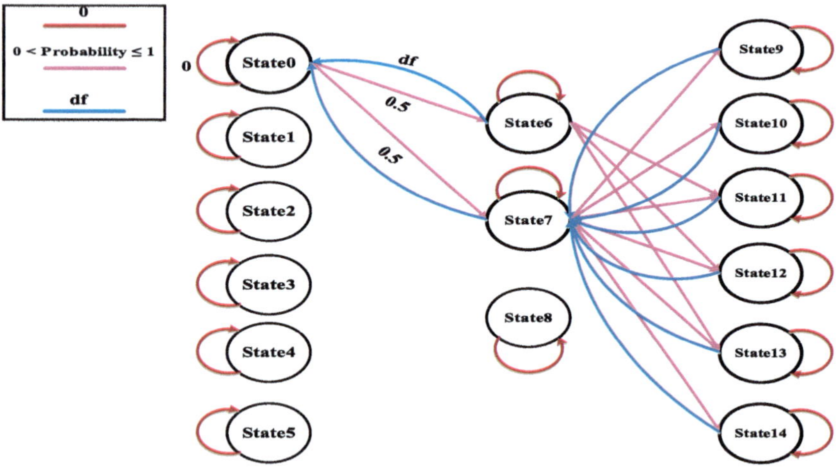

$G_Q = (15, n)$

$$Q = \begin{array}{c} \text{State0} \\ \text{State1} \\ \text{State2} \\ \text{State3} \\ \text{State4} \\ \text{State5} \\ \text{State6} \\ \text{State7} \\ \text{State8} \\ \text{State9} \\ \text{State10} \\ \text{State11} \\ \text{State12} \\ \text{State13} \\ \text{State14} \end{array} \begin{bmatrix} \text{State0} & \text{State1} & & & & & & \cdots & & & & & \text{State14} & & \text{State14} \\ 0 & 0 & 0 & 0 & 0 & 0 & 0.5 & 0.5 & 0 & 0 & 0 & 0 & 0 & 0 & 0 \\ 0 & 0 & 0 & 0 & 0 & 0 & 0 & 0 & 0 & 0 & 0 & 0 & 0 & 0 & 0 \\ 0 & 0 & 0 & 0 & 0 & 0 & 0 & 0 & 0 & 0 & 0 & 0 & 0 & 0 & 0 \\ 0 & 0 & 0 & 0 & 0 & 0 & 0 & 0 & 0 & 0 & 0 & 0 & 0 & 0 & 0 \\ 0 & 0 & 0 & 0 & 0 & 0 & 0 & 0 & 0 & 0 & 0 & 0 & 0 & 0 & 0 \\ 0 & 0 & 0 & 0 & 0 & 0 & 0 & 0 & 0 & 0 & 0 & 0 & 0 & 0 & 0 \\ 0 & 0 & 0 & 0 & 0 & 0 & 0 & 0 & 0 & 0 & 0 & 0.4 & 0.2 & 0.4 & 0 \\ 0 & 0 & 0 & 0 & 0 & 0 & 0 & 0 & 0 & 0 & 0.15 & 0.2 & 0.2 & 0.15 & 0.2 \\ 0 & 0 & 0 & 0 & 0 & 0 & 0 & 0 & 0 & 0 & 0 & 0 & 0 & 0 & 0 \\ 0 & 0 & 0 & 0 & 0 & 0 & 0 & 0 & 0 & 0 & 0 & 0 & 0 & 0 & 0 \\ 0 & 0 & 0 & 0 & 0 & 0 & 0 & 0 & 0 & 0 & 0 & 0 & 0 & 0 & 0 \\ 0 & 0 & 0 & 0 & 0 & 0 & 0 & 0 & 0 & 0 & 0 & 0 & 0 & 0 & 0 \\ 0 & 0 & 0 & 0 & 0 & 0 & 0 & 0 & 0 & 0 & 0 & 0 & 0 & 0 & 0 \\ 0 & 0 & 0 & 0 & 0 & 0 & 0 & 0 & 0 & 0 & 0 & 0 & 0 & 0 & 0 \\ 0 & 0 & 0 & 0 & 0 & 0 & 0 & 0 & 0 & 0 & 0 & 0 & 0 & 0 & 0 \end{bmatrix}$$

$$[Q]_{i \times j} = \begin{cases} i = 15 \\ j = 15 \end{cases}$$

The variables m and n represent the number of vertices and edges in the Q graph, which captures the relationship between states based on the estimated probability of transactions between two nodes (states). The probability of transactions can be estimated using the received discount factor value or by following the initialization and approximation values. The Q matrix, as depicted in the Markov model's state relationships, reflects the status of application 1 at time t when only sensor node 0 (S0) is sensing and reporting information.

The highlighted points of Q-learning approaches are the entity definition of learning rate and discount factor that indicate the current situation node and its impact on deciding the next state. When setting the discount factor (df) to a value in the range of $0 < \text{df} \leq 1$, the lookup table is updated with the new information (states and their activations). The issue can identify the security services and malicious nodes that can improve decision-making about dedicating an appropriate HSP to the requester. By joining new devices and users, the memory capacity and bandwidth requirements make it challenging to update the initial information and store the extended lookup tables via recent activations. Due to detected inappropriate states (devices), we face the static power consumption problem of the useless and ineffective components, besides the probability of leaking malicious information by faulty MIoT nodes. A neural network (NN) can overcome the problem and improve the efficiency of Q-learning via pruning the deactivated neurons and their weights and re-training the NN in addition to solving the data fusion and overfitting challenges. Figure 4a, b show a multilayer neural network that was trained by the

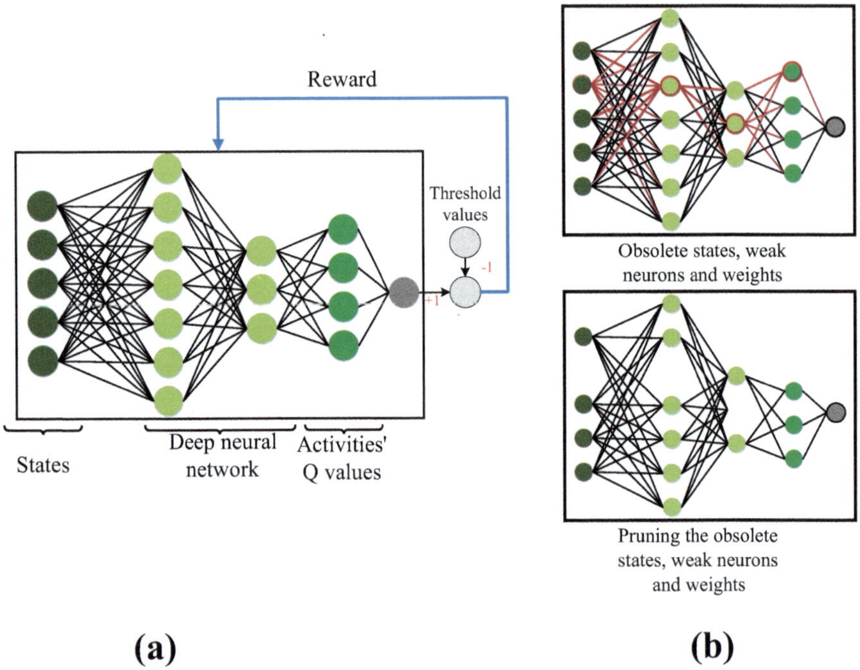

Fig. 4 *Q*-learning by the deep neural network before and after pruning; (**a**) Deep Q-learning before pruning the weak neurons and weights; (**b**) The pruned DNN after imposing rewards and identifying the ineffective states and activities

lookup table information of states and activations before and after pruning the weak neurons and weights.

Due to the application 1 priority, Q-learning and NN improve timely decision-making about detecting new cases of COVID-19 by adapting the primary symptoms (fever and oxygen level) and novel information on the sensors' outputs. When identifying the infected people with COVID-19, the combined method (Q-learning and NN) can successfully provide proper healthcare service to patients with background diseases by monitoring blood sugar and pressure, oxygen level, and heart rate. To support availability as one of the service priorities of application 1, Q-learning leads to a fall in the efficiency of MIoT where df is set to a value close to zero for a state (as a service provider node), and a risky patient has to wait for timely receiving a healthcare service. The issue applies to application 2 and confronts a similar problem when detecting a patient with background diseases in dangerous accidents and natural disasters. In application 3, the method can appear successful in diagnosing Alzheimer's and its level with high accuracy by analyzing Amyloid-beta aggregation and the destroyed area of the Hippocampus in medical images. It proves the direct dependency between the idea and image processing and its quality, which also defines a weak point of its performance.

The combined method's highlighted role is justified by its relevance in the context of emerging technologies such as the Internet of Vehicles (IoV), autonomous systems, and Electric Vehicle (EV) devices, including mobile health services and biosensors. In the metaverse system, the communication platform manages many EVs and IoV-based applications, creating a real and physical world of the vehicles, people, and their activations via the digital twins and mixed realities. Due to the mentioned feature of the metaverse, Q-learning and NN have an efficient role in supporting real-time applications and mobile devices, where some case studies followed the issue as a solution for the system [22, 23].

3 Neural Network-Based Approach

In this section, multilayer perceptron (MLP) and neural networks are targeted to analyze their efficiency in deteriorating or improving the performance of MIoT in timely decision-making, predicting, diagnosing, and availability. A pure neural network cannot support the purposes of Medical IoT-based applications with high accuracy when employing supervised learning approaches to select a dataset to train NN. The issue demands statistics, fuzzy logic, and other efficient methods to utilize them in collecting two datasets (for training and testing) to impose into the input neuron for training NN and following the purposes. In multidisciplinary topics, the researchers employed neural networks to decide about a matter and predict and forecast a situation from various angles of economic, medical, weather, and environmental factors, in addition to hiring the statistics (correlation coefficients, statistics tests), Fuzzy logic methods, etc. [24–27]. We investigate the role of neural networks in the three defined applications (Fig. 1a–c) to support their priority and their efficiency in aiding MIoT to handle the people who joined the infrastructure for receiving electronic healthcare services. Figure 5 demonstrates a fully connected neural network with one input and output layer, where the number of hidden layers and neurons are determined using the trial-and-error method.

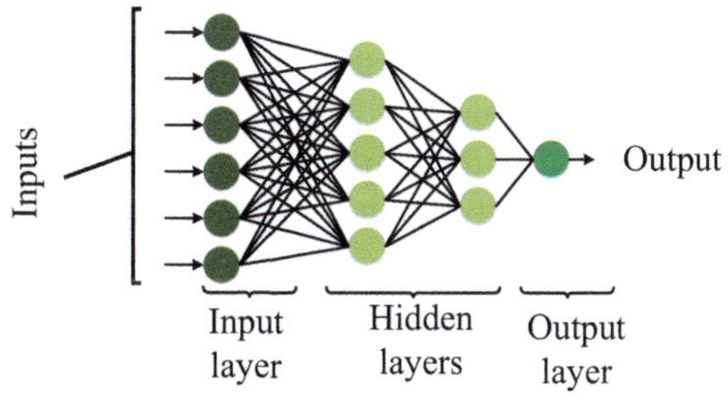

Fig. 5 A fully connected neural network based on the inputs of application 1

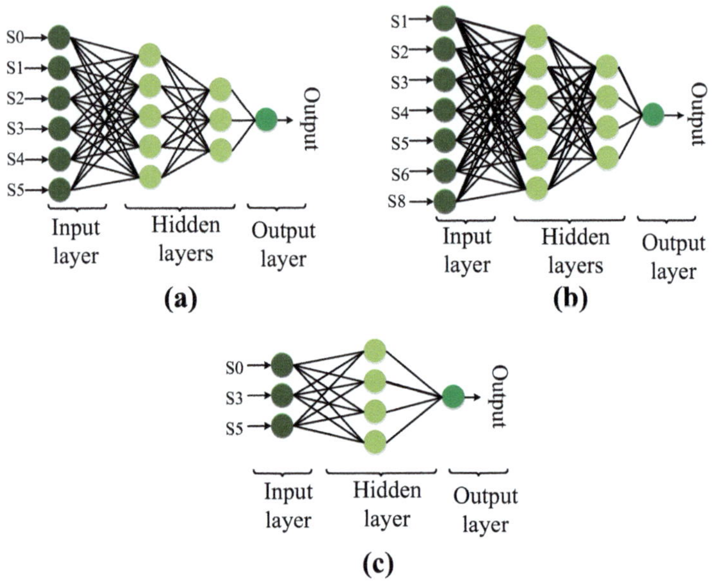

Fig. 6 Data collection and determining the inputs of the neural network via ARM; (**a**) ARM in selecting inputs of the NN on implementing application 1; (**b**) ARM in selecting inputs of the NN on implementing application 2; (**c**) ARM in selecting inputs of the NN on implementing application 3

The successful impact of associated rule mapping (ARM) on predicting and diagnosing diseases and determining appropriate healthcare services can be achieved by accessing proven medical information and employing Fuzzy logic. In particular, ARM can be applied to COVID-19 patients with infected lungs to determine their level of risk and forecast their condition over the next few days. Application 1 demonstrates how ARM can define rules using the Mamdani function and train a neural network to identify COVID-19 patients with background diseases. This approach is illustrated in Fig. 6a. It is also planned to recognize the grade of infecting their repository systems with the virus and the deterioration of the patient's health status by monitoring their symptoms and background information. The method is applied in application 2 for identifying the patients with background diseases facing critical situations, which helps to provide timely service by considering the jeopardy priority of the infected people. ARM leads to complicated operations due to specifying a massive number of rules where some of their cases are not clarified and stable because of unlimited and indistinctive situations of different accidents and natural disasters. Figure 6b indicates training the neural network (for application 2) and determining the efficient inputs after passing Fuzzy logic processes and rule mining, which have weak efficiency in identifying the dangerous conditions for risky patients. ARM on application 3, the comprehensive information and documentation of Alzheimer's can create an opportunity to define the stable rules of the efficient characteristics (Amyloid beta aggregation and demolished space of the Hippocampus) of the disease to train NN for predicting and diagnosing its level by an appropriate dataset. We demonstrate the efficient information of the sensors' outputs (inputs of the neural network) that directly depend on diagnosing and predicting Alzheimer's after rule mining in Fig. 6c.

According to the characteristics of MIoT, ARM can only successfully emerge when accessing proven and valid medical information and a particular situation for a specific application (diagnosing and predicting a disease). The issue has been addressed through researchers detecting lung cancer and other hazardous diseases to tackle them and remotely controlling the vital signs of patients and their electronic care via connecting specialists (doctors and nurses) [28]. In generalized applications of Medical IoT, the method leads to complexity enhancement to define the comprehensive and credible rules and not an efficient role in collecting a dataset for a supervised learning-based NN to cover the mentioned purposes.

In the statistics-based approaches, the first step consists of identifying the type of data distribution (after converting the sensors' outputs to data format) to determine the correlation coefficient matter by employing parametric and nonparametric methods (such as Kolmogorov–Smirnov and Shapiro-Wilk Test, etc.) [29, 30]. Due to the type of data distribution, the relationship between NN's inputs (sensor nodes) and outputs (service providers and application priorities) is estimated using the Spearman or Pierson-based correlation coefficient method. Application 1 applies to identifying the patients with COVID-19 and other risky viruses (different types of Influenza), in which the symptoms variations of a virus-based disease almost demonstrate the monotonic relationships between its variables. The issue proves that ARM is more efficient for application 1 and a similar case in comparing the statistical approaches to determine the proper inputs of an NN and support the purposes of MIoT. The method can successfully recognize the efficient variables (sensor nodes) of application 2 by employing their related data to define the inputs of the neural network when dealing with the various conditions of unpredictable events. The outcomes of an electroencephalogram (EEG), the blood factor (β protein aggregating), and medical imaging indicate the expected routine variations for the patient with Alzheimer's, and the statistical approaches can help to determine the efficient inputs of an NN for timely diagnosis on application 3. When following prediction priority, the method has less efficiency in comparing ARM because of facing a massive number of highlighted parameters (such as diet, lifestyle, genetics, etc.) that increase the probability of infection with the disease.

As we analyze the role of ARM and statistical methods in three different applications, the approach depends on the types of data distributions, parameters' variations, and priorities to cover a neural network for supporting the perception layer of MIoT. The metaverse consists of the Avatars, their activities, and their behaviors. It employs Fuzzy logic and defines many rules to create a real and physical world for them and their management, besides analyzing statistics of various events. Avatars cover the role of patients and doctors with the details of the communication between them, where they describe different MIoT-based applications and satisfy their purposes in the metaverse systems [31, 32].

4 Role Mapping and Clustering Efficiency on MIoT Performance

This section focuses on improving the efficiency of neural networks, learning methods, and other aspects of achieving the goals of MIoT for its users. After discussing the main efficient approaches, we address specific solutions that can enhance the efficiency of MIoT. Our approach targets the defined approaches (Fig. 1a–c) to describe the ideas and their roles in ameliorating the efficiency of MIoT while addressing their weaknesses. In introducing these ideas, we prioritize application efficiency and consider the appropriate allocation of HSPs to the requester for timely decision-making, which has been overlooked in previous research.

Some case studies focused on combining forward and backward-chain methods and applying them to the online training of a neural network to increase the efficiency of timely decision-making in IoT-based applications [26]. The idea can significantly impact MIoT-based applications to manage human medical requirements when employing a neural network and applying service priority to handle HSPs and patients. Role mapping can successfully speed up decision-making and support service availability by transferring the application nodes to the neural network's neurons by exerting a penalty-based approach. Each neuron of an NN behaves as a device for MIoT application, and neural network weights aim to impose penalties on weak components by receiving feedback from the output node and service provider availability. Figure 7a–c illustrate role-mapping the nodes of applications 1–3 onto the neurons of neural networks and pruning operations based on a backward chain and penalty imposing.

The perception layer gathers the appropriate information from lower levels (sensor layer) to speed up decision-making in medical and healthcare applications. This can be performed via processing elements and neurons. We define its role (perception layer) onto the neurons of an additional middle level of NN's hidden layers to recognize the correct and faulty perception nodes through a backward chain, as shown in Fig. 8a, b.

Due to the application priorities, a threshold value is defined to investigate the validation of the NN output for deciding a service provider where the condition of (Output value $\geq V_{\mathrm{Thr}}$) is met. When analyzing the legitimacy of the perception layer nodes, the defective components are identified by employing a backward chain and pruning the neurons of the next layer, as shown in Fig. 8b. The backward chain covers the operations and processes of imposing the penalty onto the related weights and neurons to the defective node of the MIoT application by detecting the active

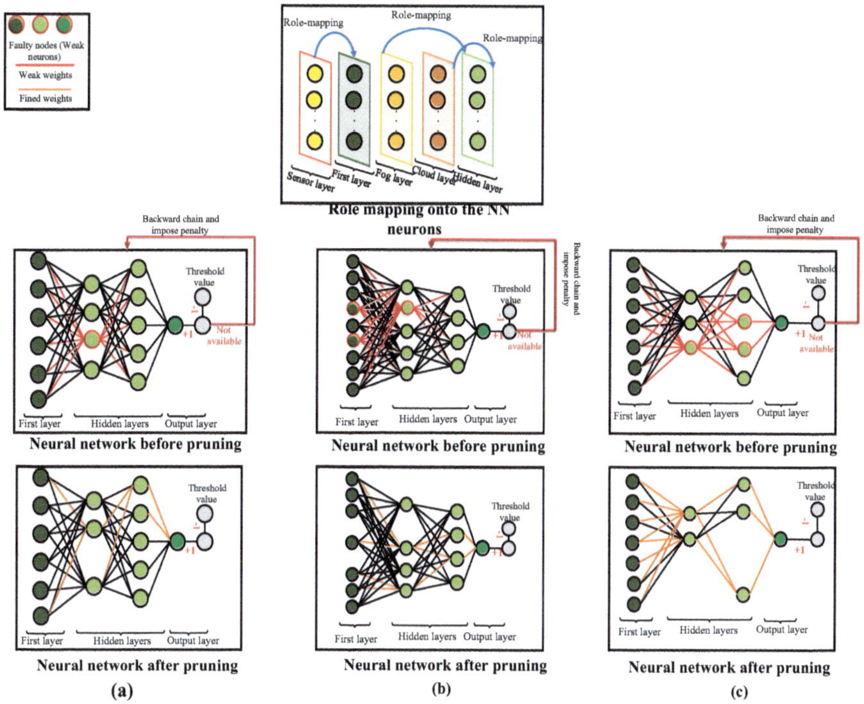

Fig. 7 Role mapping of applications 1–3 nodes onto the NNs' neurons before and after pruning process by backward chain and inserting penalty value; (**a**) Mapping the nodes of application 1 onto the neurons before and after pruning via backward chain; (**b**) Mapping the nodes of application 2 onto the neurons before and after pruning via backward chain; (c) Mapping the nodes of application 3 onto the neurons before and after pruning via backward chain

nodes and the invisibility of the output neuron (Not available) at *t* time. The method involves removing the faulty devices or stopping them via imposing the penalty value on the neural network weights, which leads to improving decision-making and energy efficiency. The failed node detection is complicated when only employing a backward chain and investigating the components' activities at *t* time. This demands total delay problems to perform related algorithmic steps for fault recognition. To overcome the issue, we propose hiring a forward chain to detect defective nodes to improve time complexity and utilizing a backward chain to impose penalties. Figure 9 gives a schematic of employing backward and forward chains together to clarify the operations of the combined method in faulty node detection and its pruning to improve the efficiency of the application. The forward chain can successfully inject rewards on the neural network's weights by joining new nodes to the application or recovering defective components.

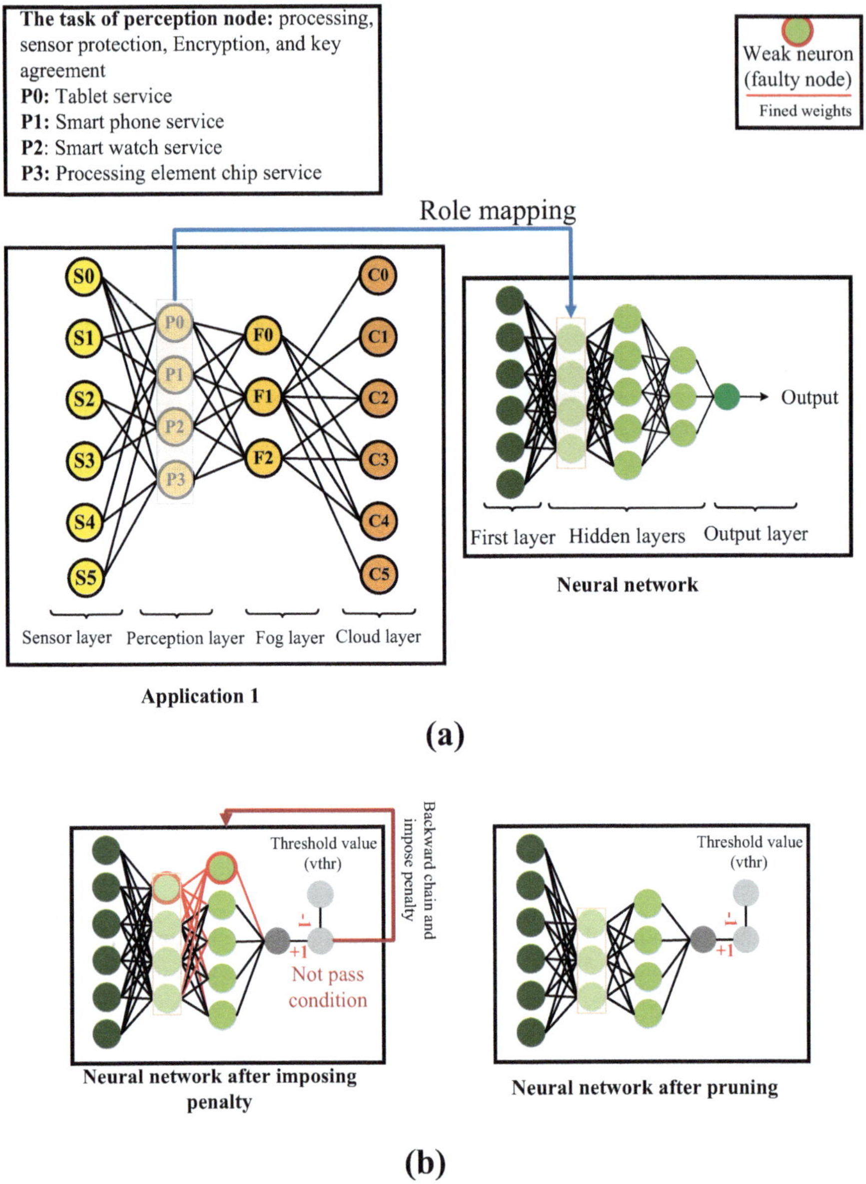

Fig. 8 The role mapping of the perception layer's nodes onto the neurons of an NN before and after the pruning approach; (**a**) Mapping the role of the perception layer's nodes onto the neurons of the hidden layer of the NN; (**b**) Penalty injecting onto the neurons and pruning weak nodes and weights

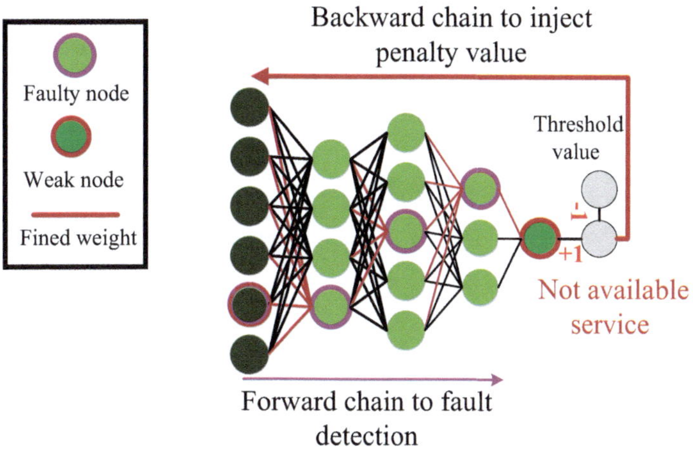

Fig. 9 A schematic of forward and backward chains to fault detection and penalty injection on a NN (for application 1)

The advantages of the combined method can prove the role of a flexible clustering approach to replace the faulty nodes and cover their operations by a neighbor service provider after identifying the proper HSPs with similar characteristics. In the flexible clustering, the neighboring applications and nodes are first recognized to analyze their efficiency in covering HSPs and other components via mapping them onto the neurons of an NN, as shown in Fig. 10a, b.

The role of the method is analyzed to cover the nodes' tasks of the perception and cloud layers of MIoT applications, whose efficiency was investigated by the healthcare service providers at the application level of the Internet of Medical Things (IoMT) [33]. To define a categorization of the nodes and map them onto a graph's vertices, the activities of the previous layers' devices are accumulated on a vertex, and the edges define their relationships with the devices of the next layer. We narrate the mentioned processes to clarify the concept of the clustering method in the area by aiming to cover perception nodes where the elements of the P matrix define the relationship between the vertices of the GP graph. The sn and p vertices describe the accumulated role of the sensor layer's nodes and perception level's components in an MIoT-based application, respectively.

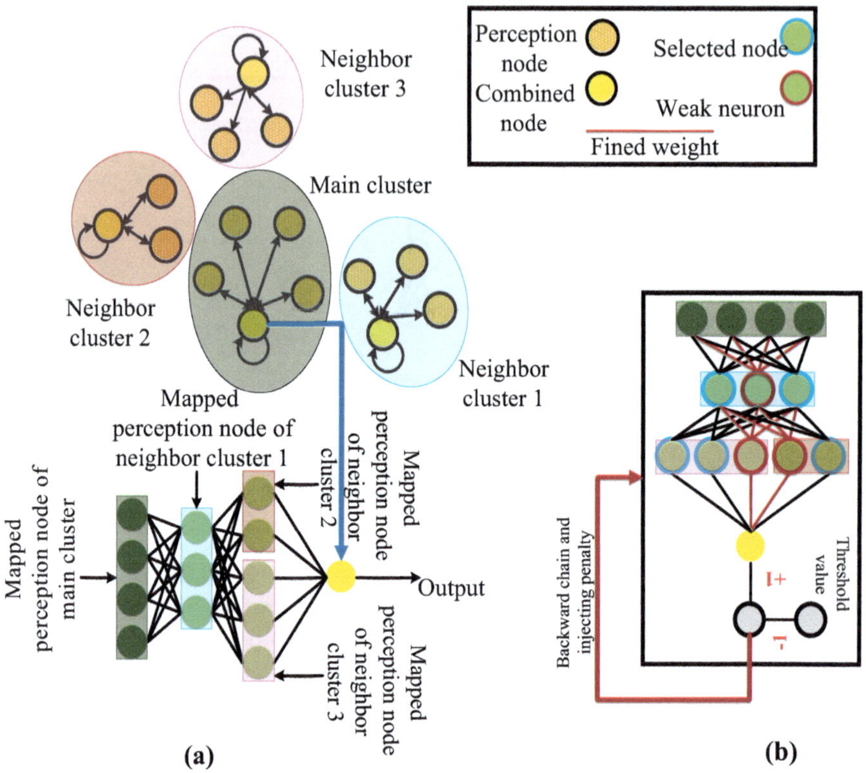

Fig. 10 Mapping the neighbor perception nodes onto the neurons of NN and identifying the appropriate devices; (**a**) Mapping the neighbor perception nodes onto the neurons of NN when targeting fault detection on the perception layer; (**b**) Recognizing the proper neighbor nodes to cover the tasks of the failed or faulty component by injecting penalty value via backward chain

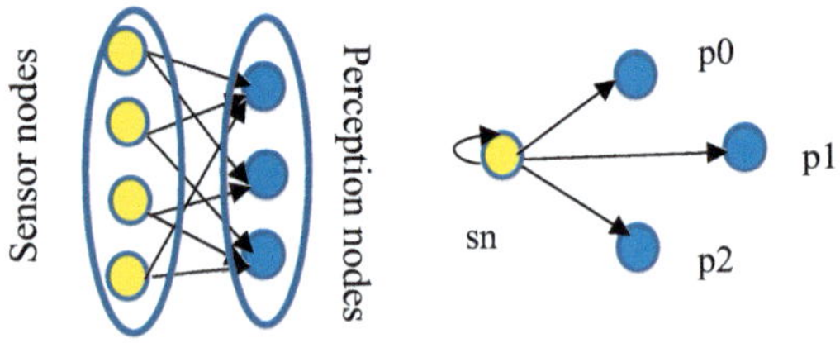

$$G_p = (V, E)$$

$$[P]_{i\times j} = \begin{cases} i = V \\ j = V \end{cases} \quad P = \begin{matrix} \\ sn \\ p0 \\ p1 \\ p2 \end{matrix} \begin{bmatrix} sn & p0 & p1 & p2 \\ 1 & 1 & 1 & 1 \\ 0 & 0 & 0 & 0 \\ 0 & 0 & 0 & 0 \\ 0 & 0 & 0 & 0 \end{bmatrix}$$

When detecting the failed components in the perception layer and overtaking the threshold value of the acceptable number of occurring faults, they are substituted by the proper neighbor nods recognized via NN and node mapping. The threshold values explain two different measures based on application priority and target layer of MIoT, in which the neural network identifies the appropriate neighbor node and cluster by analyzing them on the output neuron. The combined approach of node mapping and flexible clustering can improve the efficiency of the MIoT application by stopping faulty devices and covering their operations via the neighboring nodes. The issue improves timely decision-making, service, and application availability and dependability by considering the priorities and employing EVs to support the operations of the failed devices.

The application clustering methods help the metaverse systems support real-time devices, their management, and timely decision-making, where the property has a highlighted role in handling medical-based components and users (Avatars). A metaverse system handles Avatars and their activities and different intelligence applications and devices, which are expected to manage all the requirements of the patients by monitoring their situation. The flexible clustering can improve the efficiency of the metaverse in covering medical-based applications by identifying neighbors, efficient nodes, and EVs to support the tasks of invisible components.

5 The Efficiency of the Metaverse on MIoT-Based Applications

Due to the clarified various methods for improving and deteriorating the efficiency of MIoT, this section presents a comprehensive analysis of the positive and negative roles of the metaverse in supporting medical-based applications in timely decision-making, diagnosing, and predicting, besides satisfying availability and dependability. Before evaluating the upper exiting methods, the section gives an overview of the characteristics of the metaverse and its specific and advanced devices and technologies of AV, VR, mixed reality (MR), and Extended reality (XR) to create an opportunity for linked virtual and physical spaces of the different applications and Avatars. The technologies and devices can help patients and doctors diagnose and predict the disorders and dangerous variations in the different body's cells (the related cells to immune systems) and tumors without employing risky biopsy and x-ray-based approaches on susceptible people. We clarify the role of the metaverse in MIoT efficiency to handle medical devices, users, patients, doctors,

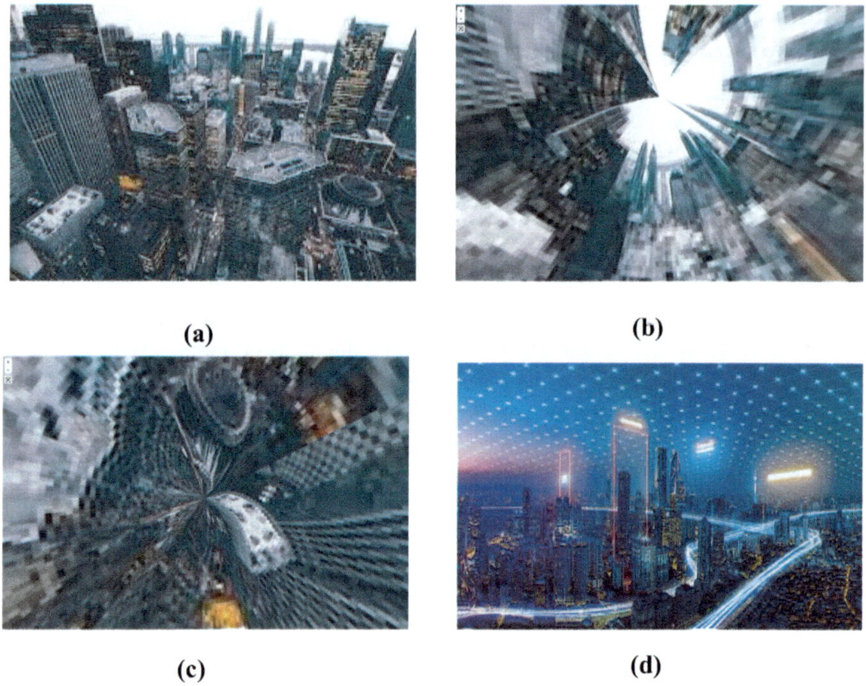

Fig. 11 AV efficiency on the reality of the picture and actual world; (**a**) An original picture of a city; (**b**) The upper view of the city by AV technology and rotating 360-degree; (**c**) The lower view of the city by AV technology and rotating 360-degree; (**d**) A schematic of a defined city by the metaverse

and other related healthcare services by analyzing its performance on the three addressed applications (Fig. 1a–c) though following different priorities. Due to creating a second real world and integrating virtual and physical facts, the system and its technology are based on the mapping concept to emulate the actual people, their characteristics, activities, diseases, and problems for managing them out of the principal life. The metaverse includes a complicated system of various information and data types, describing all activities joined and simulated by the technology. The issue leads to a massive burden of data and applications where Q-learning and DNN help in timely decision-making and detecting faulty devices and malicious chains. Blockchain-based methods prepared a secure platform for the metaverse to protect private information and communications, employing clustering, learning, and neural networks to satisfy other purposes. Figure 11a–d indicate a facing of the Metaverse platform and its components to clarify the actual and physical spaces of the system in facing various devices and applications through playing the main roles of the information and data. As shown in Fig. 11b, c, MR and AR can create a deep and real space of the physical world that covers and investigates it in 360-degree rotation.

5.1 Metaverse in Diagnosing

The chapter tried to present all explanations on three defined MIoT applications, which follow the real purposes of Medical IoT in decision-making, predicting, and diagnosing by addressing recent high-risk diseases (COVID-19 and other dangerous viruses, brain disorders, and background diseases). The AV and VR devices have a highlighted role in diagnosing Alzheimer's, Parkinson's, and acute depression diseases when joined to the metaverse and combined reality and virtual concepts of diseases. The three addressed brain disorders, multiple sclerosis (MS) and carotid occlusion, are almost challenging for doctors and treatment staff to detect due to their similar symptoms, medical-based images, and brain behaviors. The dependable medical-based method focuses on advanced blood tests to identify the type of released placks (α, β, and GPR56 proteins, etc.) besides analyzing the medical imaging thought demonstrating the status of the connected proteins to neurons with high accuracy. Alzheimer's starts with a disturbance of fair cholesterol distribution in the human brain's neurons of the Hippocamp, aggregating Aβ42, increasing the temperature of cells, and accumulating β protein, which leads to destroying the core of neurons. Due to application 3 inputs and the mentioned characteristics of the disease, the metaverse system can emerge effective to timely diagnose Alzheimer's via employing AV and VR devices to deep-monitoring the temperature of the brain's neurons of the Avatars (in the role of the patients) through removing the long delay to pass the laboratory tests. Figure 12a, b illustrate the situation of the human brain's neurons and AV/VR devices' role in detecting aggregating Aβ42 amino acid in the Hippocamp when starting the disease and increasing the cells' temperature.

Due to the intricate nature of the brain's layers and operations, technology significantly impacts the timely diagnosis of diseases with similar characteristics and symptoms. Medical imaging can often lead to misdiagnosis, but technological advancements can help solve this problem.

By adding a reality of the upper and lower respiratory systems, the metaverse can be an efficient act to detect COVID-19 and the situation of the patients with the diseases to timely dedicate an appropriate healthcare service via separating it from bronchitis and cold (on application 1 and its inputs). The system can prevent the spreading of virus-based diseases and reduce the number of new cases and death rates by supporting MIoT applications, their management, and timely decision-making in remote-controlling vital signs and symptoms, drug recommendations, and remote-checkup. The features create a suitable condition for the patients to take at home and receive healthcare services to hamper their movements in the outside environment to cater to requirements, which reduces the probability of transferring the virus to other people. In application 2 and similar cases, the metaverse can define a virtual reality of the different accidents and natural disasters to identify the Avatars (patients) in risky situations and provide healthcare services based on scheduling priority by detecting them via citing their previous records or online sensing the vital signs. To manage the injury of unforeseen events, the routine

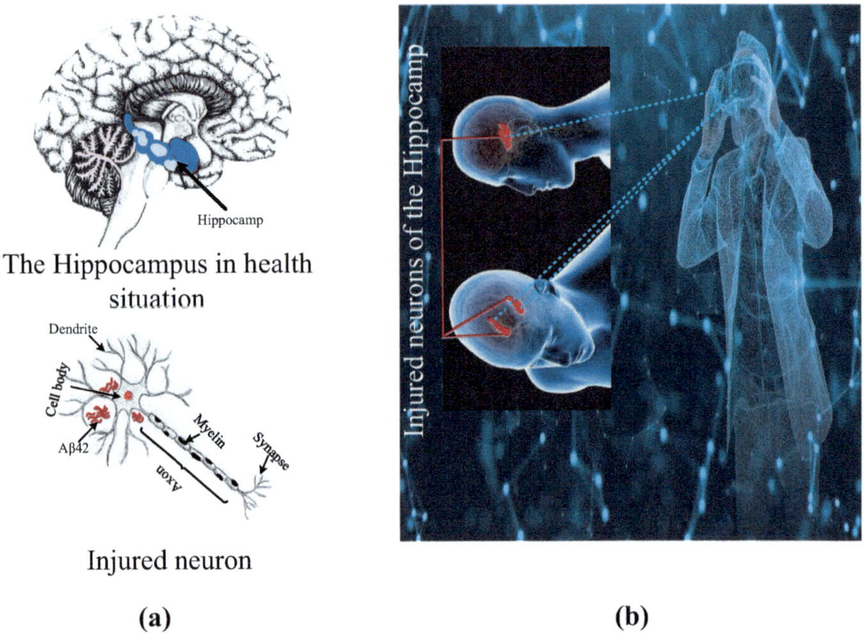

Fig. 12 A schematic of the human brain's structure and the role of AV glasses in timely diagnosing Alzheimer's; (**a**) The Hippocamp in health situation and aggregating Aβ42 and increasing the neuron temperature (red-color cell body); (**b**) Monitoring increasing the temperature of the Hippocamp's neurons by AV device

approaches face a long delay in finding the people and providing suitable medical-based services, besides the complexity of priority decision-making. In MIoT, AI can overcome some problems of routine methods and speed up decisions about HSP for the injured through various approaches that must be integrated for handling accidents and natural disasters. The metaverse platform is established on AI to emulate all routine behaviors and challenges of people's lives and their environment around and events, which utilizes the DNNs and other advanced machine learning algorithms to create an intelligent second world and manage various applications. The characteristics prove the efficiency of the metaverse in confrontation with unpredictable happenings and timely decision-making based on priority scheduling (the injured patients with background diseases, children, and disabled people) by online monitoring all events and Avatars' vital signs and their background recorders. Figure 13 shows a metaverse system process to tackle accidents and natural disasters (earthquake, flood, etc.) by finding the injured and making timely decisions about dedicating a proper HSP after detecting people with risky health situations.

A virtual reality of a City's maquette

Augmented reality of the city by AV device

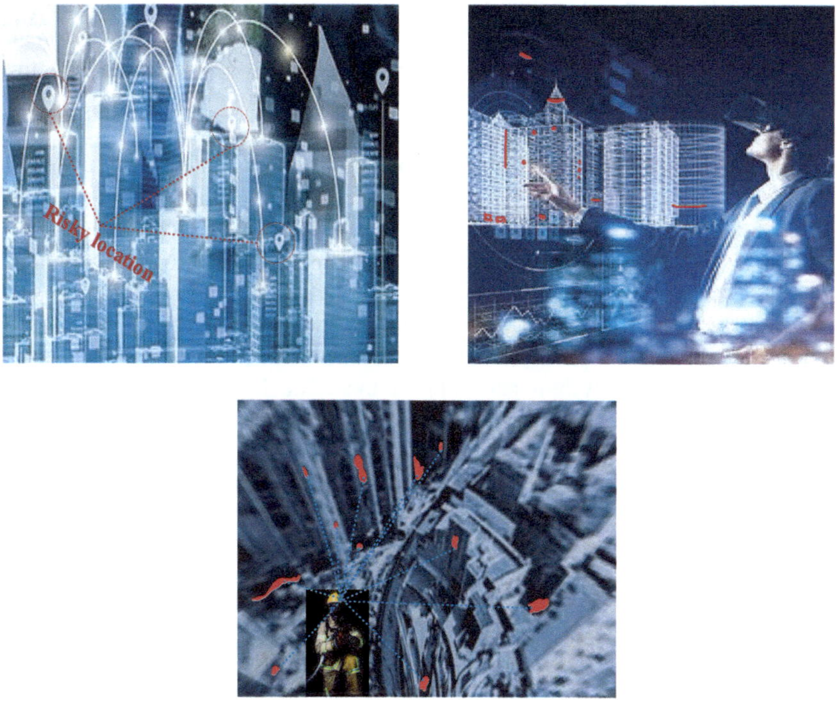

Augmented reality of the city by AV device after an earthquake

Fig. 13 Metaverse in identifying the risky locations and timely providing healthcare service when facing earthquake (as a natural disaster)

5.2 *Metaverse in Predicting*

To predict the risk of infection with a disease, the main issue is recognizing the efficient parameters to increase the probability of getting sick and investigating their particulars and impact factors on susceptible people. The issue seems simpler for virus-based diseases than other maladies, which put at risk the infected people with a low immune system (infected people with different cancers, background diseases, acquired immunodeficiency syndrome (AIDS), and autoimmune diseases). Prediction of the probability of infecting people with COVID-19 and serious injury can be solved by simply analyzing and alarming patients with low immune systems to self-caring and obeying the rules of the World Health Organization (WHO). The risky patients and prone people can join the MIoT applications to alert them (especially for the elderly and patients with Dementia and Alzheimer's at the initial level), which can be well supported by the metaverse. In application 1 and similar cases, the metaverse can detect risky locations and their surroundings via estimating the number of patients with the virus in various local positions and reporting them where Avatars (in the role of healthcare security officers) and sensors alert the people to avoid entry, as shown in Fig. 14. The approach helps to prevent the virus outbreak and reduce death rates by predicting its dangers in special cases and recognizing the risky locations to timely locking them in.

Table 1 presents three scenarios for Fig. 14, where a deep Q-learning algorithm predicts risky locations based on the background information of individuals involved in accidents.

The prediction method significantly prevents patients with background diseases and covers the susceptible people based on diet, lifestyle, and activity recommendations. To successfully pass the process of prediction and satisfy its purposes, the efficient factors first have to be identified in the diseases, though hereditary factor has a highlighted role in infecting with Diabetes mellitus and cardiovascular disorders. A metaverse system can support the issue by analyzing the output information of the sensors (inputs of application 2), which can monitor their impacts on the Avatars and their behaviors on the body cells for one month later and more via doctors. The technology can record the situation of the different locations and their information about the people who have transactions on here and the traffic

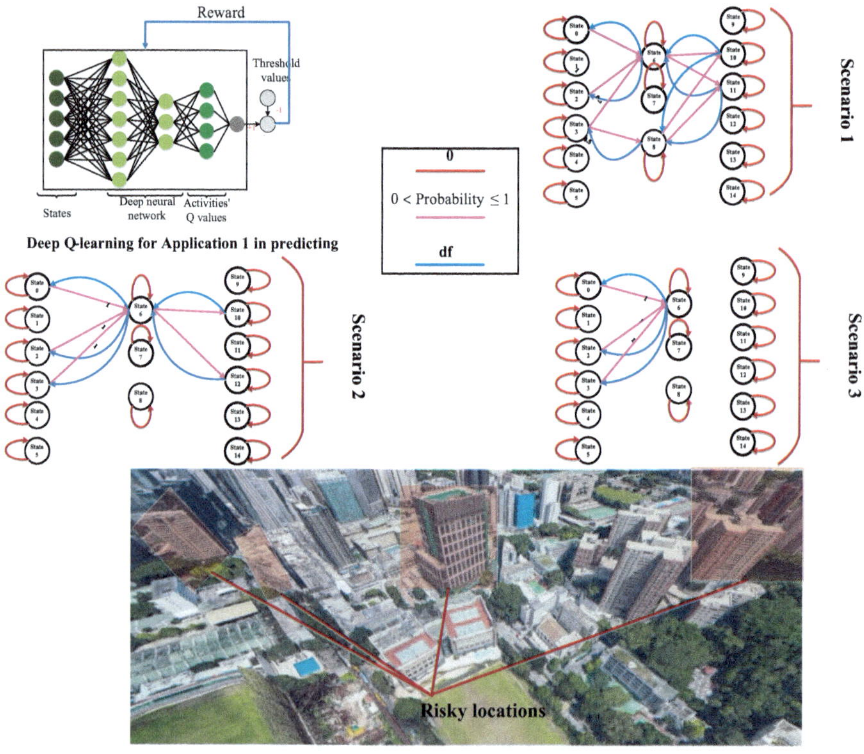

Fig. 14 Metaverse in predicting the risky locations by employing deep Q-learning approach on application 1 when facing the outbreak of COVID-19 and similar cases

Table 1 Scenario description for Fig. 14

Scenario		Purposed application	Activated state		Activity	
1	Patient with COVID-19	Application 1	State0	High temperature	Activity1	Register location
			State2	Normal blood sugar		
			State3	Low oxygen level	Activity2	Register new case
			State6	Active mobile and its location		
			State8:	Active emergency service		
			State10	Active statistics center		
			State11	Active hospital service		
2	Patient with COVID-19 and background diseases	Application 1	State0	High temperature	Activity1	Register location
			State2	Normal blood sugar		
			State3	Normal oxygen level	Activity2	Register new case
			State6	Active mobile and its location		
			State10	Active statistics center		
			State12	Active homecare service		
3	Patients with background diseases	Application 1	State0	Normal temperature	Activity1	Register location
			State2	High blood sugar	Activity2	Mobile alarming
			State3	Normal oxygen level	Activity3	Police officers alarming
			State6	Active mobile and its location		
			State10	Active statistics center service		

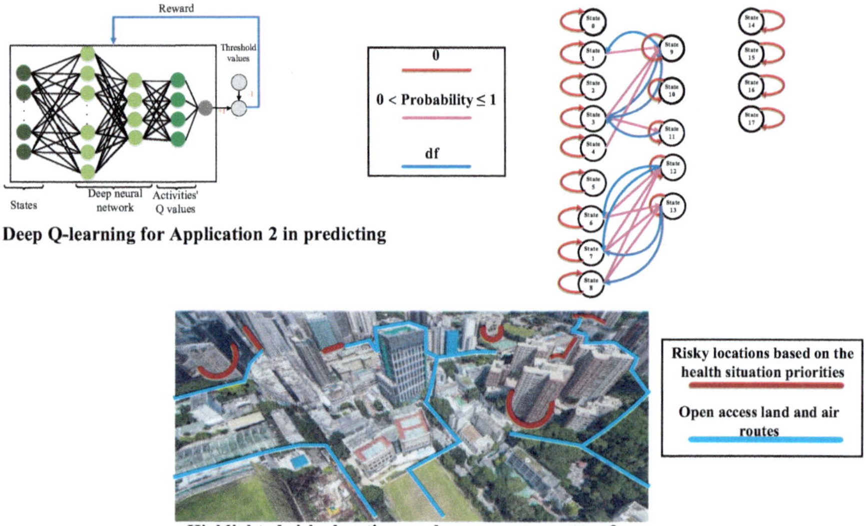

Highlighted risky locations and open access routes after earthquake simulation

Fig. 15 Metaverse in predicting the related risky locations to the patients with background diseases and open access land and air routes by employing deep Q-learning approach on application 2 after simulating earthquake with high-intensive

of various devices. It positively impacts predicting dangerous locals and positions to prioritize scheduling and timely decision-making during accidents and natural disasters (such as widespread road accidents, floods, earthquakes, tornadoes, storms, etc.). When facing the mentioned events, the HSPs can quickly deploy in the close positions to the predicted high-risk locations (school, kindergarten, hospital, nursing home, locations of transaction people, patients with background diseases, etc.) and decide about dedicating appropriate services to the injured by considering their vital signs and background information. AV devices help simulate the different natural disasters in a city with low, medium, and high intensities to predict the destruction rate and determine the air and road crossings for rescuing the injured people, besides accessing the paths of the buildings. In Fig. 15, the prediction process indicates the role of simulating a high-intensive earthquake based on the nodes of application 2 by employing AV and deep Q-learning. The two mentioned features of a metaspace lead to the successful appearance of its platform in rapidly providing healthcare services to injured people based on their health situation priorities.

Table 2 outlines a scenario that utilizes the deep Q-learning method to identify access routes for healthcare service providers during earthquake simulations. This approach aims to aid patients with background diseases who are considered to be in risky situations.

Some diseases do not have treatment methods and progress for a long or short duration (depending on the patients' age, diet, and lifestyle), and the patients will lose their routine and daily activity and need round-the-clock care, which their

Table 2 Scenario description for Fig. 15

Scenario	The purpose application	Activated state		Activity	
Earthquake simulation with high-intensive	Application 2	State1	Hurt rate anormal (Avatar information)	Activity1	Register the location of the patients with background diseases and risky locations.
		State3	Low oxygen level (Avatar information)	Activity2	Road mapping
		State4	Blood pressure anormal (Avatar information)		
		State6	Weather (simulated earthquake in weather's critical situation)		
		State7	Road-camera (simulated earthquake)		
		State8	Car (simulated earthquake)		
		State9	Mobile		
		State12	Active police		
		State13	Active relief group		

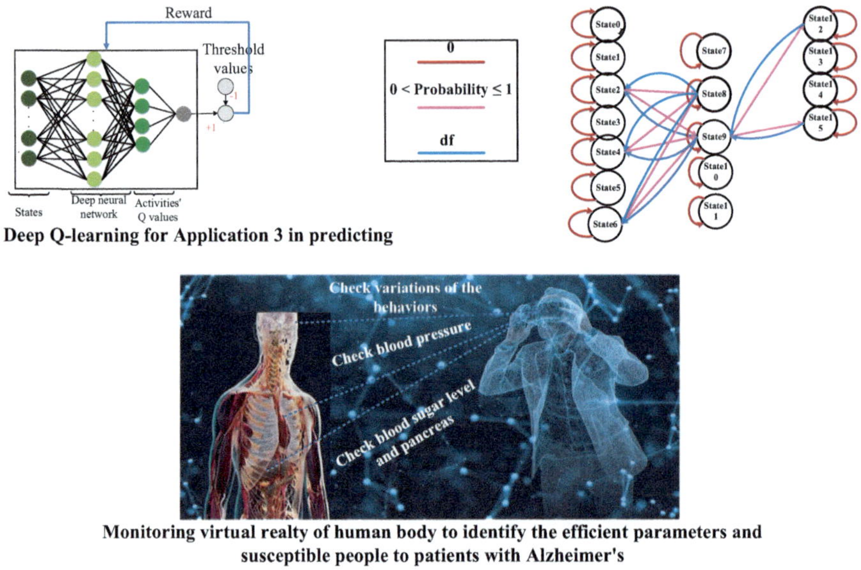

Fig. 16 Metaverse in recognizing the susceptible people to infect with Alzheimer's to prevent infecting the disease by employing a deep Q-learning approach on application 3 after monitoring the digital twins of persons and their records

prediction leads to prevent infecting them. All types of dementia and Alzheimer's embrace the addressed characteristics where the statistics demonstrate a pick up in the number of patients with the diseases and impose the hard cost for their relatives and governments to care for them. In application 3, we define all efficient parameters in Alzheimer's diagnosis and prediction via the information of the sensor layer (outputs of the indicated sensors) when medical imaging only helps its detection. Metaverse can handle the application and similar cases to predict the disease with high accuracy (not precision) by defining all individual and social habits and cultures, diets, geographical locations, and activities of the Avatars (inspired by the physical personality of each person). The characteristics were analyzed by doctors, nutritionists, geneticists, chemists, and expert persons to define comprehensive rules for employing in the metaverse to timely prediction, besides utilizing the Evolutionary computation (EC) to find the defective stands for identifying hereditary factors in susceptible people. After predicting the diseases and identifying the prone people, the technology can present an intense recommender system to prevent or reduce the probability of infecting the disease by creating variations in the diets (vegetables, nuts, reducing sugar and red meat consumption), lifestyle, habits, activities (recommending study, solving table, outdoor sports, learning a new language, etc), and periodic checkups. Figures 14, 15, and 16 are targeted to clarify the metaverse operations for predicting COVID-19, risky situations of unforeseen events, and Alzheimer's based on the three defined applications 1–3, which give a schematic of their actions, respectively.

We provide a scenario description in Table 3 that illustrates the reorganization of individuals susceptible to Alzheimer's disease by using a deep Q-learning method in the metaverse-based applications.

To support the prediction operations of the MIoT-based applications, various subset methods of AI (deep Q-learning, DNN, ARM, EC, etc.) have to be employed to improve the efficiency of Medical IoT in the research area where the metaverse can make available an artificial intelligence platform for integrating the mentioned approaches and satisfying the purposes.

5.3 *Metaverse in Drug Recommendation*

Pharmacist doctors and chemists must pass many laboratory tests and simulate times to investigate the drugs and their chemical interactions on mice, rats, and other animals and organisms for recommending a proper drug for therapy or controlling the disease. It is a time-consuming process and can lead to the spread of viruses, bacteria, and other laboratory contaminants besides facing the probable drug's severe side effects on the patients and hurting them. The metaverse can utilize the digital twin technique for defining virtual cells and drug interactions to analyze its efficiency on the Avatars (the digital twins of the patients) and predict the side effects in the patients with different conditions of allergies, background, and autoimmune diseases, cancers, and other risky health statuses for recommending it for treatment or control. After finding an appropriate drug to tackle a disease, AV/VR devices can help specialist doctors monitor and analyze the current and future situation of the body and cells by augmenting a virtual reality of the infected parts in facing medical interactions. In Alzheimer's disease, the doctor can monitor the situation of the neurons and neutralize their acidosis area after recommending a related drug to control the disease (such as Yasnal, etc.) by investigating aggregating and attaching β protein, as shown in Fig. 17a, b.

This feature enables doctors to make informed decisions about the most effective drug for slowing down the destruction of neurons and determine whether to continue with the current treatment method using the medication, adjust the dosage, or switch to a different type of medication if the patient's health does not improve or stabilize.

5.4 *Metaverse in Energy Efficiency*

In Medical IoT, energy efficiency and its management have the highlighted roles in the performance of MIoT-based applications and their availability and dependability by supporting real-time tasks and online accessing the sensors' outputs. Smart grid handles energy balancing and monitoring its distribution between electronic devices of IoT. It supports total power demands of the communication infrastructure, though supporting EV and IoV is challenging for the technology. A meta space can

Table 3 Scenario description for Fig. 16

Scenario	The purpose application	Activated state		Activity	
Identifying the susceptible people to patients with Alzheimer's	Application 3	State2	Blood sugar (Avatar records)	Activity1	Register the location of the patients
		State4	Blood pressure (Avatar records)	Activity2	Diet and lifestyle recommendations
		State6	Homecare sensor (Avatar records)		
		State8	Mobile active		
		State9	Doctor active		
		State12	Hospital active		
		State15	Drugstore active		

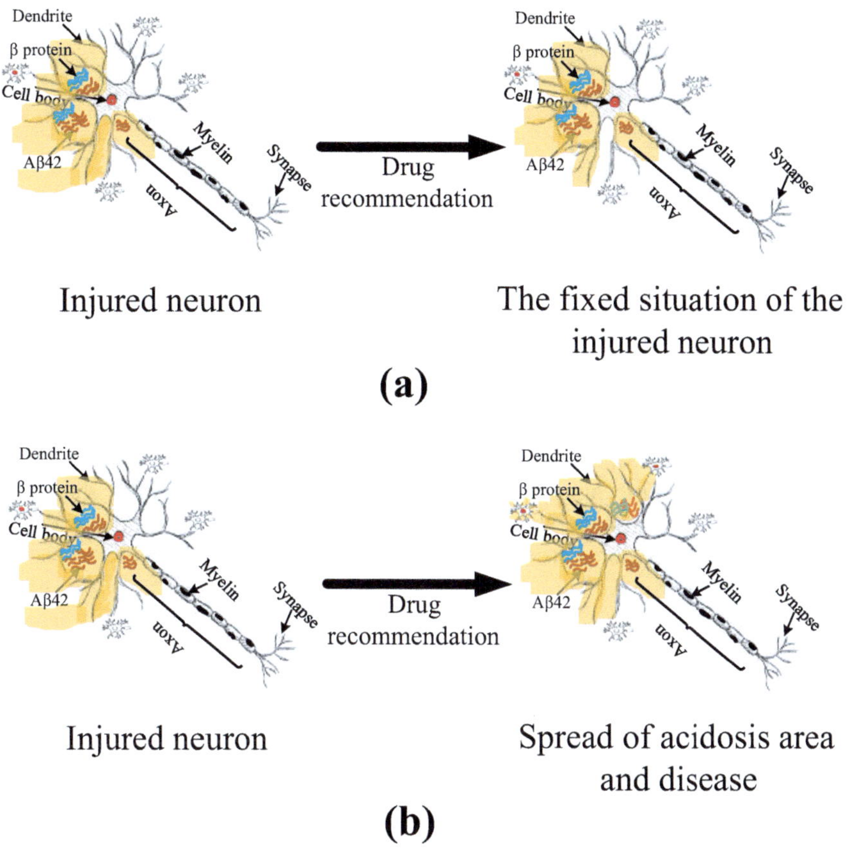

Fig. 17 The situation of neurons and Alzheimer's after recommending a drug; (**a**) The positive impact of a proper drug in fixing the neuron situation and neutralizing acidosis area; (**b**) Predicting (via an augmented reality) the negative impact of an inappropriate drug in the spread of acidosis area, aggregating Aβ42, absorbing β protein, and destroying more neighbor neurons

allow defining all details of the smart grid via the digital twins, which can analyze the energy efficiency and power demand of MIoT and Medical IoV to find the solutions to tackle their challenges in the virtual world. The metaverse also has a comprehensive definition of the purposed actual persons and their physical life and devices (medical, industrial, personal, social, and other devices) to describe their Avatars where the issue helps to analyze the energy efficiency of wearable and biosensors and the power demands of mobiles. Analyzing the energy efficiency of a network with a massive number of devices (such as smart cities) leads to the problem of handling and managing its nodes when some of them are wasting static power. A meta-based virtual reality and digital twin space can estimate the dynamic and static power consumption of different nodes (Avatars, their attached and related devices, and independent components) and their leakage energy to decide about their manufacturing technology (in transistor level) and load balancing.

6 The Relationship Between AI, Metaverse, and MIoT

The section investigates the background of the metaverse technology, where the artificial intelligence methods handle the complexity of its platform to cover the different applications with various priorities and create a real second world. Due to the properties of the mentioned AI approaches in MIoT, we clarify their roles in the metaverse to support medical IoT and explain their dependency to satisfy the purposes of decision-making, diagnosis, prediction, recommendation, and energy management.

The chapter is planned to indicate the role of a meta space, AV/VR device, MR, XR, and digital twin techniques in overcoming the challenges of MIoT and prove that the metaverse can emerge successful in improving the efficiency of medical and healthcare-based applications compared with the other technologies. As shown in Fig. 18a, a Metaverse platform creates a simple, popular, and friendly user space to present an attractive and practical environment when a complicated system of integrated different AI approaches manages its background.

6.1 Deep Q-Learning in Metaverse

The technology consists of seven main layers for scheduling the tasks and services for supporting its purposes in different aspects of industrial, management, social, game, and medical applications of the physical world. At the decentralization level, deep Q-learning is employed for timely decision-making and passing edge computing in the level and communications with the upper (spatial computing) and lower (human interface) layers. Figure 18b demonstrates the layers of the metaverse infrastructure, where the dataflow of the requests and resource allocations are defined in the upper level to lower and vice versa, respectively. The decentralization level performs the tasks of the perception layer of MIoT, while flexible clustering also has an impressive role in covering the tasks of the faulty processing elements, as reviewed in Sect. 4. The blockchain method is established on deep Q-learning to protect the private information (patients' records, doctors' recommendations, etc.) in the decentralization layer, which pruning and employing forward and backward chain approaches can lead to improving its efficiency via imposing penalties and rewards.

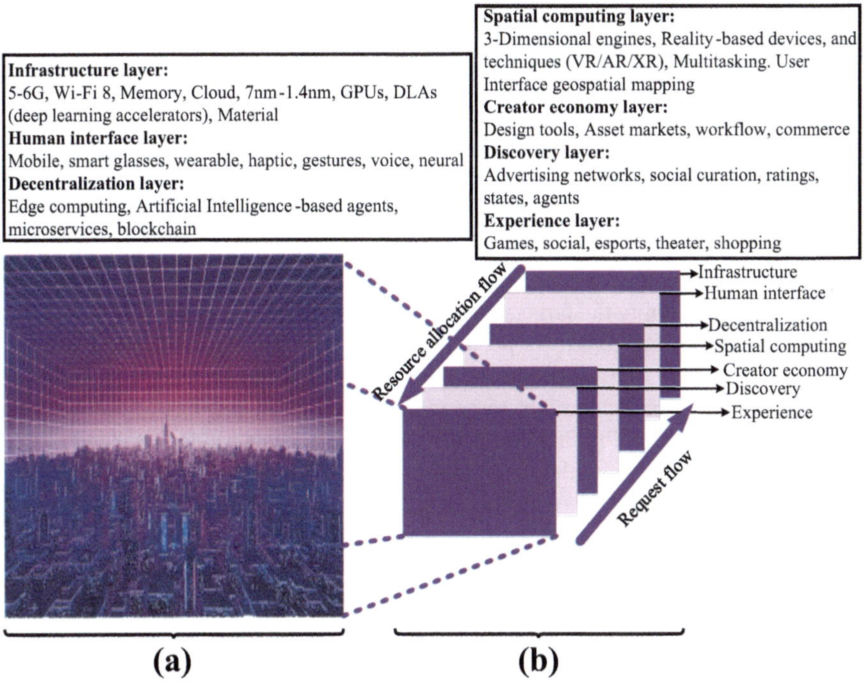

Fig. 18 A metaverse-based system and its layers to support the purposes; (**a**) Augmented reality of a metaverse-based city; (**b**) Seven main layers of the metaverse technology

6.2 *Neural Networks in Metaverse*

DNNs are popular machine learning algorithms for prediction, detection, and deciding about the various services, applications, and devices where the metaverse was developed to handle the mentioned purposes in the wide range of request variety. The data collection approach is featured at employing the DNNs and improving their efficiency to support the tasks. However, the issue applies to the metaverse technology to detect the appropriate and efficient parameters (as DNN's inputs) among the many received information and requests. To support the prediction and diagnosis demands of MIoT, the metaverse can appear successful in collecting an appropriate training and testing dataset by employing ARM methods and expert persons who are specialists in the aimed research area (based on applications and diseases). Rule mapping processes can be performed in the human interface layer before allocating resources to the upper level (decentralization layer) for edge computing and deciding about employing the devices.

6.3 Mapping and Clustering in Metaverse

The main body of the technology follows the mapping concept due to the transfer of the physical reality of the persons, their activities, habits, cultural, geographical locations, and devices to a meta-virtual space and create a second-world of human life and environment. The concept can be found in the spatial computing layer of the metaverse, where the AV/VR and XR have joined the platform to augment the reality of the emulated model. In the centralization and spatial layers, role mapping can improve the timely decision-making and service availability of MIoT-based applications by defining the targeted nodes (Avatars, sensors, devices, etc.) onto the neurons and imposing rewards or penalties on NN's weights based on the feedback of the output value. The process can also improve energy efficiency and the total delay of the failed nodes thought to be identified as weak neurons of the mapped neural network by pruning them after imposing the penalty value. To increase the efficiency of role mapping, the metaverse can support a flexible clustering method to identify the proper digital twins of healthcare service providers to cover the tasks of the faulty nodes, which are stopped by pruning operations.

In this chapter, we aim to explore the role of flexible clustering and mapping techniques in the metaverse technology for improving the efficiency of MIoT in timely decision-making about dedicating appropriate HSPs to patients in risky situations. To achieve this, we report on the total energy and delay of the communication between nodes of Application 1 for three scenarios, as depicted in Table 1. We employ a deep Q-learning algorithm to identify risky locations and consider three assumptions for the scenarios to clarify the concept of mapping and flexible clustering for Application 1. We use Table 4 to illustrate how decision-making can be used to dedicate the appropriate HSPs to patients after identifying risky locations. To analyze the efficiency of mapping and flexible clustering in improving the performance of MIoT applications, we utilize the CupCarbon tool to simulate Application 1. We describe each node of the application by c family co-designs in CupCarbon and run the application for three scenarios before and after applying mapping and flexible clustering techniques. By comparing the results, we can depict the impact of these techniques on the overall efficiency of MIoT in healthcare applications.

The proposed idea for improving the efficiency of MIoT-based applications through mapping and flexible clustering techniques has been assessed by estimating

Table 4 Assumption description for three scenarios of Table 1

Scenario number	Assumption	
1	1	Distance between patients and HSPs is reported in a similar range
2	2	Distance between patients and HSPs are not similar, and detecting a faulty HSP
3	3	Distance between patients and HSPs is not similar and are received available services from two HSPs

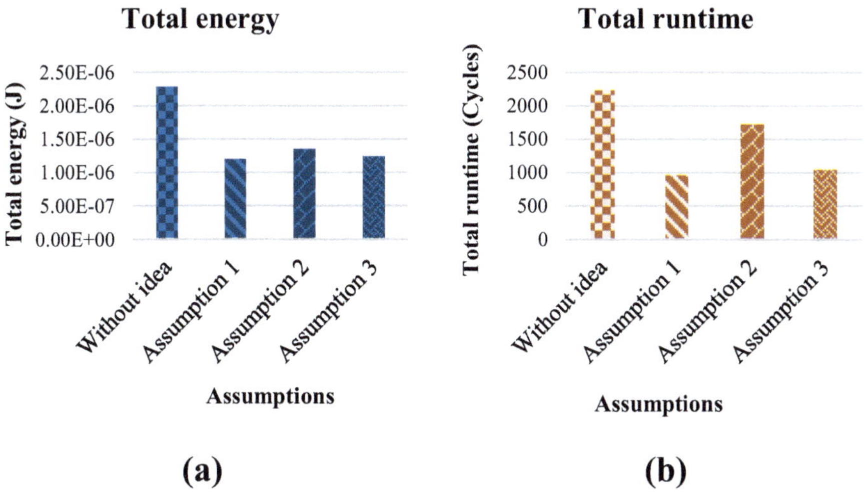

Fig. 19 Comparing total energy and total runtime between Assumption 1, Assumption 2, and Assumption 3; (**a**) Comparing total energy between Assumption 1, Assumption 2, and Assumption 3; (**b**) Comparing total runtime between Assumption 1, Assumption 2, and Assumption 3

latency and energy consumption. The results show that assumption 3 leads to a 39.36% improvement in total energy and an 8.20% improvement in total runtime compared to assumption 2, due to the removal of queue delay for releasing shared HSPs, as shown in Fig. 19a, b. In contrast, decision-making without performing these techniques results in a 41.17% increase in total energy and a 29.9% increase in delay. These simulation results demonstrate the effectiveness of mapping and flexible clustering in enhancing the performance of MIoT applications, particularly in healthcare settings. By identifying best practices for utilizing the metaverse technology and these techniques, we can ensure the delivery of high-quality healthcare services while maintaining security and privacy.

7 Concise Recent Survey

Numerous recent studies have focused on the various intelligence methods, devices, and applications required to integrate smart cities and IoT-based infrastructures into different research areas such as medical, industrial, environmental, social, management, political, economic, engineering, and basic sciences. In light of the high sensitivity of medical applications and devices, researchers have created a separate area to define Medical IoT and its priorities for planning e-healthcare ideas and addressing its challenges, in addition to the problems related to the Internet of Things. This section examines recent studies on supporting MIoT-based applications and offers suggestions for improving its efficiency in terms of security, availability, dependability, decision-making, detection, and prediction.

To improve the security of Medical IoT, categorizing the data transaction channel between the communication platform's different layers created an opportunity to protect privacy by classifying data into four groups with similar sizes. The approach confused the intruders with the passive and active attacks to access a complete data format and made it incomprehensible to devastators [34]. The main body of blockchain structure attracted researchers to apply it to provide security-based methods, where the cryptography-Merkle signature scheme emerged successfully to handle the authentication process in healthcare IoT (as one of the blockchain-based techniques) [35]. The zero-knowledge proof protocol joined the authentication-based methods to verify the legitimacy of the doctors connected to the infrastructure and monitor the patients' records [36]. It improved communication security between patients and healthcare service providers by defining authentication and private keys. However, employing the approach on the side of the doctor's legitimacy is challenging when facing intruders in the role of sicky. The cryptography protocols impose additional processing time and energy efficiency on the targeted devices where the mentioned demands are difficult for MIoT by increasing the traffic and span of data. APHAC (as an advanced method of hidden access control) reduced the total time of crypto and encrypting processes for the users of the Medical IoT to access the information in comparison with CP-ABE, besides protecting their private records [5]. In following the addressed feature, the authentication keys were targeted to protect the privacy of the patient's records and verify the legitimacy of HSPs who joined the infrastructure, in addition to improving the cost overhead of cryptography processes by reducing the length of signatures [6]. When targeting the medical applications on service reliability, the trust-based approaches prepared a secure communication platform by employing a bee colony to identify malicious components and implementing a fault tolerance routing mechanism in the fog layer [7, 8]. Due to the problems of satisfying the security of mobile communications and EVs, it appeared successful to overcome the challenge by using a trust-aware method to protect the private information in the fog layer instead of the cloud level, balancing the cost of the communication platform [7]. The decentralization layer of the metaverse was planned to establish the technology on the blockchain technique to support the security of the end devices at the edge level, where covering the decentralized components is challenging for IoV-based applications [37]. The AI-based decentralization method is impressive in protecting patients' private records when facing many vehicle healthcare sensors (wearables, biosensors, smart watches, etc.) in medical applications.

Due to the growth of smart applications and devices, machine learning algorithms have become prominent in the various sciences and industries to handle the complexity of communications and data transactions between intelligence components and decision-making about different statuses. The combined method of Q-learning, deep neural networks, and Markov model processes was targeted to implement crypto and encrypt processes for authentication protocols and identifying anomalies in MIoT applications with high accuracy and minimum cost, which the issue helps to reduce latency of timely diagnosing and decision-making in risky situations [9, 10]. The idea proved its efficient role in the actual application of rapid providing healthcare services during the duration of the COVID-19 pandemic and raising new cases by presenting a reinforcement learning-based framework when targeting covering the priorities of reliability and availability [10]. In high-risk diseases, the proposed method has to support timely diagnosis, where the artificial neural networks (as one of the machine learning algorithms) emerged successful as the efficient approach to detecting breast cancer at the initial level promptly [13]. To reduce the risky conditions of patients with chronic obstructive pulmonary disease, MIoT-based applications were developed to join them on the platform for online monitoring of their vital signs and timely provision of healthcare services by attending to cases that stopped the treatment process [14]. It supported the patients and rapidly provided healthcare services by employing a DNN to identify the inattentive cases by remotely controlling their symptoms. When facing brain disorders with specialized symptoms, the supervised machine learning algorithms could be affected in timely diagnosing Parkinson's, besides employing the advanced intelligent wearable sensors to monitor the physical examination and the condensation of the proteins in the blood [15]. In a meta space of massive numbers of digital twins, deep Q-learning was employed to reduce the communication delay between EVs and stations and handle IoV-based applications with minimal cost, where the growing data span of connections between the virtual and physical worlds is challenging for the metaverse [22]. It can overcome the challenges of all IoV-based applications, which also consist of vehicle medical devices (wearable and biosensors, vehicle healthcare stations, mobile, etc.), and improve the efficiency of MIoT in timely decision-making. The resource allocation and power management were supported by an intelligent metaverse system in the decreolization layer, where edge computing aimed at the devices and wireless communications between them via deep Q-learning to decide about total energy demands [23]. When inspiring the metaverse by fully AI-based methods, it was driven toward supporting the medical-based applications with different priorities of health care, diagnosing, predicting, surgery, and deciding where AV/VR, XR, and Digital twinges had an efficient role in covering MIoT [17, 18]. The issue proved the efficient role of the meta space of digital twins and the augmented realities in timely diagnosing skin diseases and pulmonary nodules to treatment them by employing AV, VR, expert doctors, and healthcare staff who were adapted to the metaverse platform and Avatar (digital twin of a patient) [16], [38, 39].

Recent studies have highlighted the growing trend toward integrating multidisciplinary medical sciences with the metaverse technology to support their applications at minimal cost and high accuracy. This technology provides an integrated platform that adapts different techniques and methods to establish a secure communication infrastructure based on the blockchain concept, with a minimized authentication key for reducing the total time and power demands of the crypto and decrypt processes. Overcoming the challenges of timely decision-making, diagnosing, and predicting in MIoT removes the overhead of authentication keys and reduces signature length. Augmented realities and digital twins aid doctors and treatment staff in gaining a deeper understanding of various disorders in the human body and predicting disease status for short- or long-term treatment plans. However, the technology poses a significant risk to patients when expert persons make mistakes in rule mapping due to the direct dependency between actual characteristics and their virtual definition in a meta space.

References

1. Kishor, A., & Chakraborty, C. (2022). Artificial intelligence and internet of things based healthcare 4.0 monitoring system. *Wireless Personal Communications, 127*(2), 1615–1631.
2. Mishra, S., & Tyagi, A. K.. (2022). The role of machine learning techniques in internet of things-based cloud applications. In *Artificial intelligence-based internet of things systems* (pp. 105–135). Springer, Cham.
3. Schnell, B., Moder, P., Ehm, H., Konstantinov, M., & Ismail, M. (2022). Challenges in smart health applications using wearable medical internet-of-things—A review. In *Proceedings of sixth international congress on information and communication technology* (pp. 283–296). Springer, Singapore.
4. Smys, S., & Raj, J. S. (2022). Future challenges of the internet of things in the health care domain-an overview. *Journal of Trends in Computer Science and Smart Technology., 3*(4), 274–286.
5. Wang, K., Xie, S., & Rodrigues, J. (2022). Medical data security of wearable tele-rehabilitation under internet of things. *Internet of Things and Cyber-Physical Systems., 2*(2), 1–1.
6. Rasslan, M., Nasreldin, M. M., & Aslan, H. K. (2022). Ibn Sina: A patient privacy-preserving authentication protocol in medical internet of things. *Computers & Security, 1*(119), 102753.
7. Haseeb, K., Saba, T., Rehman, A., Ahmed, Z., Song, H. H., & Wang, H. H. (2022). Trust management with fault-tolerant supervised routing for smart cities using internet of things. *IEEE Internet of Things Journal, 9*(22), 22608–22617.
8. Gali, S., & Nidumolu, V. (2022). An intelligent trust sensing scheme with metaheuristic based secure routing protocol for internet of things. *Cluster Computing, 25*(3), 1779–1789.
9. Kathamuthu, N. D., Chinnamuthu, A., Iruthayanathan, N., Ramachandran, M., & Gandomi, A. H. (2022). Deep Q-learning-based neural network with privacy preservation method for secure data transmission in internet of things (IoT) healthcare application. *Electronics, 11*(1), 157.
10. Almagrabi, A. O., Ali, R., Alghazzawi, D., AlBarakati, A., & Khurshaid, T. (2022). A reinforcement learning-based framework for crowdsourcing in massive health care internet of things. *Big Data, 10*(2), 161–170.
11. Badshah, A., Waqas, M., Muhammad, F., Abbas, G., & Abbas, Z. H. (2022). A novel framework for smart systems using blockchain-enabled internet of things. *IT Professional, 24*(3), 73–80.
12. Choo, K. K., Dehghantanha, A., & Parizi, R. M. (Eds.). (2020). *Blockchain cybersecurity, trust and privacy*. Springer.
13. Ogundokun, R. O., Misra, S., Douglas, M., Damaševičius, R., & Maskeliūnas, R. (2022). Medical internet-of-things based breast cancer diagnosis using Hyperparameter-optimized neural networks. *Future Internet, 14*(5), 153.
14. Yang, D., Li, K., Chua, D. M., Song, Y., Bai, C., & Powell, C. A. (2022). Application of internet of things in chronic respiratory disease prevention, diagnosis, treatment and management. *Clinical eHealth, 5*, 10–16.
15. Anbalagan, B., Karnam Anantha, S., & Kalpana, R. (2022). Novel approach to prognosis Parkinson's disease with wireless technology using resting tremors. *Wireless Personal Communications, 24*, 1–5.

16. Yang, D., Zhou, J., Chen, R., Song, Y., Song, Z., Zhang, X., Wang, Q., Wang, K., Zhou, C., Sun, J., & Zhang, L. (2022). Expert consensus on the metaverse in medicine. *Clinical eHealth, 1*(5), 1–9.
17. Sun, M., Xie, L., Liu, Y., Li, K., Jiang, B., Lu, Y., Yang, Y., Yu, H., Song, Y., Bai, C., & Yang, D. (2022). The metaverse in current digital medicine. *Clinical eHealth, 5*, 52.
18. Zeng, Y., Zeng, L., Zhang, C., & Cheng, A. S. (2022). The metaverse in cancer care: Applications and challenges. *Asia-Pacific Journal of Oncology Nursing, 5*, 100111.
19. Liu, W., Zhang, H., Dong, X., & Sun, Y. (2022). Composite of gold nanoclusters and basified human serum albumin significantly boosts the inhibition of Alzheimer's β-amyloid by photo-oxygenation. *Acta Biomaterialia, 1*(144), 157–167.
20. Song, C., Shi, J., Zhang, P., Zhang, Y., Xu, J., Zhao, L., Zhang, R., Wang, H., & Chen, H. (2022). Immunotherapy for Alzheimer's disease: Targeting β-amyloid and beyond. *Translational Neurodegeneration, 11*(1), 18.
21. Rahmani, A. M., Ali Naqvi, R., Ali, S., Hosseini Mirmahaleh, S. Y., Alswaitti, M., Hosseinzadeh, M., & Siddique, K. (2021). An astrocyte-flow mapping on a mesh-based communication infrastructure to defective neurons phagocytosis. *Mathematics, 9*(23), 3012.
22. Chua, T. J., Yu, W., & Zhao, J. (2022). Resource allocation for mobile metaverse with the Internet of Vehicles over 6G wireless communications: A deep reinforcement learning approach. arXiv preprint arXiv:2209.13425.
23. Kim, S. (2022). Auction, learning and bargaining based control scheme for edge assisted metaverse system. *Computer Networks, 11*, 109462.
24. Rahman, M. Z., Akbar, M. A., Leiva, V., Tahir, A., Riaz, M. T., & Martin-Barreiro, C. (2023). An intelligent health monitoring and diagnosis system based on the internet of things and fuzzy logic for cardiac arrhythmia COVID-19 patients. *Computers in Biology and Medicine, 24*, 106583.
25. Hosseini, A. M., & Mirmahaleh, S. Y. (2022). An intelligent algorithm to predict GDP rate and find a relationship between COVID-19 outbreak and economic downturn. *Computational Economics, 26*, 1–20.
26. Rahmani, A. M., Ali Naqvi, R., Ali, S., Hosseini Mirmahaleh, S. Y., & Hosseinzadeh, M. (2021). Quasi-mapping and satisfying iot availability with a penalty-based algorithm. *Mathematics., 9*(24), 3286.
27. Rahmani, A. M., Mirmahaleh, S. Y., & Hosseinzadeh, M. (2020). An intelligent algorithm to recommend percent vegetation cover (ARVC) for PM 2.5 reduction. *Air Quality, Atmosphere & Health., 13*, 859–870.
28. Ramkumar, M. P., Mano Paul, P. D., Maram, B., & Ananth, J. P. (2022). Deep maxout network for lung cancer detection using optimization algorithm in smart internet of things. *Concurrency and Computation: Practice and Experience., 34*(25), e7264.
29. Goodman, L. A. (1954). Kolmogorov-Smirnov tests for psychological research. *Psychological Bulletin., 51*(2), 160.
30. Royston, J. P. (1983). Some techniques for assessing multivarate normality based on the Shapiro-Wilk W. *Journal of the Royal Statistical Society Series C: Applied Statistics., 32*(2), 121–133.
31. Ali, S., Armand, T. P., Athar, A., Hussain, A., Ali, M., Yaseen, M., Joo, M. I., & Kim, H. C. (2023). Metaverse in healthcare integrated with explainable AI and Blockchain: Enabling Immersiveness, ensuring trust, and providing patient data security. *Sensors, 23*(2), 565.
32. Deng, Y., Weng, Z., & Zhang, T. (2022). Metaverse-driven remote management solution for scene-based energy storage power stations. *Evolutionary Intelligence., 13*, 1–2.
33. Rahmani, A. M., & Hosseini Mirmahaleh, S. Y. (2022). Flexible-clustering based on application priority to improve IoMT efficiency and dependability. *Sustainability, 14*(17), 10666.
34. Adil, M., Attique, M., Jadoon, M. M., Ali, J., Farouk, A., & Song, H. (2022). HOPCTP: A robust channel categorization data preservation scheme for industrial healthcare internet of things. *IEEE Transactions on Industrial Informatics., 18*(10), 7151–7161.

35. Mehbodniya, A., Webber, J. L., Neware, R., Arslan, F., Pamba, R. V., & Shabaz, M. (2022). Modified Lamport Merkle digital signature blockchain framework for authentication of internet of things healthcare data. *Expert Systems., 39*(10), e12978.
36. Yadav, V. K., Yadav, R. K., Verma, S., & Venkatesan, S. (2022). CP2EH: A comprehensive privacy-preserving e-health scheme over cloud. *The Journal of Supercomputing., 1*, 1–31.
37. Cao, L. (2022). Decentralized ai: Edge intelligence and smart blockchain, metaverse, web3, and desci. *IEEE Intelligent Systems., 37*(3), 6–19.
38. Kumari, J., Das, K., & Goldust, M. (2022). Metaverse in diagnosis of skin diseases. *Journal of Cosmetic Dermatology., 22*, 698.
39. Menon, D., Anand, B., & Chowdhary, C. L. (2023). Digital twin: Exploring the intersection of virtual and physical worlds. *IEEE Access, 11*, 75152.

The Metaverse and Mental Well-Being: Potential Benefits and Challenges in the Current Era

Sreeraag Govindankutty and Shynu Padinjappurathu Gopalan

1 Introduction

The metaverse is a cooperative virtual shared space that lives parallel to the actual world. This virtual environment is accessible via technology like virtual reality, augmented reality, or other favorably immersive and interactive digital media tools. In the contemporary world, the concept of the metaverse has attracted massive interest among different communities since it delivers new types of entertainment, social connections, and education to societies. The metaverse concept was initially proposed in Neal Stephenson's 1992 science fiction novel *Snow Crash*, which envisaged a virtual reality universe in which people may interact with each other and virtual objects in a shared digital environment. Since then, the notion has expanded to include a diverse range of digital experiences, which include online social networks, virtual and online gaming, virtual commerce, and online virtual events, which include several entertainment activities, including the dissemination of news and information. People can lead a second life in this new virtual world by purchasing land and properties, accepting the new environment, and following the laws and regulations defined in this new world.

The metaverse is an immersive and interactive experience where users can create their avatars, explore virtual environments and landscapes, interact in real time with other users, and create friendships with them. It is a place where users can do things that are not probable or possible in the real world, which includes exploring fictional and adventurous landscapes, trying on various identities, and participating in sophisticated virtual games and challenges [1, 2].

S. Govindankutty · S. P. Gopalan (✉)
School of Computer Science Engineering and Information Systems, Vellore Institute of Technology, Vellore, Tamil Nadu, India
e-mail: pgshynu@vit.ac.in

C. L. Chowdhary (ed.), *The Metaverse for the Healthcare Industry*,
https://doi.org/10.1007/978-3-031-60073-9_7

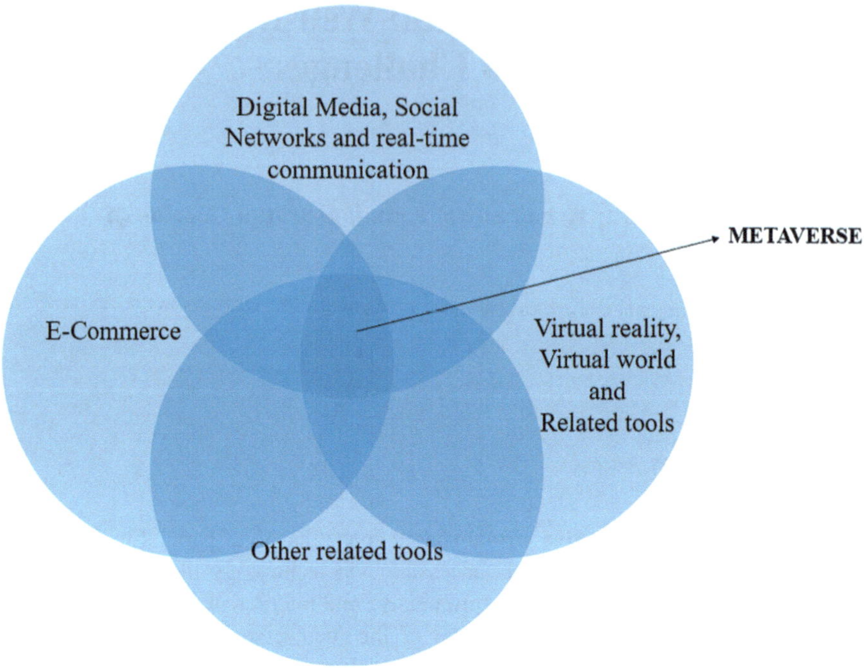

Fig. 1 The metaverse comprises digital and social media combined with virtual world aspects and other tools with a payment interface

One of the essential characteristics of the metaverse is its ability to connect people worldwide in new ways. With the advent of remote employment, distant schooling, online classes, and virtual events, the metaverse may provide a unique chance for people to gather together in a shared virtual area, regardless of their actual location. However, the metaverse, like any new technology, has potential hazards that can jeopardize one's personal life and identity in the real world. This includes privacy, security, mental well-being, and digital addiction concerns. Spending too much time in a virtual world, for example, may lead to neglect of real-world obligations and relationships, which may negatively influence mental health [3]. Studies have also showcased that the metaverse could affect the emotional well-being of individuals with long-term frequent usage (Fig. 1).

When it comes to mental well-being, it is evident that the metaverse has the potential to have both positive and harmful effects on mental health. Additionally, it may open new avenues for social connection, support, and therapy. For example, those dealing with mental health issues may find it easier to interact with people with similar experiences and struggles in virtual communities within the metaverse. Students may also be able to participate in virtual therapy sessions with professional therapists from anywhere in the world without traveling physically [4].

Nevertheless, some hazards linked with the metaverse could influence mental health. For example, the immersive and potentially addictive nature of the metaverse could increase digital addiction difficulties, leading to concerns such as social isolation, anxiety, and depression. Furthermore, there may be issues with the quality and accuracy of material exchanged within virtual communities, which could potentially impair individuals' mental health if they get incorrect or harmful advice or assistance [5, 6].

The future of the metaverse is still uncertain. However, the metaverse and virtual world concepts are gaining considerable significance and will likely play an increasingly crucial part in our daily lives shortly. Several experts in this field believe that the metaverse and virtual reality will likely become significant platforms for social relations, entertainment, education, and commerce, opening up new possibilities for collaboration, creativity, and innovation. However, as mentioned before, like with any new technology, there are risks and obstacles involved with the metaverse, which include privacy, security, and ethical considerations [7, 8]. As the metaverse evolves, it is critical for developers and stakeholders to carefully consider these dangers and act to mitigate them for the betterment of the future society.

2 Metaverse and Online Social Networks

In today's world, the term "metaverse" refers to a virtual environment where users may engage in activities such as chatting, gaming, buying, and generating content. Online social networks are essential to the metaverse since they enable users to interact and communicate in this virtual reality. Facebook, Twitter, and Instagram are already utilized for online social involvement among civilizations and communities. The metaverse, on the other hand, takes this concept to the next level by offering a fully immersive and interactive virtual environment in which users may create avatars, explore virtual worlds, and communicate with other users in real time [9].

Individuals in the metaverse can interact and engage with others using online social networks. Individuals can create virtual firms or organizations, join clubs or communities with people of similar interests, and even create virtual businesses or societies. The metaverse delivers a richer and more engaging social experience than standard and traditional social networks since it provides a more immersive and dynamic platform for social interaction [10]. Additionally, people can create and share virtual content in the metaverse, such as virtual clothing, furniture, and even entire virtual worlds. People can even purchase a home or land and even lease a house or apartment within this digital world. Inside the metaverse, online social networks enable users to trade and discover material that may be used to customize their virtual avatars and surroundings. In short, people can live a second life within the metaverse and conduct activities that push their physical and mental boundaries with the support of social networks (Fig. 2).

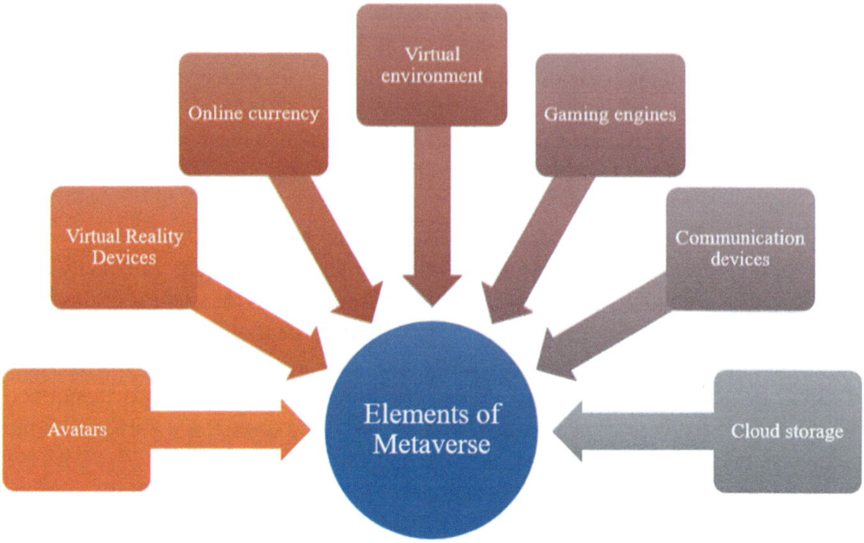

Fig. 2 Key elements of the metaverse environment

2.1 The Connection with Online Social Networks

The metaverse and online social networks are inextricably linked since both offer a platform for social interaction and content creation [11]. The metaverse, on the other hand, takes this concept to the next level by providing a more immersive and dynamic social experience that has the potential to change the way we connect and interact with one another online.

Shared identities: Users in the metaverse can build their avatars to represent them in the virtual world. This is analogous to how people create social network profiles that act as their online identities. In the metaverse, however, users have considerably more significant control over their avatar's look, behavior, and interactions, making the social experience more customized and immersive as per the interest of each individual. They can choose an identity and even an appearance of interest and likes.

Communities and groups: The metaverse, like traditional social networks, features groups and communities where users can connect with people who have common interests or hobbies. These organizations, however, can be more interactive and immersive in the metaverse since users can participate in virtual events and activities with other individuals within the virtual world.

Content creation and sharing: The capacity for people to produce and share their stuff, which includes virtual clothes, furniture, and even whole virtual lands, is a vital aspect of the metaverse. The metaverse allows individuals to trade material that can be used to customize several elements within this digital world.

Real-time communication: Similar to traditional digital networks, people inside the metaverse can communicate instantly. However, the metaverse provides more immersive communication since users can engage with each other via voice chat, gestures, and body language. Using metaverse, alternate face-to-face digital communication with the help of avatars is possible.

Privacy and security: They are essential aspects of the metaverse, just as they are in traditional social networks. Users must be aware of the risks and take appropriate actions to protect their personal information and prevent unauthorized access to their accounts. Users must understand the privacy and ethical concerns while using metaverse and the implications of their actions.

Ultimately, the metaverse and online social networks are inextricably linked since both seek to provide users with a platform for social engagement and content creation. While typical social networks are limited to a two-dimensional interface, the metaverse offers a more immersive and engaging social experience that has the potential to change the way we connect and participate online [12].

3 The Impact of Mental Health in General

The metaverse's impact on mental health is a growing topic with possible advantages and concerns [13, 14]. Some possible known effects of the metaverse on mental health are as follows:

Social interaction: The metaverse may foster a sense of social connection and community, which may benefit mental health. For example, it might connect people with others who share their interests and hobbies or provide a venue to mingle and participate in social events. Studies have advocated that the increase in connection and friend circle can benefit the mental well-being of an individual.

Escapism: The metaverse may offer an escape from real-world stressors with positive and negative mental health implications. Virtual online games may relieve the individual from their hectic schedule. On the one hand, it could help people relax and unwind, reducing stress and enhancing mental health. On the other hand, it may cause people to avoid dealing with real-world issues and worsen feelings of social isolation and separation.

Addiction: The metaverse, like other types of technology, has the potential to be addictive and hurt mental health. Excessive use may result in social isolation, disregard for real-world duties, and other undesirable consequences. Adding social and virtual networks can adversely impact the mental well-being of individuals.

Mental health support: The metaverse could also be used for support and therapy. Virtual reality treatment, for example, is already being used to treat mental health conditions, including posttraumatic stress disorder (PTSD), depression, and phobias.

Generally, the metaverse's impact on mental health is still an area under research and a topic of debate. It is critical to thoroughly assess virtual environments' possible risks and benefits before designing them to encourage healthy mental health outcomes.

3.1 Risks Faced by Young Adults

The metaverse, like any new technology, has the potential to have an impact on adolescents' mental health in both positive and negative ways. Some of the potential threats [15–18] to adolescents' mental health are:

Addiction and overuse: Several features within the metaverse have an addictive nature, which includes real-time communication to online virtual gaming sessions. Teens may become so immersed in this that they overlook real-life duties and relationships. This can lead to issues with impulse control and a lack of balance in their lives, which can harm their mental health. Teenagers who spend much time in virtual settings may grow socially alienated and find it difficult to form and sustain real-life interactions. This might result in feelings of isolation, melancholy, and anxiety.

Cyberbullying and harassment: The metaverse can serve as a platform for cyberbullying and harassment, which can be particularly harmful to adolescents who are still establishing their sense of self and social skills.

Disconnection from reality: Spending too much time in virtual settings can cause the lines between reality and imagination to blur, which can hurt an adolescent's sense of identity and comprehension of the world around them.

Exposure to explicit content: The metaverse can allow access to diverse content, some of which may be offensive or explicit. Teenagers exposed to this stuff may have unpleasant emotional reactions or acquire incorrect expectations of relationships and sexuality.

To promote healthy involvement with this new technology, it is critical for parents, educators, and mental health experts to be aware of these possible concerns and to supervise the usage of metaverse among adolescents. This includes raising awareness of the potential risks and benefits, providing education and tools on responsible use, and emphasizing in-person social interactions and self-care.

3.2 A Case Study with Online Social Networks During the COVID-19 Pandemic

A study conducted during the COVID-19 pandemic to investigate the impact of social media use on the quality of life of young adults in South India discovered that increased social media use was associated with decreased physical activity and negative emotions among adolescents [19]. Moreover, among young adults, it was identified that cyberbullying through social media is negatively associated with the quality of life. On the other hand, social media is an effective medium for connecting people across the globe.

Nonetheless, it is essential to note that social media can significantly benefit mental well-being, such as enhancing social relationships and information access when the world was isolated during the lockdown measures. These potential benefits may differ depending on how individuals use social media. Also, a favorable relationship between QoL (quality of life) and using social media to receive information and news was discovered. Furthermore, this study focused on a specific population and location, and further research is needed to investigate the possible consequences of social media use on quality of life in diverse people and contexts.

3.3 *Positive Impacts of the Metaverse*

Every innovation around us was developed for the betterment of society and the world; however, it should be used wisely and with proper and adequate knowledge. The metaverse has several positive effects on people's mental health. One of the possible benefits is the expansion of social interactions, as the metaverse allows individuals to communicate and interact with others in virtual environments. This is especially useful for persons who experience social anxiety or have little social support in their physical environment, and this helped individuals during the COVID-19 pandemic when the world was isolated under strict lockdown measures. The metaverse also allows for self-expression, encouraging and improving individuals' creativity, self-expression, and personal growth [20]. It can also provide access to mental health resources and support in virtual environments, benefiting those with difficulty accessing mental health services in their immediate surroundings. Moreover, the virtual settings in the metaverse can allow people to engage in stress-reduction and relaxation activities and practices.

The metaverse has the potential to improve mental health in various ways. It can generate a therapeutic setting for those suffering from mental diseases, especially those with problems accessing standard therapy. Virtual reality treatment is highly beneficial in treating cognitive conditions like anxiety disorders and posttraumatic stress disorder (PTSD) [21]. The metaverse can also serve as a valuable setting for exposure therapy, allowing individuals to expose themselves to stimuli that cause anxiety or terror gradually.

Furthermore, the metaverse can offer social support and a sense of community to people suffering from mental illnesses, particularly those who may feel isolated or ostracized in their actual world. It can give a place for people to speak with others who have had similar experiences and offer mutual support. The metaverse can also promote mental health and well-being by providing a platform for mental health education and awareness [22, 23]. It can allow mental health experts to reach a larger audience and give psychoeducation, coping skills training, and support. Ultimately, the metaverse can provide fresh and innovative ways to mental health care and support. We will discuss the advances that the metaverse can contribute to people's mental well-being in the upcoming section.

4 Metaverse for Improving Mental Well-Being

The metaverse has the potential to provide numerous benefits for the healthcare sector, especially in mental health. Several aspects of the metaverse are used for surgeries, fitness, medical education, and related virtual sessions. It can create a secure and immersive setting for mental health treatment and therapy, such as exposure therapy, cognitive behavioral therapy (CBT), and virtual reality therapy. Those with mental health disorders who feel lonely or stigmatized in their physical environment may find social support and community in the metaverse (Fig. 3).

Furthermore, the metaverse can promote mental well-being by providing possibilities for mental health education and awareness-raising among all categories of people. Even though some features of the metaverse are addictive, it can help adolescents control their usage and allow parents to keep track of their wards. It helps mental health experts by providing a platform to reach a larger audience and provide psychoeducation, coping skills training, and support [24]. Moreover,

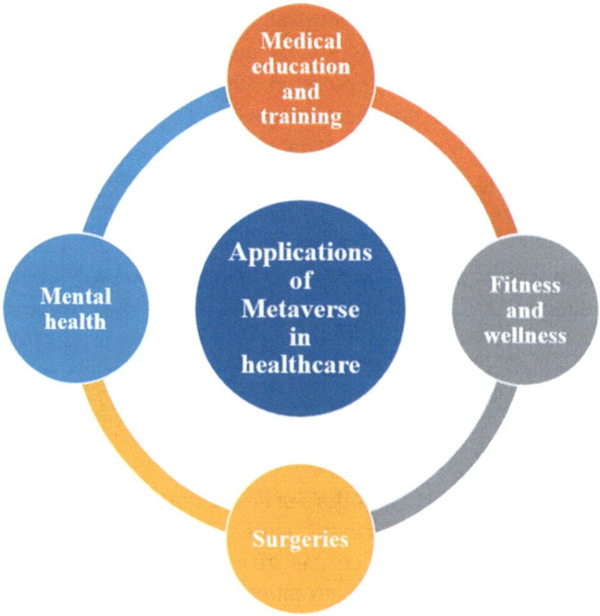

Fig. 3 Key applications of the metaverse in the healthcare sector

the metaverse technology can provide a variety of novel and effective kinds of mental therapy. One example is exposure treatment, a cognitive behavioral therapy in which individuals are gradually exposed to the source of their fear or anxiety in a safe and controlled environment [25]. The metaverse technology can provide a secure and controlled virtual environment in which people can be exposed to various stimuli that cause anxiety or fear, such as public speaking, heights, or spiders. The metaverse is an effective medium for treating irrational mental phobias like arachnophobia, katsaridaphobia, ophidiophobia, etc.

Virtual reality therapy is another potential application of the metaverse technology for mental therapy. This therapy simulates real-life situations that cause anxiety or terror using virtual environments. Virtual reality therapy has been used to treat various mental health conditions, including anxiety disorders, phobias, and posttraumatic stress disorder (PTSD). The metaverse technology can help and educate individuals about mental health concerns. It can provide virtual support groups and therapy sessions for persons suffering from mental diseases, particularly those who cannot attend in-person counseling [26]. People may also gain access to psychoeducation, coping skill training, and mental health resources via the metaverse, which also acts as a platform for mental health practitioners to interact with and assist their clients.

4.1 Treatment for Depression

The metaverse technology has the potential to be used to cure depression. Several researchers have advocated using immersive virtual environments to deliver cognitive behavioral therapy to people suffering from depression. As part of a CBT intervention, a virtual reality setting might imitate a user's bedroom and then gradually incorporate positive adjustments, such as adding more light or colorful decor [27].

Another way the metaverse technology could be used to alleviate depression is through social contact. Many people who suffer from depression experience social isolation and detachment from others, yet virtual worlds can offer chances for social interaction and assistance. Within the metaverse, virtual support groups and therapy sessions can be formed, and users can connect with avatars representing mental health experts or peers who share similar experiences [28]. According to research, engaging in virtual experiences that create a sense of presence, agency, and social connection can boost mood and minimize depression symptoms. One study, for example, discovered that partaking in a virtual reality activity that replicated strolling in nature reduced self-reported symptoms of despair and anxiety [29].

While more research is needed to thoroughly examine the metaverse technology's potential for treating depression, its capacity to create immersive and interactive experiences that promote positive cognitive and emotional states makes it an attractive subject for future investigation.

4.2 Treatment for PTSD and Other Disorders

PTSD (posttraumatic stress disorder) is a mental health condition that can develop in those who have witnessed or experienced a terrible event, such as military combat, sexual assault, natural disaster, or accident [30]. PTSD can cause several symptoms, such as intrusive memories or flashbacks, avoidance of stimuli, changes in mood or cognition, and heightened arousal or reactivity.

The metaverse has been used as an exposure treatment technique for PTSD (posttraumatic stress disorder). Exposure therapy aims to progressively expose the individual to the traumatic incident or condition in a safe and controlled setting to diminish fear and anxiety reactions. PTSD patients can be exposed to traumatic situations or stimuli in a controlled and safe environment, helping them to confront and overcome their phobias [31].

Virtual reality software may simulate a military scenario or natural disaster, allowing the user to experience the situation safely while guided by a qualified therapist. The therapist can help people process their emotions and create coping strategies for their PTSD symptoms. In trials, virtual reality exposure therapy is an effective treatment for PTSD, particularly in individuals who have not reacted well to traditional therapies [32]. Additionally, virtual reality exposure treatment may be beneficial for persons who cannot engage in conventional exposure therapy owing to logistical or safety concerns.

4.2.1 Treating Anxiety and Eating Disorders

With the help of the metaverse, a virtual environment that matches the feared condition or stimulus is created in virtual reality exposure treatment, allowing the individual to confront and conquer their anxieties in a controlled and safe atmosphere. The therapist can help clients navigate the virtual world and develop coping strategies to regulate their anxiety. Virtual reality exposure therapy has been shown in trials to be an effective treatment for anxiety disorders such as specific phobias, social anxiety disorder, and panic disorder. For example, research published in the *Journal of Anxiety Disorders* revealed that virtual reality exposure treatment was more successful than regular exposure therapy in reducing the fear of heights in patients with acrophobia (fear of heights) [33].

The metaverse can aid in treating eating disorders such as anorexia, bulimia, and binge eating disorder. Eating disorders are complex mental diseases that can be challenging to treat with traditional therapeutic approaches. On the other hand, the Metaverse provides a novel and effective method for treating eating disorders.

Exposure therapy is also effective for employing the metaverse to treat eating problems in this case. Exposure treatment is used to treat food-related cues that produce anxiety or discomfort. Exposure therapy entails progressively increasing the intensity of the exposure over time. In a metaverse setting, virtual food cues may be supplied to the user in a regulated and safe manner, enabling them to progressively overcome their fear and negative emotions connected with eating [34].

The metaverse can also be used to teach people coping skills and solutions for dealing with the symptoms of an eating disorder. Virtual reality, for example, can recreate real-world circumstances that trigger an individual's eating problem habits, such as grocery shopping or dining out. Individuals can practice coping strategies such as mindfulness, cognitive restructuring, and problem-solving in these settings to help them regulate their emotions and behaviors.

Moreover, the metaverse can help provide social support for people suffering from eating disorders. Social support is an essential aspect of the therapy of eating disorders, and online virtual support groups may be helpful when interacting with others experiencing similar challenges. People can join virtual support groups to gain mental support, share their experiences, and learn from others who have recovered from similar issues.

However, it must be noted that virtual reality exposure therapy should only be administered by qualified experts in this area and even in a controlled and safe environment. Virtual reality exposure therapy is not appropriate for everyone, and treatment plans should be tailored to the individual's unique needs.

4.3 Relaxation and Mindfulness Practices

Creating virtual landscapes that mimic quiet and relaxing areas such as beaches, woods, or gardens is possible. People can practice relaxation techniques such as deep breathing, meditation, and visualization while immersed in a visually and audibly immersive experience in these circumstances [35].

One method the metaverse might be utilized for relaxation and awareness is guided meditation. Guided meditation is a meditation in which a narrator takes the user through relaxation exercises and visualization strategies to help them attain a feeling of serenity and relaxation [36]. In a metaverse environment, the individual can be immersed in a pleasant and calm setting, which increases the benefits of guided meditation.

In addition to guided meditation, the metaverse may be used for mindfulness-based stress reduction (MBSR) activities [37]. The MBSR method is a systematic approach to stress, anxiety, and other emotional problems that combines mindfulness meditation, body awareness, and yoga. People can engage in MBSR activities while immersed in a visually and acoustically immersive setting that increases their attention and relaxation in a Metaverse environment. The metaverse may also be used for biofeedback training, a therapy that teaches patients how to manage biological functions such as heart rate, breathing, and muscular tension via electrical sensor feedback. People in a metaverse environment can be educated to use biofeedback techniques to manage stress and anxiety while immersed in a tranquil setting that increases their ability to focus and concentrate.

Finally, we can conclude that the metaverse offers a distinct and immersive environment where users may engage in relaxation and mindfulness activities that can assist in treating stress, anxiety, and other emotional challenges.

4.4 Challenges Faced by the Metaverse for Mental Health Treatments

The metaverse technology has the potential to open up a new path for treating mental health issues but to become effective, it must overcome several challenges. The metaverse faces significant challenges in mental healthcare treatments [37].

Standardization: The creation and implementation of the metaverse-based mental health interventions are not standardized. This makes evaluating the effectiveness of various approaches and ensuring that they satisfy established standards of care difficult.

User engagement: Some patients, mainly those uncomfortable with technology or unfamiliar with immersive digital environments, may find the metaverse-based interventions insufficiently engaging.

Concerns about ethics: The metaverse technology creates various ethical difficulties, including privacy and informed consent, that must be addressed in developing and implementing mental health interventions.

Cost: Designing and executing the metaverse-based interventions may be too expensive for many patients and healthcare professionals.

To solve these challenges, it is necessary to perform ongoing research and development of the metaverse-based mental health therapies and incorporate patients, healthcare professionals, and other stakeholders in the development process. Setting care standards and ensuring that therapies comply with recognized ethical norms will also be crucial in guaranteeing the efficacy and safety of these treatments.

5 Misinformation in the Metaverse

Fake news used to have a significant influence on the metaverse in a variety of ways [38]. It may affect the trustworthiness of information transmitted in virtual communities and organizations. Inaccurate data may quickly spread across the metaverse, confusing and distrusting users. This could harm the reputation of virtual communities and the organizations that manage them [39].

Moreover, false news can be used to influence the metaverse user behavior. False news within social networks and the metaverse can be used to influence virtual communities' attitudes and behavior. This is especially concerning regarding social and online digital media platforms, where erroneous information can spread disinformation, incite violence, or instigate conflict. Several mob killings in various parts of the world showcase the impact of fake news on the community. Continuous exposure to hateful content in the metaverse can also harm persons' mental health.

Fake news can also influence the financial models of the Metaverse firms. Several Metaverse systems rely on user-generated content and social engagement to generate revenue. If consumers begin to doubt the information provided in these communities, it can result in the decline of user engagement and, as a result, can collapse these firms.

5.1 Problems with Mental Health Induced by Constant Exposure to Fake News in the Metaverse

Frequent exposure to fake news, hate speech, conspiracy theories, and cyberbullying may harm mental health [40, 41]. Fake news may spread rapidly and reach a broader audience because of the emergence of the Metaverse platforms and the rise of citizen journalism. Fake news is usually produced to be spectacular or shocking to garner hits and views.

1. *Stress and anxiety*: Fake news reports may be created to generate an emotional response, such as fear or indignation. Constant exposure to such stories might lead to chronic anxiety and stress. False news stories may be intended to evoke an emotional response, such as fear or indignation. When people are repeatedly exposed to stories that elicit a strong emotional reaction, chronic anxiety and tension might develop. Those with anxiety or mood problems may find this extremely challenging.
2. *Confusion and mistrust*: When presented with contradicting evidence, people may struggle to decide what to accept and what not to believe. This leads to a general sense of bewilderment and mistrust, which hurts one's mental health and cognitive ability. Such incidents might even lead to widespread distrust of reputable news outlets. People may begin to question the authenticity of whatever information they hear, leading to feelings of fear and mistrust. This might affect both their personal and professional life. The implication of losing trust in reputable organizations is too high as it can adversely impact the organization and communities.
3. *Paranoia and delusions*: Some people may have paranoid or delusional thinking due to frequent exposure to false news. People continuously exposed to conspiracy theories will likely become convinced of a cover-up or conspiracy. This is especially dangerous when people begin acting on their beliefs or become increasingly alienated due to their ideals. Several groups like "flat earthers" often tend to pollute the thinking nature of ordinary individuals and young adults.

4. *Desperation and hopelessness*: False news broadcasts may be especially dangerous when they are meant to spread harmful or depressing information. Exposure to such stories regularly might leave one feeling powerless and unhappy. This is especially true for climate change, poverty, or crime topics. Several instances of panic while people had been exposed to false news are recorded in history.
5. *Isolation and withdrawal*: When people are overwhelmed or perplexed by information, they may withdraw from social activities or stop reading the news. This might result in feelings of isolation and loneliness, which harm one's mental health. People frequently exposed to misinformation fail to trust society and even organizations around them, which can gradually isolate them from the rest of the world.

Generally, it is best to assume that fake news in digital media, including the metaverse, can significantly impact mental health and that we must exercise caution while consuming information. Finding reliable sources based on facts and evidence might help mitigate some negative repercussions of false news. Pauses from the news and social media are also required to allow our brains to relax and repair. By adopting these actions, individuals may help preserve their mental health and well-being in an age of continual information overload. Interventions in a post-truth society should consider older people's changing social expectations and gaps in their digital literacy [42].

As the metaverse faces challenges related to fake news and misinformation, the use of epidemic models can be a valuable tool for understanding and managing virtual communities and analyzing the spread of misinformation within the networks, especially with the increasing importance of the metaverse in our daily lives.

6 Epidemic Models

Epidemic models, which are mathematical models designed to analyze the transmission of infectious illnesses, can help understand the spread of information and behaviors inside the metaverse, a virtual shared environment generated by virtual reality and the internet [43–45]. Here are some examples of how epidemic models might be helpful in the metaverse:

1. *Understanding misinformation spread*: Epidemic models can assist academics in understanding how disinformation and rumors spread within virtual communities in the metaverse. This can aid in developing measures to combat the spread of misleading information and promote the dissemination of genuine information.
2. *Modeling the adoption of new behaviors*: Epidemic models can mimic the adoption of novel behaviors within virtual communities, such as masking or social distance [46] . This can help researchers better understand the key people within the community and the factors that influence the adoption of certain habits and devise ways to encourage them. These models can also help the researchers to identify the influencers and their behaviors within the metaverse.

3. *Creating management strategies for virtual communities*: Epidemic models may be used to develop management strategies for the metaverse virtual communities. Models, for example, might help researchers decide how to allocate resources to minimize the spread of infectious behaviors or information.
4. *Prediction of contagious behaviors and information spread*: Epidemic models can anticipate the spread of infectious behaviors and information. This can help virtual community administrators and politicians build effective preventive techniques for disseminating contagious behaviors and information.

6.1 Traditional Epidemic Models

Epidemic models are mathematical models used to study the spread of infectious diseases or behavioral trends within a population. Virtual and social networks are ideal environments for exploring the spread of infectious diseases or behaviors because they allow us to reflect on the connections between individuals in a community [47]. Several basic epidemic models may be used to investigate the spread of infectious illnesses or behaviors inside social networks. Three of the most fundamental models are SI, SIS, and SIR.

The *SI model* is the most fundamental epidemiological model, assuming everyone within the community is susceptible (S) or infected (I). When a person becomes infected, they remain infected forever. The SI model posits that in social networks, people can get infected by interacting with other infected nodes within their network [48]. The model can be mathematically expressed as follows:

$$\frac{ds}{dt} = -\beta si \tag{1}$$

$$\frac{di}{dt} = \beta si \tag{2}$$

β is the infection rate with s and i referring to the susceptible and infected state, respectively. Figure 4 shows the compartmental representation of the SI model.

The SIR model is a more complicated epidemiological model that includes a third compartment – those who have recovered – in the SI model (R). In social networks, the SIR model predicts that those infected will ultimately recover and become immune to the infection. A person who has recovered cannot become infected again. The SIR model is commonly employed for pathogenic epidemics to study infectious

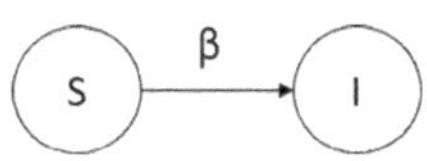

Fig. 4 The SI model

Fig. 5 The SIR model

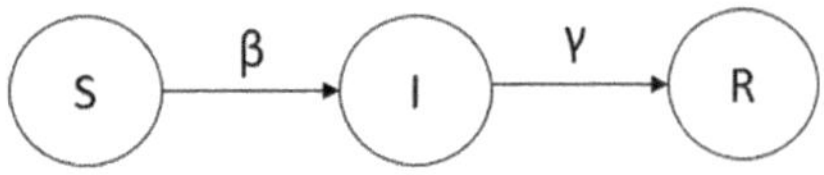

Fig. 6 The SIS model

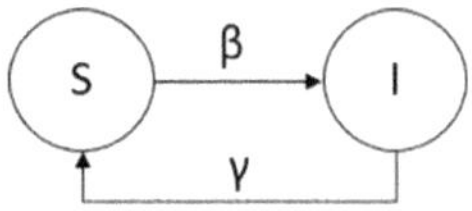

illnesses like measles and chickenpox. The compartmental representation of the SIR model is shown in Fig. 5.

In the SIS model, individuals can become infected and return to the susceptible state. This means that the individuals who recover from an infectious behavior might become vulnerable again if they come into touch with infected others in their social network. Figure 6 represents the compartmental diagram for the SIS model.

These three models are generally used to study the transmission of fake news and rumors through social networks, and the spread of misinformation can be controlled by using necessary intervention mechanisms.

6.2 Epidemic Models by Considering the Human Mental Well-Being

6.2.1 The SEDIS Model

The SEDIS model is based on the SEIR (Susceptible-Exposed-Infected-Recovered) model, but with the inclusion of a new "Doubter" state to reflect persons who have been exposed to the rumor but are not yet persuaded of its veracity [49]. The model considers both users' social contacts and their selection behavior, with different levels of susceptibility and chance of accepting or rejecting information based on their social status, trustworthiness, and content quality. The model also explains the pandemic aspect in digital networks, including the metaverse [50]. The model considers all fake news and misinformation in all digital networks as a single disease, showcasing the pandemic nature of misinformation in digital and social networks. Figure 7 depicts the SEDIS model's discrete compartmental representation.

Mathematically, the model can be defined as

$$\frac{ds}{dt} = \mu_1 e + \mu_2 d + \mu_3 i - \alpha s \tag{3}$$

$$\frac{de}{dt} = \alpha s - \beta_1 e - \beta_2 e - \mu_1 e \tag{4}$$

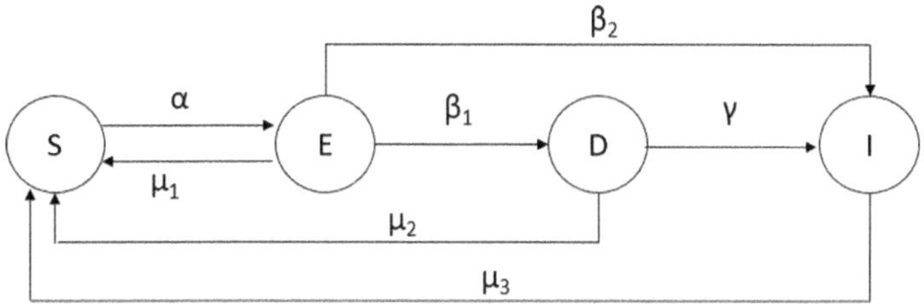

Fig. 7 The SEDIS model

$$\frac{dd}{dt} = \beta_1 e - \gamma i - \mu_2 d \tag{5}$$

$$\frac{di}{dt} = \gamma i + \beta_2 e - \mu_3 i \tag{6}$$

Here, α is the likelihood of an exposed node being exposed, β_1 and β_2 are the probabilities of an exposed node entering the Doubter and Infected states, respectively, and is the probability of a Doubter node getting infected. Similarly, μ_1 represents the likelihood of an exposed node returning to a susceptible state, μ_2 describes the probability of a Doubter node returning to the Susceptible state, and μ_3 3 represents the probability of an Infected node returning to the Susceptible state.

While the model primarily focuses on spreading rumors on social networks, it has implications for psychology and mental health. Rumors and misinformation have been found to impact people's mental health significantly, and the SEDIS model attempts to capture the psychological and behavioral factors that determine how individuals absorb and respond to information. For example, the model considers the importance of social position and trustworthiness in determining whether individuals are inclined to accept or reject the information they encounter. This is consistent with social psychological research, which has shown that people are more likely to receive information from credible and trustworthy sources.

Moreover, the SEDIS model's Doubter state acknowledges that people may be exposed to misinformation but are not immediately convinced of its reality. This is consistent with cognitive psychology, which has shown that people evaluate information based on their prior views and preconceptions and that new knowledge may take many exposures before acceptance. By better understanding the psychological components that influence how individuals perceive and respond to information, the SEDIS model can help build viable solutions for limiting rumors and disinformation that consider people's mental well-being. The model demonstrates that targeting influential users and restricting untrustworthy sources may help regulate the spread of rumors and fake news and lessen the negative impact on people's mental health.

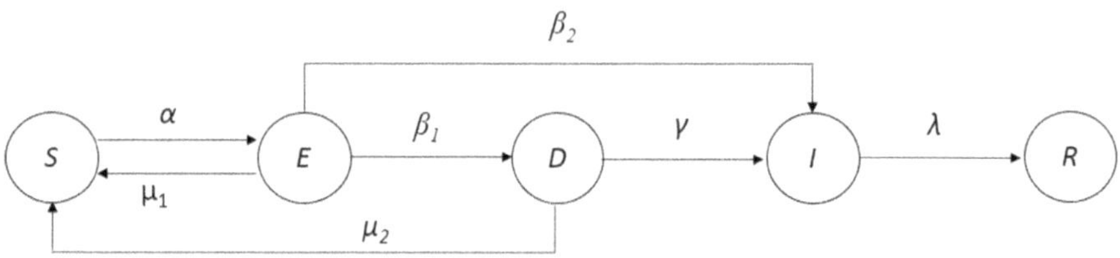

Fig. 8 The SEDIR model

6.3 The SEDIR Model

The SEDIS model has one drawback: it cannot consider a single viral misinformation being propagated through the metaverse. The SEDIR (Susceptible–Exposed–Doubter–Infected–Recovered) model, which focuses on a single viral misinformation being propagated through the metaverse, can counter this drawback [51]. The model is similar to the former SEDIS model with an addition of a restrained state node where restrained individuals refer to the ones who are no longer actively sharing the misinformation. They may still hold some residual doubts or beliefs about the misinformation, but they no longer actively promote its spread (Fig. 8).

The SEDIR model captures the harmful nature of the information system by enabling people to move from one place to another over time. For example, some people risk being exposed after hearing false information, becoming skeptical after their integrity is questioned, and avoiding biting. By developing and improving this model, we can learn essential lessons on reducing the negative impact of misinformation and creating a more informed learning and consumption environment.

6.4 Future of Epidemic Modeling in the Metaverse

The modeling of fake news epidemics in the metaverse is a relatively new topic of study, and its future is likely to be determined for several reasons. One cause is the advancement of technology and techniques that allow for more efficient data collecting and processing. As the metaverse technology advances, new avenues for collecting and analyzing data on the propagation of fake news in virtual environments may emerge. The metaverse and social network research might help analyze information flow, especially during a crisis or pandemic [52]. Many studies have advocated how individuals frequently respond in times of distress. Such analyses can assist governments in taking the required actions to prevent public fear and disinformation spread. Another reason is the adoption of data-sharing and collaboration standards and protocols. Researchers will need to exchange data and interact with other specialists in the area to construct effective epidemic models of false news in the metaverse. Creating standards and norms for data exchange and cooperation might aid this process. Finally, the future of epidemic modeling of fake news in the metaverse may also depend on the willingness of stakeholders to engage in this research. This could include virtual platform owners, policymakers, and members of the public. Suppose stakeholders are willing to engage with this research and use its insights to inform their decisions. In that case, there may be significant opportunities to mitigate the spread of fake news in virtual environments. Overall, the future of epidemic modeling of fake news in the metaverse will likely depend on technological advancements, collaboration and data sharing, and stakeholder engagement.

7 Conclusion

In recent years, there has been a surge of interest in the concept of the metaverse, which refers to a virtual shared space that people occupy, inhabit, and interact with others using virtual reality and other technologies. While forecasting the future of these immersive technologies with certainty is impossible, numerous potential patterns and challenges related to expanding the metaverse in our environment and society may be recognized. In the future, the metaverse may become an increasingly important part of our social and economic life. People are highly likely to lead a double life between the natural and virtual worlds by giving equal importance to both worlds. As virtual reality and other technologies advance, more individuals may spend time in virtual environments for work, recreation, or socializing. The metaverse may also open up new opportunities for innovation and business, such as developing new virtual goods or services. Nevertheless, potential issues and risks are associated with the metaverse's expansion. For example, the metaverse can exacerbate current socioeconomic imbalances if not carefully created and regulated. There may also be concerns about privacy and data security, as well as the likelihood of addiction or negative impacts on mental health. Another major worry is the effect of the metaverse on our physical reality. The growth of virtual environments, among other things, might impact energy use, resource consumption, and carbon emissions. It will be vital to ensure that the expansion of the metaverse is sustainable and does not damage our physical environment.

The metaverse may have significant implications for mental health in the future. Virtual reality treatment might treat mental diseases like anxiety disorders or PTSD by imitating real-life circumstances and experiences. Persons can communicate with others in the metaverse and obtain peer support and encouragement through online support groups and virtual communities. Moreover, the metaverse might be utilized to educate and raise awareness about mental health issues through virtual simulations, instructional games, and interactive tools. Finally, the metaverse might offer unique and personalized approaches to rehabilitation, such as virtual reality exposure therapy. Therefore, it is vital to guarantee that the development and deployment of new technologies are ethical, responsible, and aware of potential risks and benefits.

References

1. Zhang, X., Chen, Y., Hu, L., & Wang, Y. (2022). The metaverse in education: Definition, framework, features, potential applications, challenges, and future research topics. *Frontiers in Psychology, 13*, 1016300. https://doi.org/10.3389/fpsyg.2022.1016300
2. Trunfio, M., & Rossi, S. (2022). Advances in Metaverse investigation: Streams of research and future agenda. *Virtual Worlds, 1*, 103–129. https://doi.org/10.3390/virtualworlds1020007
3. Turkle, S. (2011). *Alone together: Why we expect more from technology and less from each other*. Basic Books.
4. Yawised, K., Apasrawirote, D., & Boonparn, C. (2022). From traditional business shifted towards transformation: The emerging business opportunities and challenges in 'Metaverse' era. *INCBAA, 162*, 175.
5. Griffiths, M. D., Kuss, D. J., King, D. L., & Griffiths, D. (2012). Video game addiction: Past, present and future. *Current Psychiatry Reviews, 8*(4), 308–318.
6. King, D., Delfabbro, P., & Griffiths, M. (2010). Video game structural characteristics: A new psychological taxonomy. *International Journal of Mental Health and Addiction, 8*, 90–106.
7. Liu, Y., Castronovo, F., Messner, J., & Leicht, R. (2020). Evaluating the impact of virtual reality on design review meetings. *Journal of Computing in Civil Engineering, 34*(1), 04019045.
8. Narula, H. (2022). *Virtual society: The metaverse and the new frontiers of human experience*. Random House.
9. Narin, N. G. (2021). A content analysis of the metaverse articles. *Journal of Metaverse, 1*(1), 17–24.
10. Oh, H. J., Kim, J., Chang, J. J., Park, N., & Lee, S. (2023). Social benefits of living in the metaverse: The relationships among social presence, supportive interaction, social self-efficacy, and feelings of loneliness. *Computers in Human Behavior, 139*, 107498.
11. Liang, H., Li, J., Wang, Y., Pan, J., Zhang, Y., & Dong, X. (2023). Metaverse virtual social center for the elderly communication during the social distancing. *Virtual Reality & Intelligent Hardware, 5*(1), 68–80.
12. Shi, F., Ning, H., Zhang, X., Li, R., Tian, Q., Zhang, S., et al. (2023). A new technology perspective of the metaverse: Its essence, framework and challenges. *Digital Communications and Networks*.
13. Usmani, S. S., Sharath, M., & Mehendale, M. (2022). Future of mental health in the metaverse. *General Psychiatry, 35*(4), e100825.
14. Han, D. I. D., Bergs, Y., & Moorhouse, N. (2022). Virtual reality consumer experience escapes: Preparing for the metaverse. *Virtual Reality*, 1–16.
15. Bottino, S. M. B., Bottino, C., Regina, C. G., Correia, A. V. L., & Ribeiro, W. S. (2015). Cyberbullying and adolescent mental health: Systematic review. *Cadernos De Saude Publica, 31*, 463–475.
16. Kobayashi, L. C., & Steptoe, A. (2018). Social isolation, loneliness, and health behaviors at older ages: Longitudinal cohort study. *Annals of Behavioral Medicine, 52*(7), 582–593.
17. Laranjo, L., Arguel, A., Neves, A. L., Gallagher, A. M., Kaplan, R., Mortimer, N., et al. (2015). The influence of social networking sites on health behavior change: A systematic review and meta-analysis. *Journal of the American Medical Informatics Association, 22*(1), 243–256.
18. Paquin, V., Ferrari, M., Sekhon, H., & Rej, S. (2023). Time to think "meta": A critical viewpoint on the risks and benefits of virtual worlds for mental health. *JMIR Serious Games, 11*, e43388.
19. von Lieres, J. S., & Cauvery, G. (2022, September). The impact of social media use on young adults' Quality of life during the COVID-19 pandemic in South India. In *2022 IEEE global humanitarian technology conference (GHTC)* (pp. 318–324). IEEE.
20. Gorini, A., Pallavicini, F., Algeri, D., Repetto, C., Gaggioli, A., & Riva, G. (2010). Virtual reality in the treatment of generalized anxiety disorders. *Annual Review of Cybertherapy and Telemedicine, 2010*, 39–43.

21. Kramer, T. L., Pyne, J. M., Kimbrell, T. A., Savary, P. E., Smith, J. L., & Jegley, S. M. (2010). Clinician perceptions of virtual reality to assess and treat returning veterans. *Psychiatric Services, 61*(11), 1153–1156.
22. Gaggioli, A., Pallavicini, F., Morganti, L., Serino, S., Scaratti, C., Briguglio, M., et al. (2014). Experiential virtual scenarios with real-time monitoring (interreality) for the management of psychological stress: A block randomized controlled trial. *Journal of Medical Internet Research, 16*(7), e3235.
23. Bouchard, S., Dumoulin, S., Robillard, G., Guitard, T., Klinger, E., Forget, H., et al. (2017). Virtual reality compared with in vivo exposure in the treatment of social anxiety disorder: A three-arm randomised controlled trial. *The British Journal of Psychiatry, 210*(4), 276–283.
24. Maples-Keller, J. L., Bunnell, B. E., Kim, S. J., & Rothbaum, B. O. (2017). The use of virtual reality technology in the treatment of anxiety and other psychiatric disorders. *Harvard Review of Psychiatry, 25*(3), 103.
25. Freeman, D., Haselton, P., Freeman, J., Spanlang, B., Kishore, S., Albery, E., et al. (2018). Automated psychological therapy using immersive virtual reality for treatment of fear of heights: A single-blind, parallel-group, randomised controlled trial. *The Lancet Psychiatry, 5*(8), 625–632.
26. Bohil, C. J., Alicea, B., & Biocca, F. A. (2011). Virtual reality in neuroscience research and therapy. *Nature Reviews Neuroscience, 12*(12), 752–762.
27. Grenier, S., Forget, H., Bouchard, S., Isere, S., Belleville, S., Potvin, O., et al. (2015). Using virtual reality to improve the efficacy of cognitive-behavioral therapy (CBT) in the treatment of late-life anxiety: Preliminary recommendations for future research. *International Psychogeriatrics, 27*(7), 1217–1225.
28. Quackenbush, D. M., & Krasner, A. (2012). Avatar therapy: Where technology, symbols, culture, and connection collide. *Journal of Psychiatric Practice®, 18*(6), 451–459.
29. Jimenez, M. P., DeVille, N. V., Elliott, E. G., Schiff, J. E., Wilt, G. E., Hart, J. E., & James, P. (2021). Associations between nature exposure and health: A review of the evidence. *International Journal of Environmental Research and Public Health, 18*(9), 4790.
30. Yehuda, R., Hoge, C. W., McFarlane, A. C., Vermetten, E., Lanius, R. A., Nievergelt, C. M., et al. (2015). Post-traumatic stress disorder. *Nature Reviews Disease Primers, 1*(1), 1–22.
31. Rizzo, A., Pair, J., Graap, K., Manson, B., McNerney, P. J., Wiederhold, B., et al. (2006). A virtual reality exposure therapy application for Iraq War military personnel with post-traumatic stress disorder: From training to toy to treatment. *NATO Security Through Science Series E Human and Societal Dynamics, 6*, 235.
32. Reger, G. M., Holloway, K. M., Candy, C., Rothbaum, B. O., Difede, J., Rizzo, A. A., & Gahm, G. A. (2011). Effectiveness of virtual reality exposure therapy for active duty soldiers in a military mental health clinic. *Journal of Traumatic Stress, 24*(1), 93–96.
33. McCann, R. A., Armstrong, C. M., Skopp, N. A., Edwards-Stewart, A., Smolenski, D. J., June, J. D., et al. (2014). Virtual reality exposure therapy for the treatment of anxiety disorders: An evaluation of research quality. *Journal of Anxiety Disorders, 28*(6), 625–631.
34. Riva, G., Malighetti, C., & Serino, S. (2021). Virtual reality in the treatment of eating disorders. *Clinical Psychology & Psychotherapy, 28*(3), 477–488.
35. Riches, S., Azevedo, L., Bird, L., Pisani, S., & Valmaggia, L. (2021). Virtual reality relaxation for the general population: A systematic review. *Social Psychiatry and Psychiatric Epidemiology, 56*, 1707–1727.
36. Kosunen, I., Salminen, M., Järvelä, S., Ruonala, A., Ravaja, N., & Jacucci, G. (2016, March). RelaWorld: Neuroadaptive and immersive virtual reality meditation system. In *Proceedings of the 21st international conference on intelligent user interfaces* (pp. 208–217).
37. Wang, X., Mo, X., Fan, M., Lee, L. H., Shi, B. E., & Hui, P. (2022). Reducing stress and anxiety in the metaverse: A systematic review of meditation. *Mindfulness and Virtual Reality*. arXiv preprint arXiv:2209.14645.

38. Lindner, P., Miloff, A., Hamilton, W., Reuterskiöld, L., Andersson, G., Powers, M. B., & Carlbring, P. (2017). Creating state of the art, next-generation virtual reality exposure therapies for anxiety disorders using consumer hardware platforms: Design considerations and future directions. *Cognitive Behaviour Therapy, 46*(5), 404–420.
39. Fernandez, M., & Alani, H. (2018, April). Online misinformation: Challenges and future directions. In *Companion proceedings of the the web conference 2018* (pp. 595–602).
40. Siebenhaar, K. U., Köther, A. K., & Alpers, G. W. (2020). Dealing with the COVID-19 infodemic: Distress by information, information avoidance, and compliance with preventive measures. *Frontiers in Psychology, 11*, 2981.
41. Quandt, T., Klapproth, J., & Frischlich, L. (2022). Dark social media participation and well-being. *Current Opinion in Psychology, 45*, 101284.
42. Brashier, N. M., & Schacter, D. L. (2020). Aging in an era of fake news. *Current Directions in Psychological Science, 29*(3), 316–323. https://doi.org/10.1177/0963721420915872
43. Dwivedi, Y. K., Hughes, L., Baabdullah, A. M., Ribeiro-Navarrete, S., Giannakis, M., Al-Debei, M. M., et al. (2022). Metaverse beyond the hype: Multidisciplinary perspectives on emerging challenges, opportunities, and agenda for research, practice and policy. *International Journal of Information Management, 66*, 102542.
44. Wang, J., Makowski, S., Cieślik, A., Lv, H., & Lv, Z. (2023). Fake news in virtual community, virtual society, and metaverse: A survey. *IEEE Transactions on Computational Social Systems.*
45. Kermack, W. O., & McKendrick, A. G. (1927). A contribution to the mathematical theory of epidemics. *Proceedings of the Royal Society of London Series A, Containing Papers of a Mathematical and Physical Character, 115*(772), 700–721. https://doi.org/10.1098/rspa.1927.0118
46. Schelling, T. C. (2006). *Micromotives and macrobehavior*. WW Norton & Company.
47. Törnberg, P. (2018). Echo chambers and viral misinformation: Modeling fake news as complex contagion. *PLoS One, 13*(9), e0203958.
48. Albert, R., & Barabási, A. L. (2002). Statistical mechanics of complex networks. *Reviews of Modern Physics, 74*(1), 47.
49. Govindankutty, S., & Gopalan, S. P. (2023). SEDIS – A rumor propagation model for social networks by incorporating the human nature of selection. *Systems, 11*(1), 12.
50. Govindankutty, S., & Gopalan, S. P. (2023). From fake reviews to fake news: A novel pandemic model of misinformation in digital networks. *Journal of Theoretical and Applied Electronic Commerce Research, 18*(2), 1069–1085.
51. Govindankutty, S., & Padinjappurathu Gopalan, S. (2023). Modeling rumor spread and influencer impact on social networks. *IEEE Access, 11*, 121617–121628. https://doi.org/10.1109/ACCESS.2023.3327863
52. Sreeraag, G., & Shynu, P. G. (2022, June). A comparative analysis of tweets from the south Indian states based on COVID-19 omicron wave. In *2022 international conference on computing, communication, security and intelligent systems (IC3SIS)* (pp. 1–7). IEEE.

Metaverse-Enabled Internet of Medical Things: A New Paradigm for Personalized and Precision Medicine

B. Anudeep and B. K. Tripathy

1 Introduction

Virtual reality (VR) and augmented reality (AR) glasses should be used to access the Internet of Medical Things (IoMT), which is thought to be the next-generation mobile computing platform that will be widely used in the future. A detailed discussion on applications of IoMT in the healthcare industry along with the concepts involved are presented in [1]. Recently, the concept of the metaverse has drawn a lot of interest. As the next-generation mobile computing platform that will extensively be utilized in the future, it depicts the internet that is accessible with VR and AR eyewear. Others contend that the metaverse is a ternary digital universe that combines the virtual and real worlds and that individuals enter using their digital identities. It is built on digital technology. In all fields and vocations, including the production of video games and other types of leisure and entertainment, the development of the metaverse has created infinite opportunities.

The phrase "metaverse in medicine" refers to IoMT made possible by AR and VR glasses, when personal computers were still in use. Nearby clinics and hospitals could not propose high-quality services to customers who were more than a few kilometers away. Now, however, with the help of smartphones' precise location capabilities, they are able to do just that. Based on the new platform, it creates an entirely new user experience that may also be utilized for disease prevention and control during pandemics like COVID-19. By acquiring VR and AR technologies, the metaverse enables face-to-face virtual interactions between users and their digital avatars. As a result of technology developments that have

B. Anudeep · B. K. Tripathy (✉)
School of Computer Science Engineering and Information Systems, Vellore Institute of Technology, Vellore, Tamil Nadu, India
e-mail: bhattaram.anudeep2021@vitstudent.ac.in; tripathybk@vit.ac.in

C. L. Chowdhary (ed.), *The Metaverse for the Healthcare Industry*,
https://doi.org/10.1007/978-3-031-60073-9_8

already revolutionized e-commerce, the applications for comprehensive healthcare and medical services may change.

1.1 The Internet of Things (IoT)

The concept of tethering real-world devices to the internet was in existence for many years. The coining of the term "Internet of Things" is frequently credited to British technology pioneer Kevin Ashton, who did it in 1999. However, prior advancements in machine-to-machine communication can be used to trace back the idea of linking common things to the internet and enabling them to gather and exchange data. The advancement of sensors, communication protocols, and cloud computing have all contributed to the considerable growth and development of IoT technology throughout the years. Healthcare is one of the many fields where it has been used. The naming services of IoT are presented in [2]. Evolution of social IoT world and its security issues are presented in [3], along with its research challenges. Applications of IoT to address the solutions for children affected by autism spectrum disorders (ASDs) are presented in [4]. Embedding IoT into artificial intelligence (AI) has created a new road to the future digital world. This has been discussed in [5]. Several concepts related to IoT, applications in various directions, challenges involved, and their possible solutions are presented in several chapters in the treatise [6].

1.2 IoT for Medicine

IoMT is the term used to describe how IoT technology has been incorporated into the healthcare industry. To track patients' health, gather information, and enhance healthcare delivery, this entails the use of linked medical devices, wearables, and sensors. Continuous Monitoring: IoMT has made it possible to track health-related data such as medication adherence, vital signs, and other parameters continuously. It may improve patient care, lessen readmissions to hospitals, and give healthcare professionals insightful data.

1.3 The Medical Metaverse

The metaverse is a shared, virtual world that is connected to other digital worlds, allowing users to interact with each other and other virtual things in real time. Despite having its origins in science fiction literature and VR, the idea really started to gain traction in the 2020s with the development of VR technologies, AR, and blockchain [7].

The concept of integrating the metaverse into medicine entails developing virtual healthcare settings where patients, physicians, and other healthcare specialists can communicate. This can help with things like VR and robotic surgery, as well as remote consultations and training for doctors.

The COVID-19 epidemic has increased the use of telemedicine and virtual health services. These advancements fit in with the broader metaverse idea as healthcare practitioners investigated how to provide care and education in virtual settings.

The IoMT and the metaverse in medicine envision a time when healthcare is not only provided in physical locations but also in virtual worlds. Through the use of cutting-edge robots and VR, surgeons might perform surgery on patients from a distance. Immersive virtual training environments could also be used in medical education. It's important to note that these ideas were still in development as of my most recent knowledge update in September 2021, and it might take some time for the healthcare sector to gain regulatory approval before the full potential of the metaverse in medicine and the widespread integration of IoMT is realized.

2 Metaverse

2.1 Basics of Metaverse in Medicine

The origins of IoT in healthcare can be traced back to the broader IoT movement, which started gaining momentum in the early 2000s. IoT is about connecting everyday objects to the internet to collect and exchange data. In the healthcare sector, IoT applications are starting to emerge as medical devices and sensors become more complex and connected. For example, wearable fitness trackers and remote monitoring devices have become popular for tracking health metrics.

The growth of telemedicine and telehealth services, especially during the COVID-19 pandemic, has highlighted the need for virtual healthcare solutions. The telemedicine platform has formed the basis for remote consultation and patient monitoring, bridging the concept of a virtual medical environment.

Advances in VR and AR technologies have played an important role in shaping the idea of a "super universe" in medicine. VR and AR deliver immersive and interactive experiences, making them ideal for creating virtual healthcare environments. Medical simulations and VR-based training have become more common, and surgeons have begun to use VR for preoperative planning and practice.

The use of blockchain technology in healthcare has begun to address issues of data security and privacy, especially when dealing with sensitive medical information. Blockchain can ensure data integrity and provide secure access control. This technology has also laid the foundation for concepts such as decentralized management of health data in virtual environments.

The term "metaverse" gained popularity in the 2020s, mainly thanks to the video game industry and the growth of virtual worlds connecting users in a shared and enduring digital space. The concept has extended beyond gaming, sparking discussions about its potential applications in various fields, including healthcare.

The COVID-19 pandemic has accelerated digital transformation across all industries, including healthcare. The need for telehealth delivery and the adoption of telemedicine have helped create richer and connected virtual health environments. The idea of the metaverse has been actively debated since 2021. It describes the internet accessible using VR and AR goggles and is seen as the next-generation mobile computing platform that will be widely used in the future. The novel *True Names* by American mathematician Professor Vernor Vinge served as the inspiration for the concept. The author of this 1981 short tale imaginatively imagined a virtual world that might be accessed and experienced through a brain–computer interface. Later, in 1992, American science-fiction author Neal Stephenson used the phrase "metaverse" in his book *Snow Crash*, in which the characters explore a parallel internet universe to the real one while interacting with it through digital avatars of themselves.

The patient community should benefit from IoMT in a positive way. The IoMT should aid in raising the standard of healthcare. AR and VR glasses should be used to access the IoMT, which is thought to be the next-generation mobile computing platform that will be extensively utilized in the future. The metaverse should provide technical assistance to maximize the value of the IoMT.

2.2 *Objectives of Metaverse in Medicine*

Security and Privacy Data security: Ensure that all IoMT-generated healthcare data are encrypted thoroughly and stored securely. It is crucial to comply with laws governing data privacy, such as General Data Protection Regulation in the European Union and Health Insurance Portability and Accountability Act in the United States. Identity verification: Put strong identity verification measures in place to stop illegal access to medical data within the metaverse. Access control: Create systems with fine-grained access restrictions that only licensed healthcare professionals can use to access and interact with patient data. Anonymizing patient data is a good way to preserve patient privacy while also enabling research and analysis.

Interoperability Standardized protocols ensure that IoMT devices and the metaverse platform employ standardized communication protocols, including HL7 FHIR, to speed up data transfer across systems. Integration with EHRs: Connect the metaverse to electronic health records (EHRs) so that medical professionals can view a patient's whole medical history. Device compatibility: Support a variety of IoMT devices and sensors so that patients can utilize their preferred monitoring equipment.

Accessibility for VR/AR To accommodate a range of user preferences, make the metaverse usable on a variety of hardware, including smartphones, PCs, AR glasses, and VR headsets. Design user-friendly, intuitive interfaces that are simple for patients and healthcare professionals to utilize when navigating the online environment for patient care, including realistic user avatars or representations in application.

Telephonic Consultations and Telemedicine High-quality audio and video: To promote efficient communication between medical professionals and patients, make sure that telemedicine consultations stream in high-quality audio and video. Medical device integration: With seamless integration of IoMT devices, allow for the real-time monitoring of vital signs during virtual consultations. Creating tools for remote diagnostics and examinations, such as the capacity to examine X-rays and conduct virtual physical examinations, is called remote diagnostics.

Simulation and Training in Medicine Immersive training environments: Develop true-to-life digital medical training environments so that students and medical professionals can practice procedures and operations. Real-time feedback: Put in place tools that allow for objective evaluation of skills while also providing real-time feedback on medical treatments. Use the metaverse for continuing medical education so that healthcare practitioners can stay informed about the latest medical advancements.

3 Architecture

Figure 1 provides the architecture of the metaverse.

The characteristics of the metaverse are expressed in Fig. 2. In Fig. 3, a typical architecture of the metaverse is characterized by its place as an intersection of the real world and the virtual world.

The metaverse has several requirements. In Fig. 4, we depict six groups of such requirements. Also, we specify their roles with respect to the metaverse.

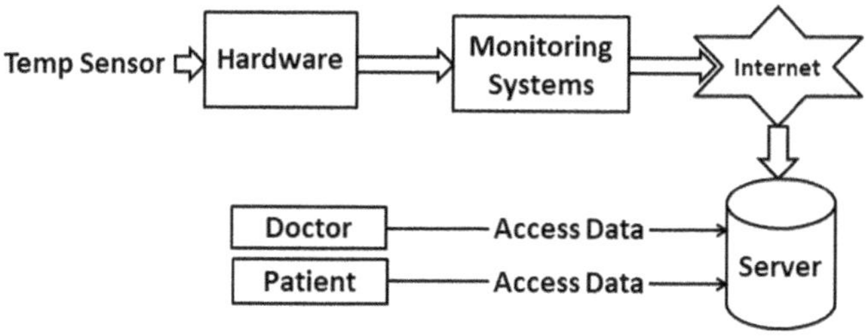

Fig. 1 Architecture of the metaverse

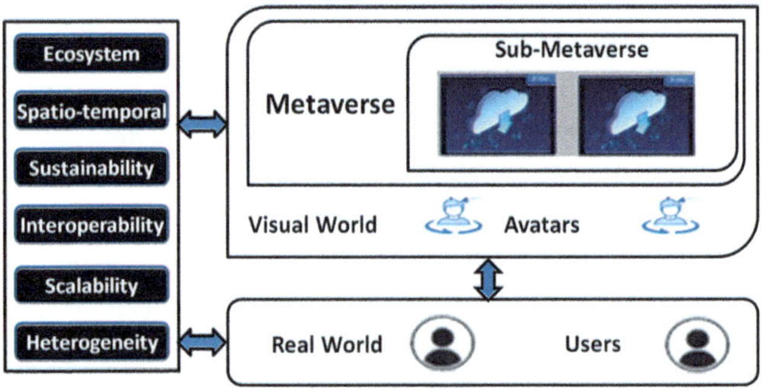

Fig. 2 Characteristics of the metaverse

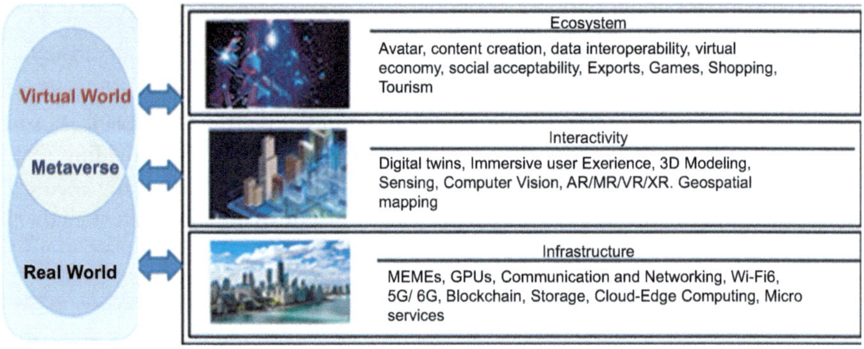

Fig. 3 Typical architecture of the metaverse

4 Metaverse in Medicine and Its Various Aspects

4.1 Metaverse in Medicine

The emergence of the IoMT has provided timely solutions to this problem as it provides effective tech support. Based on current IoMT theory, it is possible to achieve efficient and accurate tiered diagnosis and treatment through communication between physicians in large hospitals ("cloud specialists") and doctors in small hospitals ("terminal physicians") and contribute to the research and development of related technologies to improve diagnosis and treatment. Some of the problems are mentioned below.

- Cloud experts are unwilling to engage in mass science education or professional teaching, at all times and in all contexts.
- Cloud experts are unwilling to provide guidance to end-stage doctors who are responsible for diagnosing and treating patients at any time and in any location.

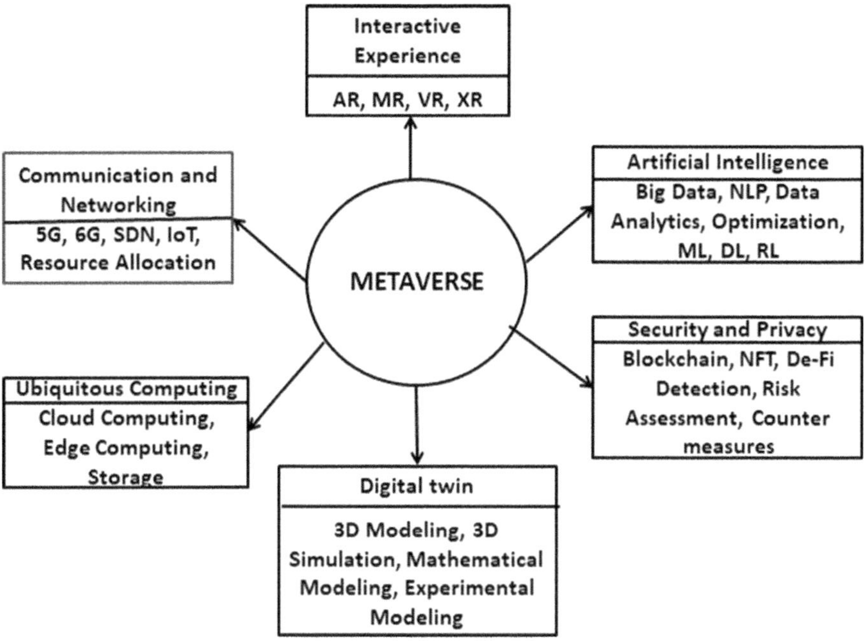

Fig. 4 Illustration of the key requirements and their role in the metaverse

- In clinical trials, researchers may not always be available to monitor research or guide groups under all circumstances.
- Because real-time quality control is not consistently available in all settings, diagnostic processes may be affected.

The craft of processing with the character of a craft workshop still exists to a large extent. The real cause lies within the limits of Internet technology itself, which cannot facilitate communication all the time and in all contexts between the cloud expert and the end practitioner regarding tiered diagnostics and analytics treatment. Therefore, IoMT-based digital platforms need to be further improved, especially in terms of human–computer communication and interaction as well as the integration and connectivity between the virtual and real worlds. It's nice that the concept of the metaverse has been established and introduced, providing possible solutions to all these problems and serving as the basis for proposed and developed the metaverse in medicine.

Prototyping, debugging, and iterating designs directly from the Unity Editor, without the bother of protracted build and deployment delays, will immediately help developers designing applications for Microsoft Hollers. Researchers have developed a program called the "human-machine MDT" that demonstrates how to systematize the virtual-real linkage-human-machine fusion problem [8].

4.2 MetaHealth – Role of the Metaverse in Changing Healthcare

We are living in a digital age, and the pandemic has accelerated innovation in healthcare, bringing new economic models and opportunities for health. Blockchain plays a crucial role in telemedicine, supply chain management, secure data sharing, and the rise of non-fungible tokens (NFTs). It allows anyone to exchange value on a decentralized network. Futurists and technologists are also exploring how the metaverse can play roles in different fields. This comment is intended to discover how the metaverse can be used in the future to change and improve healthcare. The areas where changes can occur are cooperation in work and education, clinical care, health, and finance [9].

4.3 Expert Consensus on the Metaverse in Medicine

Recently, Professor Chunxue Bai and colleagues have proposed a definition of the metaverse in medicine as the IoMT facilitated using AR and/or VR glasses.

Methods A multidisciplinary panel of doctors and IT experts from Asia, the United States, and Europe analyzed published articles regarding expert consensus on the IoMT, with reference to study results in the field of the metaverse technology.

Findings It is feasible to implement the three basic functions of the IoMT, namely, comprehensive perception, reliable transmission, and intelligent processing, by applying a metaverse platform, which is composed of AR and VR glasses and the IoMT system, and integrated with the technologies of holographic construction, holographic emulation, VR integration, and VR interconnection. In other words, through interactions between virtual and real cloud experts and terminal doctors, we will be able to carry out medical education, science popularization, consultation, graded diagnosis and treatment, clinical research, and even comprehensive healthcare in the metaverse. The interaction between virtual and real cloud experts and terminal users (including terminal doctors, patients, and even their family members) could also facilitate different medical services, such as disease prevention, healthcare, physical examination, diagnosis and treatment of diseases, rehabilitation, management of chronic diseases, in-home care, first aid, outpatient attendance, consultation, etc. Furthermore, it should be noted that security is a prerequisite for the metaverse in medicine, and a reliable security system is the basis to ensure the normal operation of that platform [10].

4.4 *Virtual Worlds and Health*

Virtual worlds offer exciting opportunities for healthcare professionals, but addressing challenges is essential for wider adoption. With decades of experience in the field of simulation, medical professionals are relatively well-versed in the virtual world. More generally, there is increasing experience and supporting evidence about the benefits of the virtual world in sharing expertise, clinical simulation, health provided, and as a research tool. The virtual world has proven the results experimentally in the form of simulation tools to advance medical knowledge and professionals, and early discoveries in healthcare delivery show promise. Key challenges for wider adoption of virtual worlds in healthcare industries include the lack of established standards for confidentiality, a disjointed approach to collaboration, and marked skepticism toward the virtual world as a platform for healthcare delivery. Recommended for formal cooperation mechanisms, agreements on standards and future research pathways are established moving forward, emphasizing the virtual world as a tool that will increasingly play a central role in professional learning and practice [11].

4.5 *The Metaverse in Cardiovascular Medicine*

The recent pandemic has caused acceleration in adoption cutting-edge technology in the healthcare industry. One of the technological advancements that flourished during this period and quickly became popular in trends is the new concept of the metaverse. The combination of VR, AR, and metaverse technology opens up exciting opportunities for creating vast online spaces where users can interact, explore, and participate in various activities. Blockchain technology further enhances security, ownership, and decentralized governance within the metaverse. Overall, the metaverse represents a transformative shift in how we engage with digital environments and each other. Various industries (from high tech and business to art and real estate) have started investing actively and exploring its potential applications. The healthcare sector will investigate this groundbreaking digital innovation, which promises to revolutionize the medical ecosystem, including cardiovascular medicine [12].

4.6 *Blockchain for Metaverse*

Since Facebook officially changed its name to Meta in October 2021, the metaverse has become the new normal. The metaverse aims to deliver immersive and personalized 3D user experience by leveraging a variety of related technologies. Despite the interest and benefits, a natural question in the metaverse is a way to secure users' digital content and data. In this regard, blockchain is a promising solution because of its distinct characteristics of decentralization, immutability, and plainness. To better understand the role of blockchain in the metaverse, we aim to provide an in-depth investigation of blockchain applications for metaverse. First, we present blockchain, metaverse preliminaries and highlight motivation behind using blockchain for metaverse. Next, we discuss in detail blockchain-based methods to the metaverse from a technical point of view, such as data collection, data storage, data sharing, data interoperability, and data security preservation. For each potential customer, we first discuss the technical aspects, diverse challenges, and then highlight how blockchain can help. In addition, we study the impact of blockchain on important metaverse technologies, including the IoT, digital twin [13], multi-sensory and immersive applications, AI, and big data. We also introduce some great features projects that demonstrate the role of blockchain in metaverse applications and services. Finally, we present some promising avenues to stimulate more innovation and research development to use blockchain in metaverse [14].

4.7 Internet of Medical Things and Big Data in Healthcare

Several technologies can reduce the overall cost of chronic disease prevention or management. These include devices that continuously monitor health indicators, devices that automatically deliver therapy, or devices that monitor real-time health data as patients self-medicate. With more and more access to high-speed Internet and smartphones, many patients have started using mobile applications (apps) to manage various health needs. These mobile devices and applications are now increasingly being used and integrated with telemedicine through the IoMT. This article reviews IoMT and big data in healthcare [15].

4.8 Security and Privacy in IoMT

IoMT, is playing an increasingly important role in improving the health, safety, and care of billions of people as it emerges. Instead of going to the hospital for help, parameters related to patient health can be monitored remotely, continuously, and in real time and then processed and transferred to a medical data center, such as cloud storage, which can greatly increase the efficiency, convenience, and cost of healthcare efficiency. The amount of data processed by IoMT devices is growing exponentially, which means more sensitive data is exposed. The security and privacy of data collected from IoMT devices, whether in transit to the cloud or when stored in the cloud, are major unresolved concerns. This document focuses on the security and privacy requirements related to data flow in IoMT. Furthermore, we thoroughly investigate existing solutions to security and privacy issues, as well as open challenges and research questions for future work [16].

4.9 Development of the Metaverse for Intelligent Healthcare

The metaverse combines the real world and the virtual world, allowing people to interact with their avatars in a setting supported by cutting-edge technologies like high-speed internet, virtual reality, augmented reality, mixed reality, extended reality, blockchain, digital twins, and AI, all of which are enhanced by practically limitless data. Recently, the metaverse has become a platform for social media and entertainment, but its expansion into the field of medicine could have a significant impact on clinical procedures and people's health. We seek special potential for metaverse techniques in the healthcare area as a team of academic, industrial, clinical, and regulatory experts. The development, prototyping, assessment, regulation, translation, and improvement of AI-based medical practice, particularly medical imaging-guided diagnosis and therapy, can be facilitated by a metaverse of "medical technology and AI" (MeTAI). Here, we provide examples of metaverse utilization, such as incorporating raw data sharing, improved regulatory science, and metaverse medical intervention. We talk about important topics like privacy, security, and inequity that pertain to the MeTAI metaverse ecosystem. Additionally, we pinpoint concrete steps that must be taken in order to establish the MeTAI metaverse, which will enhance patient satisfaction and the quality, accessibility, and affordability of healthcare [17].

4.10 A Scoping Review of the Metaverse in Emergency Medicine

As the virtual world offers chances for extremely immersive and engaging experiences, interest in the metaverse has been developing across the globe. With the development of technologies like big data, the IoT, and 5G mobile networks, the metaverse has increasingly acquired recognition in the medical industry. Due to patients with variable degrees of clinical sickness, the demand for and development of metaverse differ in various subspecialties. As a result, we evaluate published studies and patient clinical treatment in order to investigate the use of the metaverse in acute medicine. The metaverse roadmap was developed by the Acceleration Studies Foundation to explain the four different types of the metaverse in two dimensions. In order to analyze the metaverse in the context, we preserved the classification and changed the axes from earlier studies of emergency medicine [18].

4.11 Exploring Research Trends of Emerging Technologies in Health Metaverse: A Bibliometric Analysis

The next-generation internet's infrastructure, the metaverse, has drawn considerable attention as a result of the growth of the digital economy. In the metaverse, medical and health informatics have a bright future. This study uses a bibliometric analysis of over 34,000 publications on the metaverse published over 22 years to present the novel idea of the Health Metaverse. To examine the study framework, difficulties, and application of the Health Metaverse, we used the approaches of Zipf's Law, Bradford's Law, and Lotka's Law, respectively. Our investigation's findings are distilled into four perspectives: knowledge, socialization, digitalization, and intelligence. The Health Metaverse framework primarily concentrates on multi-modal medical information standards, medical and social data fusion, telemedicine and online health management, and medical AI. Additionally, it provides medical education, surgery, and fosters essential innovation in the interaction between service providers and patients. However, there are difficulties with technological advancements, gamification of medical services, patient privacy protection, and preventing individuals from escaping from reality [19].

4.12 Metaverse in Healthcare Integrated with Explainable AI and Blockchain: Enabling Immersiveness, Ensuring Trust, and Providing Patient Data Security

The impact of automation and digitization on the healthcare industry has always been significant. Every cutting-edge technology is accepted by it. The rise of the metaverse, a new digital technology, has been recently observed by people all around the world. The metaverse has enormous potential to offer patients and medical professionals a wide range of health services in a seamless manner. In order to create better, faster, and more secure healthcare facilities in VR with a realistic experience, this research suggests combining blockchain with AI in the metaverse. This is a succinct summary of our suggested architecture. It is divided into three settings: the metaverse setting, the patient setting, and the doctor setting. In a metaverse setting, blockchain technology is used to facilitate doctor–patient interaction which ensures the safety, security, and privacy of data. Our suggested architecture's primary component is the metaverse setting. Avatars serve as the doctors', patients', and nurses' representations in the metaverse environment after they register on the blockchain. The data, including photographs, speech, text, videos, clinical data, etc., will be acquired, transferred, and kept on the blockchain. All consultation actions between the doctor and the patient will be recorded. Explainable artificial intelligence (XAI) models employ these data to forecast and identify illnesses. The GradCAM and LIME techniques of XAI offer logical reasoning for disease prediction and guarantee confidence, explainability, interpretability, and transparency in relation to the diagnosis and prognosis of diseases. While offering transparency, traceability, and immutability about their data, blockchain technology offers patients data security. With relation to their data, patients can feel confident thanks to these blockchain features. As a result, the architecture that is being presented guarantees openness and confidence in terms of both disease diagnosis and patient data protection. Furthermore, we looked at the foundational technologies of the metaverse. The benefits and difficulties of the metaverse in healthcare were also studied [20].

4.13 Information and Communication Technologies Combined with Mixed Reality as Supporting Tools in Medical Education

Academic institutions are now forced to investigate nontraditional teaching modalities as a result of the volatile COVID-19 pandemic, which has disrupted education. Getting around the fact that lab experiences with hands-on learning have been found to improve student comprehension and pique their interest is one of the main problems this poses. The use of conventional visualization techniques is already constrained, and concepts like 3D molecule structures are still challenging to comprehend. In this regard, developments in information and communication technologies (ICT), such as remote meetings, AR, VR, mixed reality (MR), and extended reality (XR, or the so-called metaverse), provide tremendous potential to transform the educational landscape. In particular, how MR blends actual and virtual life in a particularly promising way and presents prospects for completely new educational applications. In this work, we provide a brief overview of and a report on our preliminary experiences using MR-based instruction for medical and pharmacy students. We also look into the potential application of MR in the teaching of pharmacy. Both online courses and conventional laboratory classes use MR to simulate real-world situations. We also suggest ICT-based programs that can be successfully used in pharmacy and medical school coursework that are created to work with Microsoft HoloLens2 MR Goggles. Autodesk Maya was used to create and implement the models before exporting them to Unity. Our results show that MR-based solutions can be a great replacement for conventional classes, especially in the fields of medicine, anatomy, organic chemistry, and biochemistry (especially 3D molecular structures), both in terms of distance learning and conventional in-person instruction. MR, thus, has the potential to become a crucial component of the medical industry in both remote learning and in-person study [21].

4.14 Dynamics of Metaverse and Medicine

The idea of a metaverse is a relatively recent development in technology. These advances have won the admiration of many industries, including finance, entertainment, and communication. The list of domains that benefit from the metaverse has recently included the study of medicine in addition to these numerous aspects of medicine, such as for academic and teaching reasons, surgical simulations, conferences, and gatherings. Research is being done on awareness campaigns, research campaigns, and many more projects. Depending on the metaverse is a flexible platform that may be modified appropriately, enabling a versatile instrument for the advancement of medicine. These fields, which have a favorable impact on the output of the medical field, are covered in detail in this review article, along with the benefits and drawbacks of each. The findings from these headings, which have all undergone only a very brief amount of research and experimentation in terms of studies, are acceptable. To provide a speculative analysis, which is the main goal of the review article [22], the domain of the metaverse is ascertained and it is shown how they will serve as a crucial tool for medical operations in the future.

4.15 What the Literature on Medicine, Nursing, Public Health, Midwifery, and Dentistry Reveals: An Overview of the Rapidly Approaching Metaverse

What research is being conducted and what themes are covered in the metaverse literature in a range of health-related fields, including medicine, nursing, public health, midwifery, and dentistry? An analysis of the studies cited in all works on health that use the term "metaverse" is offered in this paper. Studies were conducted on the materials found through searches for "metaverse" made on June 5, 2022, in Web of Science and Scopus. Data were gathered from two sources: Web of Science for 240 publications and the Scopus bibliometric database for 312 pieces. Not many direct investigations on the metaverse technology have been done in the realm of health. This is due to the fact that the metaverse technology is composed of a variety of interconnected, constantly improving technologies. Avatars, social media, blockchain technology, AR and VR are a few of these technologies. The study also informs field researchers on literature changes and metaverse studies that are crucial to the health sector. The documents were based on the research areas, and only the studies in the domain of health were examined. It is intriguing to consider how the metaverse technology will alter processes in the fields of science, medicine, and healthcare. The research examines the state of the metaverse technological literature at the moment as well as the potential of the area going forward. AR supplements reality by overlaying digital content, while VR creates entirely new virtual environments. The metaverse, on the other hand, is a broader concept that encompasses both AR and VR experiences, connecting digital spaces and interactions across various platforms. So, applications in the metaverse can indeed describe themselves as either AR or VR, depending on their specific features and functionalities. In the health industry, these applications are particularly helpful in urgent situations and during challenging, trial-and-error processes. The mechanical resolution of touch in the Nobel Peace Prize in physiology and medicine received in 2021 can be seen as one of the field's crucial turning points, in addition to the enormous technological advancements (Blockchain, computer vision, haptic devices, sensors, computer networks) with which the metaverse technology is associated in recent years. Numerous real-world applications may eventually be ported over to the metaverse realm, as seen by the field's growth and prior successes. This connection will have a significant impact on a number of industries, including the healthcare industry [23].

4.16 Metaverse Applications in Smart Cities: Enabling Technologies, Opportunities, Challenges, and Future Directions

Global interest in the metaverse has increased recently. The metaverse is a network of interconnected, immersive, digital worlds where people can communicate with one another in virtual settings. The metaverse has the power to significantly revolutionize, reshape, and transform smart cities because smart cities seek to improve the experiences of their citizens by enhancing infrastructure, modernizing government services, increasing accessibility, accelerating economic growth, and promoting sustainability. In this paper, we address the use of the metaverse in smart cities as a way to promote innovations and achieve significant advancements. We talk about the fundamental technologies that make up the metaverse, as well as the top advantages of using it and the chances it offers for applications in smart cities. To demonstrate how useful the metaverse technology is across different industries, we share ongoing projects and case studies. The realization of the full potential of the metaverse is currently hampered by important research hurdles, which we also identify and debate. In order to advance the evolution of the metaverse and its integration with smart cities, we conclude by outlining potential future research topics [24].

4.17 The Promise of the Metaverse in Mental Health: The New Era of MED Verse

There has been much discussion regarding the potential of this technology since Mark Zuckerberg announced the creation of new three-dimensional virtual worlds for social interaction. The term "metaverse," which combines the words "meta" and "universe," could usher in a new age in mental health, particularly in psychological disorders, where the construction of a full-body illusion via a digital avatar could advance healthcare and individual well-being. Patients affected by body dysmorphism symptoms (i.e., eating disorders) and social deficits (i.e., autism) could greatly benefit from this kind of technology. However, it is unclear what advantages the metaverse would have. Considering the well-known and successful use of VR in the treatment of psychological illnesses therapy, numerous researches conducted over the past 20 years have shown that VR technology is useful in lowering pain, anxiety, and stress symptoms and in enhancing cognitive and social skills. We postulate that the metaverse will present more opportunities, such as a more intricate virtual world where sensory inputs and recurring feedback can be reinterpreted for enabling a new kind of IoT and blockchain-mediated "federation" of various technologies. Today, though, a clear starting point is lacking. Due to this, it is important to establish a theoretical framework for utilizing this new type of technology in a social setting using neuroscience to provide precise answers for mental health issues in the future [25].

4.18 Metaverse: Requirements, Architecture, Standards, Status, Challenges, and Perspectives

The Internet is being replaced by a single, shared, immersive, persistent 3D virtual space called the metaverse, which is driving the next wave of innovation for new prospects. This paper outlines requirements (Fig. 4), the metaverse architecture (Fig. 1), standards, problems, and solutions. We offer the metaverse architecture and specifications, including several metaverse standards that form the foundation for the creation and application (Fig. 3). Additionally, we provide the latest state, difficulties like AI and metaverse integration, viewpoints, the security and privacy of the metaverse, and solutions (Fig. 2) [26].

4.19 The Future of Health in the Metaverse

The term "metaverse" refers to an immersive three-dimensional digital space; conceptions of its precise nature and structure have evolved over time. These changes more strongly emphasize the transition from thinking of the metaverse as a large network of an infinite number of interconnected worlds to an extended version of a single virtual world. The purpose of this essay is to discuss the potential of the metaverse in the field of healthcare. The use of VR technology to design immersive, individualized treatment environments for patients could be one potential aspect of a doctor's office in the metaverse. The doctor might also be able to employ VR equipment to show the patient different treatment options or procedures or to give them educational materials. The use of VR and other immersive technology for patient care is one of many potential uses of the metaverse in medicine. These applications include VR exposure therapy for anxiety disorders, VR–based cognitive behavioral therapy for depression, VR rehabilitation and physical therapy, VR pain management, and VR education and training. Delivering clinical treatment in the metaverse has a number of potential advantages. Particularly for patients who reside in isolated or underserved areas, the metaverse may enable more effective and accessible access to healthcare. As VR technology may be utilized to create specialized surroundings and experiences for patients, these platforms will contribute to more individualized and immersive therapeutic experiences [27].

4.20 Important Turning Points

Since 2017, related work, namely the creation of the BRM all-in-one machine, also known as the medical metaverse prototype, has been underway. The data refer to the model that comprises all of the system's data and are gathered and compiled from many sources, viewpoints, and aspects.

Various sensors such as light-sensitive elements sensor, gas-sensitive elements sensor, force-sensitive elements sensor, sound-sensitive elements sensor, radiation-sensitive elements sensor, ultrasound sensor, CT sensor, PET/CT sensor, lung function sensor, liver function sensor, kidney biochemical tests sensor, eye movement sensor, nose and airflow sensor, chest and abdominal movement sensor, blood oxygen saturation sensor, and ECG sensors are used in medical and diagnostic contexts for establishing the foundation for virtual-real connectivity. In order to provide the foundation for potential virtual-real connectivity, patients or clinicians can later have digital-twin stand-ins in the metaverse. The cloud experts are not always accessible to devote their time to teaching the general public about science or to deliver formal lectures in all circumstances. The terminal doctors cannot always and in all circumstances receive advice from the cloud experts regarding a diagnosis or course of action. In clinical trials, the lead researchers are not always present to oversee the study or direct the crew in all circumstances. Nonstandard diagnosis and treatment, with characteristics of a handicraft workshop, still persist to a significant extent since there is no real-time quality control at all times and in all locations.

The growth of the metaverse in medicine, especially during the integration of the IoMT, has seen a number of important turning points that have shaped its development. These milestones reflect progress in merging VR, IoT technology, and healthcare. Here are some important milestones:

Rise of IoT in healthcare (early 2000s): The early adoption of IoT technology in healthcare marked an important turning point. Medical devices and sensors have begun to be connected, allowing remote monitoring of patient health data. This laid the foundation for IoMT.

Popularity of mobile devices (mid-2010s): The popularity of fitness trackers and wearable smart watches has brought IoMT into the mainstream. These devices allow individuals to track their health metrics and share the data with healthcare providers.

The telemedicine boom (the 2020s): The COVID-19 pandemic has accelerated the adoption of telemedicine and telehealth services. Healthcare providers have rapidly turned to virtual consultations and remote monitoring. This transformation marks a turning point in the acceptance of virtual healthcare delivery.

VR for medical education (2010–present): The adoption of VR for medical training and simulation continues to grow. Medical students and professionals can now practice procedures, surgery, and diagnostics in a VR environment. This marks a shift in medical training and skills development.

Blockchain for healthcare (2010s–present): The use of blockchain technology to secure health data and ensure confidentiality is an important turning point. Blockchain offers the potential to create secure and decentralized healthcare data systems in the medical super universe. The emergence of the concept of the metaverse (decades of 2020): The term "metaverse" grew in popularity, initially spurred on by the video game industry. However, discussions have begun about extending the metaverse concept to other areas, including medicine. This marks the conception of a virtual and interconnected medical space.

Specific examples (decades of 2020): Several concrete examples and pilot projects have begun to show the potential of the metaverse in medicine. These range from virtual hospitals and clinics to real medical training platforms. Investment and research (ongoing): The growing investment by technology companies, healthcare organizations, and research institutions in developing the metaverse in medicine reflects its growing importance. Research initiatives aim to fully explore its applications and possibilities.

Regulatory adjustments (in progress): Regulators are adapting to the changing landscape by developing guidelines and standards for virtual healthcare environments and IoMT. Ensuring compliance with healthcare regulations remains an important turning point in the industry.

Patient-centered virtual care (in progress): A significant shift towards patient-centered virtual care is underway. Patients are increasingly participating in their healthcare using IoMT devices to monitor their health and access virtual healthcare services within the metaverse.

These turning points collectively illustrate the evolving landscape of the medical metaverse with the integration of IoMT. As technology continues to advance and healthcare practices evolve, more important moments are likely to shape the future of virtual healthcare environments.

5 Overview

Technology Road-map of the Future Trend of Metaverse explores the convergence of AI, blockchain, IoT, and immersive technologies in the Metaverse environment, presenting new opportunities for the healthcare industry. The metaverse is defined as a collection of technologies utility and the metaverse connected to IoT, blockchain, AI, and all other industries, including the medical industry area. IoT and the metaverse are digital twins; the metaverse uses the maximum number of IoT devices in its virtual workstation. These data have a tag that uniquely identifies and is used as traceable data in the metaverse and is based on blockchain. In the metaverse, this data has become a valuable resource for AI. The metaverse uses AI and blockchain technology to create a digital virtual world where you can participate freely and safely Socio-economic activities transcend the limits of the real world, and the adoption of these latest technologies will accelerate. In this article, we describe the technologies that the metaverse uses and the potential of the metaverse in healthcare.

5.1 Metaverse in Medical Domain

The training and development of future medical professionals' skill sets and knowledge bases are significantly impacted by the use of AR in the healthcare industry. Surgical technology such as the Microsoft HoloLens counts as an assistive tool that surgeons utilize to help with and speed up surgical procedures. AR headsets are used to view crucial real-time patient information, such heart rate, body temperature, blood pressure, and respiration rate, in addition to preoperative CT imaging and RI and 3D scans. Nurses and doctors are currently using AR to enhance vein detection. For many patients, this eliminates the problem of locating a vein, even if their blood vessels are tiny or their skin is strongly pigmented. The use of visual technology like X-rays and CT scans is widespread in the sector of healthcare. Simply put, these technologies assist clinicians by enabling them to identify, classify, and treat patients by allowing for more accurate observations and personalized care. Several medical facilities began utilizing the metaverse technologies (Fig. 5) [28].

5.2 Proposed Process of Patients' General Treatment Using the Metaverse Technology

Application treatments involving no fear or danger can expedite training with the help of metaverse. A wide variety of disorders are treated with it in the medical sector. The metaverse technology of the future can play a significant role in enhancing the medical profession's performance. It is a helpful and efficient technology that enhances patient training for both trainees and instructors. With the help of this technology, a practical answer is provided. The metaverse plays a vital role in the medical industry, utilizing customized technologies in hardware development and cutting-edge software.

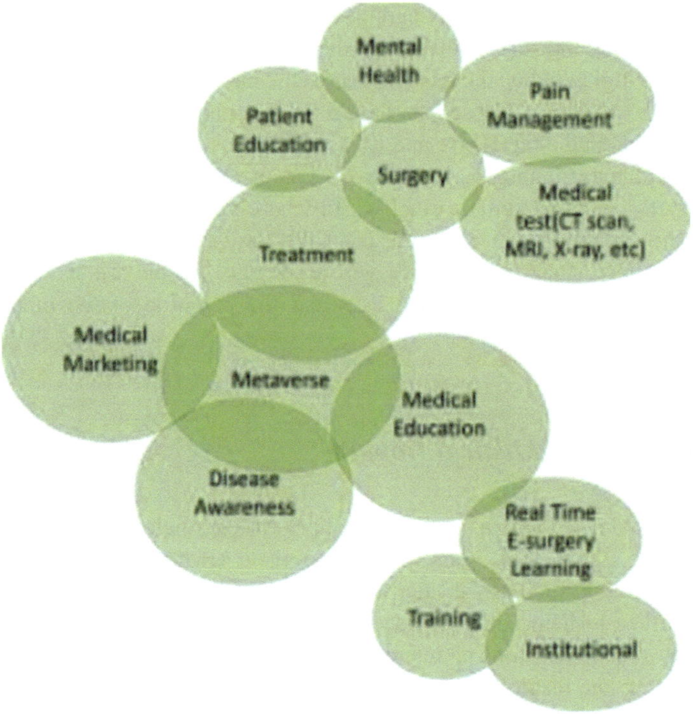

Fig. 5 The metaverse in medical domain

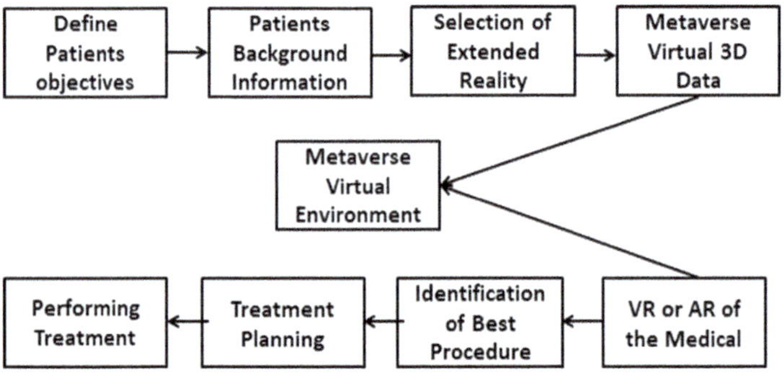

Fig. 6 The metaverse technology in the medical environment

We can gather the patient's medical history and specify the precise goal of the necessary treatment. Various hardware and software are used to create 3D virtual data that produces a 3D virtual setting. The metaverse, VR and relevant medical data are used to create AR experiences and are associated with an ideal process. This process is related to the treatment planning process and ultimately aids in carrying out the real treatment (Fig. 6) [8, 29, 30].

5.3 *Possible Further Study Related to the Metaverse in Medicine*

Future research should focus on how difficult and expensive it is to put up AR/VR systems in healthcare settings, as well as how older people tend to be less accepting of such technology. In addition to general training, quality control in accordance with regional or global standards will also be necessary in the future of metaverse in medicine.

Here are a few areas that offer opportunities for further exploration and investigation:

Usability and user experience (UX): Study UX design principles and usability for virtual healthcare environments in the metaverse. Evaluate how to optimize these interfaces for both healthcare providers and patients.

Security and privacy: Research advanced security measures, including blockchain-based solutions, to protect patient data and ensure privacy in the virtual healthcare space.

Data analytics and AI integration: Explore the application of artificial intelligence (AI) and data analysis in medical metadata. How can AI help diagnose, monitor, and predict medical conditions in a virtual environment?

Interaction standards: Seek development and implementation of standardized protocols and interoperability standards for IoMT devices and virtual healthcare platforms to improve data sharing and integration.

Analysis of patient behavior and engagement: Investigate how to improve patient engagement in virtual healthcare environments and analyze patient behavior in these environments to improve healthcare outcomes.

Telemedicine and remote monitoring: Study the scalability and effectiveness of telemedicine and telemedicine monitoring solutions in the metaverse, especially in the context of chronic disease management and postoperative care.

Medical training and simulation: Explore the evolution of the rich medical training and simulation programs in the metaverse. Assess their impact on medical education and skills acquisition.

Regulatory compliance and ethical considerations: Consider the legal challenges and ethical considerations surrounding the use of virtual healthcare environments and IoMT. How can these technologies align with healthcare regulations and ethical standards?

Global access to healthcare: Research how medical metadata can address healthcare disparities by providing access to quality health services to underserved and remote populations.

Economic and financial models: Analyze the economic viability and financial models of virtual healthcare platforms in the metaverse. Evaluate their profitability and revenue-generating potential.

6 Conclusions

In summary, through enhancing patient outcomes in diagnosis, treatment, and care, the metaverse in medicine and the IoMT have enormous potential to improve healthcare. Soft computing methods can improve the capabilities of these technologies by offering more precise, effective, and adaptable solutions. The requirement for interdisciplinary collaboration among professionals in medicine, engineering, and computer science is one of several obstacles that still has to be overcome. Others include privacy and security issues, regulatory problems, and regulatory issues.

Future research in this field may concentrate on creating new soft computing architectures and algorithms that can handle larger and more complex datasets, enhancing the precision and dependability of medical sensors and investigating the potential of cutting-edge technologies like edge computing and blockchain for secure and decentralized medical data management. Additionally, research efforts may focus on exploring the ethical and social implications of the metaverse in medicine and the IoMT, including issues related to privacy, equity, and access to healthcare. The metaverse in medicine, especially when it incorporates the IoMT, is a dynamic and rapidly evolving field with opportunities for further study and research.

References

1. Mitra, A., Roy, U., & Tripathy, B. K. (2022). IoMT in healthcare industry – Concepts and applications. In B. K. Tripathy, P. Lingras, A. K. Kar, & C. L. Chowdhary (Eds.), *Next generation healthcare informatics, studies in computational intelligence* (Vol. 1039). Springer. https://doi.org/10.1007/978-981-19-2416-3_8
2. Tripathy, B. K., Sooraj, T. R., & Mohanty, R. K. (2018). Chapter 9: Naming services in Internet of Things. In B. K. Tripathy & J. Anuradha (Eds.), *Internet of Things (IoT): Technologies, applications, challenges and solutions* (1st ed., pp. 167–188). CRC Publications.
3. Tripathy, B. K., Panda, G. K., & Padhi, M. K. (2018). Chapter 5: Evolution of social IoT world: security issues and research challenges. In B. K. Tripathy & J. Anuradha (Eds.), *Internet of Things (IoT): Technologies, applications, challenges and solutions* (pp. 77–98). CRC Publications.
4. Tripathy, B. K., & Tripathy, H. K. (2018). Chapter 14: Applications of IoT to address the solutions for children affected by autism spectrum disorders (ASDs). In B. K. Tripathy & J. Anuradha (Eds.), *Internet of Things (IoT): Technologies, applications, challenges and solutions* (pp. 295–325). CRC Publications.
5. Tripathy, B. K., & Panda, M. (2018). Chapter 3: Internet of things and artificial intelligence: A new road to the future digital world. In B. K. Tripathy & J. Anuradha (Eds.), *Internet of Things (IoT): Technologies, applications, challenges and solutions* (pp. 41–58). CRC Publications.
6. Tripathy, B. K., & Anuradha, J. (Eds.). (2018). *Internet of Things (IoT): Technologies, applications, challenges and solutions*. CRC Publications.
7. Preethi, D., Khare, N., & Tripathy, B. K. (2020). Chapter 11: Security and privacy issues in blockchain technology. In R. Agrawal, J. Chatterjee, A. Kumar, & P. S. Rathore (Eds.), *Blockchain technology and the Internet of Things, challenges and applications in bitcoin and security* (pp. 1–19).

8. Yang, D., Zhou, J., Song, Y., Sun, M., & Bai, C. (2022). Metaverse in medicine. *Clinical eHealth, 5*(1), 39–43.
9. Thomason, J. (2021). Metahealth-how will the metaverse change health care? *Journal of Metaverse, 1*(1), 13–16.
10. Yang, D., Zhou, J., Chen, R., Song, Y., Song, Z., Zhang, X., & Bai, C. (2022). Expert consensus on the metaverse in medicine. *Clinical eHealth, 5*, 1–9.
11. Holloway, D. (2012). Virtual worlds and health: Healthcare delivery and simulation opportunities. In *Virtual worlds and metaverse platforms: New communication and identity paradigms* (pp. 251–270). IGI Global.
12. Skalidis, I., Muller, O., & Fournier, S. (2022). The metaverse in cardio-vascular medicines applications, challenges and the role of non-fungible tokens. *Canadian Journal of Cardiology, 38*(9), 1467–1468.
13. Okegbile, S. D., Cai, J., Yi, C., & Niyato, D. (2022). Human digital twin for personalized healthcare: Vision, architecture and future directions. *IEEE Network.*
14. Gadekallu, T. R., Huynh-The, T., Wang, W., Yenduri, G., Ranaweera, P., Pham, Q.-V., da Costa, D. B., & Liyanage, M. (2023). Blockchain for the metaverse: A review. *Future Generation Computer Systems, 143*, 401–419.
15. Dimitrov, D. V. (2016). Medical internet of things and big data in healthcare. *Healthcare Informatics Research, 22*(3), 156–163.
16. Sun, W., Cai, Z., Li, Y., Liu, F., Fang, S., & Wang, G. (2018). Security and privacy in the medical internet of things: A review. *Security and Communication Networks, 2018*, 1–9.
17. Wang, G., Badal, A., Jia, X., Maltz, J. S., Mueller, K., Myers, K. J., Niu, C., Vannier, M., Yan, P., Yu, Z., & Zeng, R. (2022). Development of metaverse for intelligent healthcare. *Nature Machine Intelligence, 4*, 922–929.
18. Wu, T.-C., & Ho, C.-T. B. (2023). A scoping review of metaverse in emergency medicine. *Australasian Emergency Care, 26*(1), 75–83.
19. Chen D., & Zhang R. (2022). *Exploring research trends of emerging technologies in health metaverse: A bibliometric analysis*. https://doi.org/10.2139/ssrn.3998068.
20. Ali, S., Abdullah, Armand, T. P. T., Athar, A., Hussain, A., Ali, M., et al. (2023). Metaverse in healthcare integrated with explainable AI and blockchain: Enabling immersiveness, ensuring trust, and providing patient data security. *Sensors, 23*(2), 565.
21. Pregowska, A., Osial, M., Dolega-Dolegowski, D., Kolecki, R., & Proniewska, K. (2022). Information and communication technologies combined with mixed reality as supporting tools in medical education. *Electronics, 11*(22), 3778. https://doi.org/10.3390/electronics11223778
22. Kawarase, M. A., & Anjankar, A. (2022). Dynamics of metaverse and medicine: A review article. *Cureus, 14*(11), e31232. https://doi.org/10.7759/cureus.31232
23. Damar, M. What the literature on medicine, nursing, public health, midwifery, and dentistry reveals: An overview of the rapidly approaching metaverse. *Journal of Metaverse, 2*(2), 62–70.
24. Yaqoob, I., Salah, K., Jayaraman, R., & Omar, M. (2023). Metaverse applications in smart cities: Enabling technologies, opportunities, challenges, and future directions. *Internet of Things, 23*, 100884.
25. Cerasa, A., Marino, A. G. F., Riva, G., & Pioggia, G. (2022). The promise of the metaverse in mental health: the new era of MEDverse. *Heliyon, 8*(11), e11762. https://doi.org/10.1016/j.heliyon.2022.e11762
26. Rawat, D. B., & El Alami, H. (2023). Metaverse: Requirements, architecture, standards, status, challenges, and perspectives. *IEEE Internet of Things Magazine, 6*(1), 14–18. https://doi.org/10.1109/IOTM.001.2200258
27. Díaz-Chieng, L. Y., Auza-Santiváñez, J. C., & Castillo, J. I. R. (2022). The future of health in the metaverse. *Metaverse Basic and Applied Research, 1*, –1. https://doi.org/10.56294/mr20221

28. Mozumder, M. A. I., Sheeraz, M. M., Athar, A., Aich, S., & Kim, H.-C. (2022). Technology roadmap of the future trend of metaverse based on IoT, blockchain, AI technique, and medical domain metaverse activity. In *Proceedings of 24th International Conference on Advanced Communications Technology (ICACT)* (pp. 256–261).
29. Chengoden, R., Victor, N., Huynh-The, T., Yenduri, G., Jhaveri, R. H., Alazab, M., et al. (2023). *Metaverse for healthcare: A survey on potential applications, challenges and future directions*. IEEE Access.
30. Sun, M., Xie, L., Liu, Y., Li, K., Jiang, B., Lu, Y., et al. (2022). The metaverse in current digital medicine. *Clinical eHealth*.

The Metaverse in Prevention and Treatment of Disease

Dhruv Sompura and B. K. Tripathy

1 Introduction

The concept of the metaverse, a vast interconnected virtual universe, has transcended the realms of science fiction and entered the forefront of technological innovation and societal discourse. It has become a focal point for technologists, futurists, and researchers worldwide, promising to reshape the way we interact with each other and with digital environments. While it has predominantly been associated with entertainment and social connectivity, the transformative potential of the metaverse extends far beyond these domains. This chapter delves into the groundbreaking applications of the metaverse in the critical realm of disease prevention and treatment, highlighting its capacity to revolutionize health-care practices and foster innovative solutions to some of the most pressing global health challenges [1].

The concept of the metaverse, a virtual universe where users can interact with each other and digital environments, has recently gained significant traction in both technological and popular culture circles. Technological advancements in augmented reality (AR), virtual reality (VR), and blockchain technology have converged to create an environment that is poised to redefine human interaction and immersion in digital spaces [2]. As we stand on the precipice of this technological revolution, it is essential to explore the potential applications that extend beyond gaming and social interactions [3]. This exploration takes us into the realm of health care, where the metaverse holds the promise of transforming how we approach disease prevention and treatment.

D. Sompura · B. K. Tripathy (✉)
School of Computer Science Engineering and Information Systems, Vellore Institute of Technology, Vellore, Tamil Nadu, India
e-mail: tripathybk@vit.ac.in

C. L. Chowdhary (ed.), *The Metaverse for the Healthcare Industry*,
https://doi.org/10.1007/978-3-031-60073-9_9

While the metaverse has captured imaginations with its potential for entertainment and social engagement, its application in health care remains largely uncharted territory. However, the capacity of the metaverse for immersive, educational experiences opens up unprecedented possibilities in the field of disease prevention and treatment [4]. Picture a scenario where individuals can step into a virtual world to learn about the importance of vaccination, witness the consequences of unhealthy lifestyle choices, or even participate in interactive simulations of disease outbreaks. These experiences, made possible by the metaverse, have the potential to revolutionize health education and promote healthier behaviors.

The metaverse offers a multifaceted approach to health care. By leveraging immersive experiences, real-time data sharing, and telemedicine capabilities, it has the potential to transform health-care practices in several key ways [5].

One of the most promising applications of the metaverse in health care lies in its ability to educate individuals about health risks, promote healthy behaviors, and enhance public health awareness [6]. Imagine a virtual world where users can explore the human body in three dimensions, witnessing the effects of smoking on lung health or the progression of a chronic disease over time. Through immersive educational experiences, users can gain a deeper understanding of the importance of preventive measures and disease management. They can engage with interactive content that not only informs but also empowers them to make healthier choices in their daily lives. This type of experiential learning has the potential to drive significant improvements in public health outcomes.

The capacity of the metaverse to facilitate real-time data sharing and analysis stands as a critical asset in the global fight against pandemics [7, 8]. Imagine a world where health-care professionals from around the globe can collaborate in a virtual environment to monitor disease trends in real time. In such a metaverse, the early detection of disease outbreaks becomes more than a possibility; it becomes a reality. Data from various sources, including wearable health devices, hospital records, and global health organizations, can be seamlessly integrated and analyzed within the metaverse. This interconnectedness enables rapid response and the implementation of preventive measures on a global scale.

Telemedicine, remote surgeries conducted through robotic avatars, and interactive therapy sessions are just a few examples of how the metaverse can revolutionize disease treatment [9]. Imagine a scenario where a patient in a remote area can access a virtual clinic staffed by health-care professionals from around the world. Through the metaverse, patients can engage in consultations, receive diagnoses, and even undergo surgeries without the need for physical presence. Robotic avatars, controlled by skilled surgeons, can perform delicate procedures with precision, regardless of geographical barriers. This not only enhances access to health-care services but also fosters a patient-centric approach to treatment.

The role of the metaverse in medical research cannot be understated [10]. Imagine researchers collaborating in virtual laboratories, conducting experiments in a digital environment that mirrors the intricacies of the physical world. This allows them to accelerate drug discovery, simulate disease progression, and conduct experiments without the limitations of physical constraints. These virtual laboratories offer a dynamic and collaborative space where experts from different fields can come together to tackle complex medical challenges. Whether it's simulating the effects of potential drugs on a virtual organ or studying the interactions of molecules at the nano scale, the metaverse offers a sandbox for innovation and discovery.

As the metaverse integrates into health care, critical ethical and privacy concerns arise [11]. Ensuring data security, patient confidentiality, and informed consent within the metaverse framework is paramount. Additionally, addressing the potential for bias and discrimination in virtual health-care settings is essential. Researchers and policymakers must work collaboratively to establish robust ethical guidelines and regulatory frameworks that protect patients' rights and ensure the responsible use of the metaverse technologies in health care.

While the potential of the metaverse in health care is promising, it is not without its challenges [12]. Integrating this technology into the health-care sector requires addressing technological, ethical, and regulatory hurdles to harness its full potential.

The metaverse thus presents a transformative opportunity to revolutionize disease prevention and treatment, offering unprecedented possibilities for education, research, and patient care [13]. However, its successful integration into health care will require careful consideration of the associated ethical and logistical complexities [14]. This chapter serves as a comprehensive exploration of the role of the metaverse in reshaping the future of health care, offering a glimpse into the exciting possibilities and challenges on the horizon. As we proceed in this chapter, we will delve deeper into each of these aspects, providing a comprehensive overview of the potential of the metaverse in disease prevention and treatment. Through a multidisciplinary exploration of technological innovations, ethical considerations, and regulatory frameworks, we aim to provide a holistic understanding of how the metaverse can serve as a powerful tool in addressing the health care challenges of our time. From the virtual classrooms of health education to the collaborative laboratories of medical research, the metaverse holds the promise of transforming health care as we know it.

2 The Metaverse

The metaverse, a term that has permeated popular culture and technological discussions, represents a convergence of digital spaces, AR, VR, and interconnected virtual environments. Its emergence has sparked intrigue and excitement among technologists, futurists, and researchers worldwide. In this comprehensive exploration, we will delve into the multifaceted uses and applications of the metaverse across various industries, with a particular focus on its transformative role in the health-care sector.

The metaverse is a digital frontier where users can traverse interconnected virtual worlds, engage in real-time interactions, and create immersive experiences. This concept, often associated with science fiction, is increasingly becoming a reality, driven by advancements in technology and a growing demand for immersive digital experiences [14].

The gaming and entertainment industry serves as the cornerstone of the evolution of the metaverse. Virtual worlds, online games, and social platforms have pioneered the concept of interconnected digital spaces. Games like Roblox, Fortnite, and Minecraft have provided users with environments for creativity, collaboration, and social interaction, laying the foundation for broader metaverse applications [15].

The metaverse redefines social interaction and networking by offering immersive and dynamic environments. Virtual gatherings, conferences, and events have gained prominence, allowing individuals to connect and collaborate irrespective of geographical barriers. Platforms like AltspaceVR and Spatial demonstrate the potential for virtual meetings and collaborative workspaces [16].

Education and training have embraced the metaverse as a powerful tool for learning and skill development. Virtual classrooms, training simulations, and immersive experiences enable students and professionals to acquire knowledge and expertise in engaging digital environments. Medical students, for instance, can practice surgical procedures in realistic virtual settings [17].

Commerce and retail are undergoing a metaverse-driven transformation. Virtual storefronts and immersive shopping experiences offer customers new ways to explore products and make purchases. Brands are exploring the metaverse strategies to engage customers and provide interactive shopping opportunities [18].

The metaverse has extended its reach into real estate and architecture. Virtual property ownership, design simulations, and walkthroughs of architectural projects are now possible. Companies like Decentraland and Somnium Space offer users the chance to buy, sell, and build on virtual land [19].

Among the diverse array of the metaverse applications, health care stands out as an industry poised for transformation. The potential of the metaverse in health care extends to multiple facets, offering innovative solutions to some of the most pressing global health challenges [13].

The metaverse redefines health education by providing immersive, interactive experiences that educate individuals about health risks, promote healthy behaviors, and enhance public health awareness. VR simulations enable users to explore the human body, witness the consequences of unhealthy habits, and participate in interactive disease prevention scenarios [20].

Real-time data sharing and analysis within the metaverse empower health-care professionals and organizations to monitor disease trends, track outbreaks, and make informed decisions. This capability proved invaluable during the COVID-19 pandemic, enabling rapid response and global collaboration [21].

Telemedicine, remote surgeries conducted through robotic avatars, and interactive therapy sessions within the metaverse improve access to health-care services and foster a patient-centric approach to treatment. Patients can receive medical consultations and care from anywhere, reducing geographical barriers [4].

Virtual laboratories and simulations in the metaverse expedite medical research, drug discovery, and disease modeling. Researchers collaborate in digital environments, accelerating experiments, and reducing time and costs associated with drug development. These virtual laboratories are critical in advancing medical science [10].

As the metaverse integrates into health care, ethical considerations and data privacy are paramount. Ensuring data security, patient confidentiality, and informed consent within the metaverse framework is essential to maintaining trust and ethical standards in health care [22]. Regulatory bodies are adapting to the emergence of the metaverse in health care. Establishing robust ethical guidelines and regulatory frameworks is crucial to ensure responsible technology use and protect patients' rights.

The role of the metaverse in health care is poised to redefine how we approach disease prevention, treatment, and medical research. Its transformative potential holds the promise of improved patient outcomes, global collaboration, and groundbreaking discoveries. As the health-care industry continues to embrace the metaverse, it is essential to navigate the ethical, privacy, and regulatory challenges responsibly. The Metaverse represents a new frontier in health care, offering unprecedented possibilities to enhance human well-being and revolutionize the delivery of health-care services worldwide.

3 Architectures of the Metaverse

Figure 1 succinctly illustrates the seven integral layers of the metaverse. At its core, the "Experience" layer promises immersive, photorealistic environments beyond real-world limitations. The "Discovery" layer aids user navigation through inbound

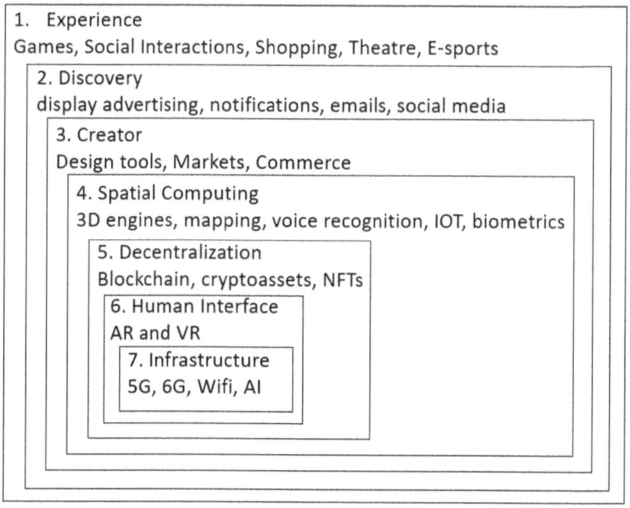

Fig. 1 Architecture layers of the metaverse

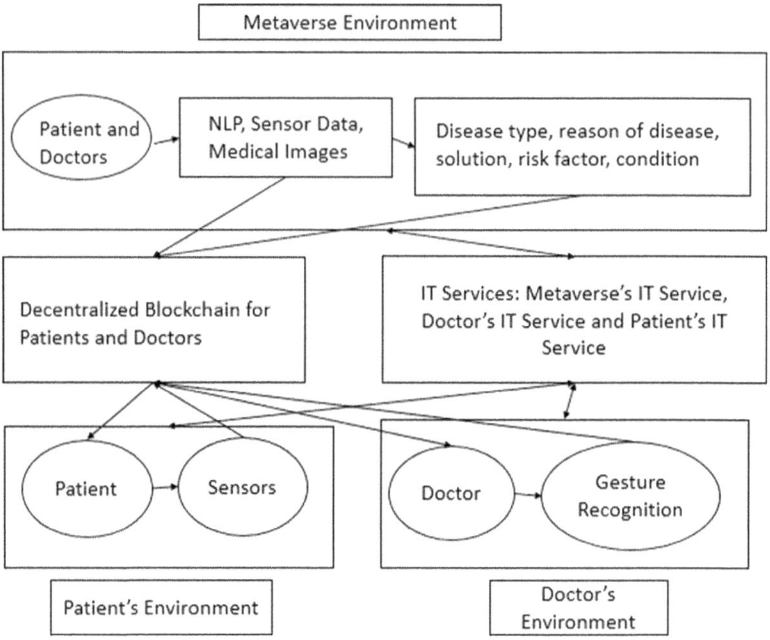

Fig. 2 Sample architecture of the metaverse being used in a health-care setup

and outbound mechanisms. The "Creator Economy" thrives as content creators monetize digital offerings, while "Spatial Computing" seamlessly merges AR, VR, and MR technologies. "Decentralization" ensures privacy via Blockchain. The "Human Interface" integrates wearables for an immersive metaverse experience. Lastly, the "Infrastructure" layer's technology clusters form the technological foundation of the metaverse. These visual helps in understanding the structure of the metaverse, emphasizing its potential to redefine human experiences.

Figure 2 shows the sample architecture of the metaverse that can be used in health-care industry. In the proposed framework, three distinct environments are integrated: the doctor's environment, the metaverse or virtual environment, and the patient's environment. This innovative system aims to deliver immersive virtual health services. Patients can receive counseling and health-care services within the metaverse. Blockchain technology is utilized to secure patient data, ensuring its integrity and transparency, while also providing unique IDs for both doctors and patients for identity tracking and medical history maintenance. The metaverse environment serves as the central hub for delivering virtual healthcare services. Consultations take place in this virtual realm, utilizing natural language processing to extract data. When necessary, additional clinical data can be provided by specialists and securely stored on the patient's Blockchain. In cases requiring surgical procedures, cobots can be employed, with doctors guiding them through real-time movements in the patient's environment, supported by video monitoring and an actual operating theater setup. This comprehensive framework represents a cutting-edge approach to health-care delivery, seamlessly merging technology and patient care.

4 The Metaverse for Disease Prevention and Treatment

The role of the metaverse in disease prevention and treatment is a rapidly evolving field with the potential to revolutionize health care. A bibliometric analysis of VR and AR highlights the promise of the metaverse in various medical domains, including diagnostic procedures, surgical interventions, and rehabilitation for conditions such as pain, stroke, anxiety, depression, fear, cancer, and neurodegenerative disorders, yielding satisfying results [23]. For instance, artificial intelligence technologies are increasingly employed in cancer care, facilitating prevention, early diagnosis, treatment, and patient rehabilitation [5, 24].

The concept of Health 4.0 represents the integration of innovative technologies into health care [25, 26]. This transformation encompasses diverse elements like the Internet of Health Things, medical cyber-physical systems, health cloud or fog, big data analytics, machine learning, blockchain, and smart algorithms [26]. VR also plays a pivotal role within Health 4.0, allowing for population monitoring and community engagement. Digital innovations present alternatives to conventional health-care delivery, including the creation of avatars to facilitate consultations and personalized care [24]. In the metaverse, health-care professionals can interact with patients in immersive 3D virtual clinics using telemedicine services and employ home-based devices like wearable sensors and smartphone applications to monitor patients' health in real time [27].

The metaverse offers a bridge between the physical and virtual worlds, enabling the monitoring of health conditions from the comfort of one's home. Various devices have emerged for this purpose, connecting individuals with their virtual health data. These devices include 12-lead electrocardiograms for heart health, blood pressure instruments to assess cardiovascular function, oxygen saturation meters for cardio-respiratory monitoring, and blood glucose calculators, particularly beneficial for individuals with diabetes [28]. Additionally, web-based tools like heart rate monitors have gained popularity for evaluating physical performance [29, 30]. Among the most prominent devices are smart watches, which integrate features like heart rate monitoring, blood oxygen measurement, pedometers, accelerometers, and GPS tracking. These devices not only monitor health status and physical performance but also aid in managing chronic diseases [30–32].

Smart watches are often connected to smartphones, which, in turn, are linked to online communities where users can share real-time health data, engage in challenges, and receive guidance from experts worldwide. The potential of smart watches in health promotion is significant, as they facilitate real-time monitoring, community participation, and expert guidance, encouraging individuals to adopt healthier lifestyles [33]. This seamless integration with virtual communities enhances the potential of the metaverse, to make individuals feel more alive within it. Moreover, continuous 24-hour health parameter monitoring allows for early prevention and intervention, even in cases like atrial fibrillation [34], contributing to the overall safety of health-care interventions. It also helps service providers increase the security of the system. Another important point to consider, in addition to monitoring, is that virtual and smart-based avatars or agents in the metadata base can provide personalized advice and motivation so that interventions can promote positive behavior change [38].

Beyond monitoring, the metaverse introduces the concept of virtual, artificial intelligence-based avatars or agents that can offer personalized feedback and motivation. These avatars interact realistically, employing natural speech, facial expressions, and body language [39]. VR extends its applications to pre-operative planning by enabling 3D analysis and collaboration among experts connected via the internet [28, 35]. Furthermore, VR can be integrated into various therapies, offering advantages in terms of customization, patient compliance, cost-effectiveness, accessibility, motivation, and convenience [25]. An example is mirror therapy, which leverages VR to create visual illusions to aid in the rehabilitation of impaired limbs, such as after a stroke [36].

One intriguing aspect is the creation of "virtual nurses" within the metaverse. These avatars can direct and monitor care, educate patients and health-care staff, and provide real-time quality and patient safety surveillance, as well as oversight of physician activities and admission and discharge processes [37]. The virtual world can serve as a time changer before the real-world experience with the doctor and accompany patients into a unique, personalized environment to enhance treatment [38]. The metaverse serves as both a transitional stage before real-world experiences, with health-care providers accompanying patients into personalized virtual environments to enhance treatment efficacy, and a platform for innovative care models, particularly for chronic diseases like hypertension, diabetes, obesity, and certain mental health conditions. These models may include psychological group support programs and remote virtual nursing care with robotic delivery units [35]. For mental health care, the metaverse offers an anonymous virtual realm where individuals can comfortably share their stories and concerns with professionals [39].

Health promotion and education in the metaverse extend beyond traditional methods. Virtual teaching rooms can simulate real-world scenarios for health-care students, facilitating experiential learning [5]. Additionally, virtual spaces can be designed for group exercise and training, encouraging physical activity and combatting sedentary behavior. A real-world example of this concept is Peloton, a virtual cycling environment that leverages VR and interactive video to enable individuals to exercise together in shared virtual spaces. Users can engage in activities such as walking, running, or pedaling on stationary bicycles, all while being monitored and guided by avatar instructors [40]. This innovative approach fosters physical activity, even within the confines of one's home or office [41]. Sensors on exercise equipment track users' training progress, and avatar instructors provide guidance to help users achieve their fitness goals [41].

The metaverse is poised to transform health care by offering innovative solutions for disease prevention, treatment, remote monitoring, and health promotion. By seamlessly blending advanced technology with health-care expertise, the metaverse has the potential to reshape the health-care landscape, making it more accessible, personalized, and engaging for individuals worldwide.

5 Scope of the Metaverse in Disease Prevention

The future scope for the metaverse in disease prevention and treatment is vast, with the potential to transform health care in numerous ways. Here are some key areas of future development and opportunities:

- Personalized Preventive Health Care: The metaverse will enable the creation of highly personalized preventive health-care experiences. AI-driven algorithms and data analytics will allow for tailored health assessments, risk predictions [30], and lifestyle recommendations, helping individuals make informed decisions to prevent diseases [42].
- Virtual Health Coaches: Virtual avatars or AI-driven virtual health coaches can guide individuals in disease prevention efforts. These virtual assistants can provide real-time feedback, motivation, and education on healthy living, helping users maintain optimal health [43].
- Disease-Specific Virtual Clinics: Disease-specific virtual clinics within the metaverse can offer specialized care and support for various medical conditions. Patients can access virtual clinics for chronic disease management, regular check-ups, and ongoing treatment plans [39].
- Remote Surgery and Procedures: Advanced telemedicine and robotic surgery technologies within the metaverse will enable surgeons to perform complex procedures remotely with precision. This can improve access to specialized care, particularly in underserved areas [43].
- Pain Management and Rehabilitation: VR-based pain management and rehabilitation programs can be tailored to individual patients. These immersive experiences can assist in pain relief, physical therapy, and post-operative recovery [44].
- Drug Development and Testing: Virtual simulations and modeling in the metaverse can accelerate drug discovery and testing. Researchers can virtually simulate the effects of new drugs on virtual patients before conducting clinical trials, potentially speeding up the development process [45].
- Global Medical Collaboration: Health-care professionals and researchers worldwide can collaborate seamlessly within the metaverse. This global collaboration can lead to more effective disease prevention strategies, treatment innovations, and shared knowledge [46].
- Health-Care Data Ownership and Security: Ensuring the security and privacy of health-care data within the metaverse will be critical. Blockchain technology

and advanced encryption methods may be integrated to protect sensitive patient information [47].

- Integration of Wearable Devices: Wearable health devices such as smart watches and fitness trackers can be seamlessly integrated into the metaverse. Real-time health data from these devices can inform preventive measures and enable early disease detection [47].
- AR Diagnostics: AR can be used for rapid and noninvasive diagnostic procedures. AR glasses or headsets can assist health-care professionals in visualizing and diagnosing medical conditions with high precision [28].
- Patient Empowerment and Engagement: The metaverse can empower patients to take an active role in their health care. Gamification, social interaction, and immersive experiences can encourage individuals to adhere to treatment plans and preventive measures [48].
- Mental Health and Wellness: Virtual mental health services will expand, providing therapy, stress management, and wellness programs. The metaverse can offer innovative solutions for addressing the growing mental health crisis [4].
- Health-Care Accessibility: The metaverse can bridge health-care accessibility gaps by providing virtual health-care services to remote and underserved populations. This can lead to more equitable health-care delivery [13].
- Health Regulation and Ethics: As the role of the metaverse in health care grows, regulations and ethical guidelines for data usage, AI, and virtual health-care practices will need to be developed and enforced [13].
- Training and Medical Education: Advanced simulations and immersive training within the metaverse can revolutionize medical education, enabling health-care professionals to practice and refine their skills in realistic virtual environments [28].
- Integration with Internet of Things (IoT): The metaverse will seamlessly integrate with IoT devices, allowing for continuous monitoring of health parameters and automated responses to health events [49].

The future of the metaverse in disease prevention and treatment holds immense potential for improving patient outcomes, increasing access to health care, and advancing medical research and innovation. However, it also presents challenges related to privacy, security, and ethical considerations that will need to be carefully addressed as this technology continues to evolve.

6 A Multifaceted Approach to Disease Treatment

The metaverse has the potential to significantly aid in disease treatment through various innovative approaches and technologies:

- Immersive Medical Environments: The metaverse enables the creation of immersive virtual medical environments, including VR and AR simulations. These environments can be used for therapy and rehabilitation, particularly in the treatment of psychological disorders such as anxiety, depression, and post-traumatic stress disorder (PTSD). Patients can engage in immersive experiences that help alleviate symptoms and improve their mental health [50].

- Behavioral Therapy and Neurodiverse Conditions: Platforms like Floreo have developed virtual worlds specifically designed for individuals with autism spectrum disorder (ASD), ADHD, anxiety, and other neurodiverse conditions. These virtual environments provide a safe space for therapy and skill development, allowing patients to learn social, behavioral, and communication skills, which can significantly enhance their quality of life [50].
- Medical Education and Training: The metaverse offers new opportunities for medical education and training. Medical professionals, including surgeons, can use AR and mixed reality technologies to visualize complex medical procedures and anatomy. This immersive training can enhance the skills of health-care practitioners and improve patient outcomes [28].
- Remote Consultations and Telemedicine: The metaverse can facilitate remote consultations between patients and health-care providers, reducing the need for in-person visits. Virtual medical consultations can be conducted in a secure and immersive virtual environment, allowing patients to receive medical advice and treatment recommendations from the comfort of their homes [43].
- Medical Simulation and Research: Medical researchers can use the metaverse to create realistic simulations of diseases and medical conditions. This can aid in drug development, treatment testing, and understanding disease mechanisms. Researchers can collaborate in virtual labs and share data and findings seamlessly across the metaverse [45].
- Brain-Computer Interfaces (BCI): The metaverse can integrate BCI technology to establish direct communication between the human brain and external devices. This has the potential to assist individuals with mobility impairments and neurological disorders, enabling them to control assistive devices and interact with the metaverse for therapeutic purposes [51].
- Advanced Medical Devices: The metaverse can incorporate advanced medical devices and technologies, such as holographic displays and organoids. These technologies can enhance the sense of immersion and provide health-care professionals with more detailed and interactive representations of patient data and medical conditions [13].
- Efficient Data Exchange: The metaverse can streamline the exchange of medical information among health-care providers, researchers, and patients. This efficient data sharing can lead to quicker diagnoses, personalized treatment plans, and better health-care outcomes [52].
- Patient Engagement and Adherence: Gamification and interactive experiences within the metaverse can encourage patient engagement and adherence to treatment plans. Virtual rewards and feedback mechanisms can motivate patients to actively participate in their health-care journey [49].
- Global Collaboration: The metaverse transcends geographical boundaries, enabling global collaboration among health-care experts and researchers. This

international collaboration can lead to breakthroughs in disease treatment, as diverse perspectives and expertise are readily accessible [53].

In summary, the metaverse offers a multifaceted approach to disease treatment, leveraging immersive experiences, advanced technologies, and global connectivity to enhance patient care, medical education, and research. It has the potential to transform the health-care landscape by making treatment more accessible, engaging, and effective across a wide range of medical conditions.

7 Exploring the Potential of the Metaverse: A Case Study

7.1 Case Study 1: A Novel Infectious Disease Outbreak

7.1.1 Background

In our hypothetical scenario, a new and highly contagious infectious disease called "Metavirus" has emerged, posing a significant global health threat. The traditional approaches to disease prevention and treatment have proven insufficient, prompting health-care authorities and technology experts to explore innovative solutions.

7.1.2 Case Study Scenario

Metaverse-Based Disease Education and Awareness

To combat the rapid spread of Metavirus, a team of health-care experts, educators, and VR developers collaborates to create an immersive metaverse experience aimed at educating the public about the virus.

- Creation of a Virtual Metavirus World: A metaverse environment is designed, representing a virtual world where users can see the virus in action, its modes of transmission, and its effects on the human body.
- Interactive Learning: Users can explore the metaverse, interact with educational content, and learn about hygiene practices, preventive measures, and vaccination importance.
- Real-Time Updates: The metaverse is updated with the latest information and statistics about the Metavirus outbreak, helping users stay informed.

Telemedicine and Virtual Clinics

Health-care institutions establish virtual clinics within the metaverse to facilitate remote diagnosis and treatment.

- Accessible Health Care: Patients experiencing Metavirus symptoms can access the metaverse from the safety of their homes and consult health-care professionals through avatars.
- Remote Monitoring: Patients' vital signs and health data are monitored in real time through wearable devices, which transmit data to the virtual clinic.
- Treatment Plans: Doctors prescribe treatment regimens, which are integrated into the metaverse platform for easy access and adherence tracking.

Collaborative Research and Development

Researchers and scientists from various fields use the metaverse to collaborate on Metavirus research.

- Virtual Research Labs: A virtual laboratory environment is created within the metaverse, allowing researchers to conduct experiments, share findings, and collaborate on vaccine and treatment development.
- Global Collaboration: Experts from around the world collaborate seamlessly in the virtual lab, accelerating research progress.
- Simulated Clinical Trials: The metaverse hosts simulated clinical trials, expediting the evaluation of potential treatments and vaccines.

Patient Support and Mental Health

Recognizing the psychological toll of the Metavirus outbreak, mental health professionals establish virtual support groups and therapy sessions.

- Virtual Therapy: Patients and individuals affected by the outbreak can attend therapy sessions and receive emotional support from mental health professionals within the metaverse.
- Support Communities: Virtual support groups allow users to connect with others facing similar challenges, fostering a sense of community and reducing feelings of isolation.

7.1.3 Conclusion

This hypothetical case study demonstrates the significant potential of the metaverse in disease prevention and treatment. Through immersive education, telemedicine, research collaboration, and mental health support, the metaverse offers innovative solutions to address complex health challenges like the Metavirus outbreak. While this scenario is fictional, it underscores the importance of exploring emerging technologies to enhance health-care delivery and mitigate the impact of infectious diseases in an increasingly interconnected world.

7.2 Case Study 2: Combating an Existing Disease

7.2.1 Background

Despite significant advancements in HIV/AIDS prevention and treatment, challenges such as stigma, access to care, and patient education persist. The metaverse offers a novel approach to addressing these issues while improving overall HIV/AIDS management.

7.2.2 Case Study Scenario

Metaverse-Based HIV/AIDS Education and Awareness

A health-care organization partners with the metaverse developers to create an immersive educational experience for HIV/AIDS prevention and awareness.

- Virtual HIV/AIDS World: A metaverse environment is designed, allowing users to explore a simulated world to understand how HIV/AIDS spreads and affects the immune system.
- Gamified Learning: Gamification elements encourage users to actively engage with the content, reinforcing key messages about safe sex, testing, and stigma reduction.
- Anonymous Information Access: Users can access information without revealing their identity, reducing the fear of discrimination.

Telemedicine and Virtual HIV Clinics

To provide accessible and stigma-free HIV care, virtual HIV clinics are established within the metaverse.

- Remote Consultations: Individuals living with HIV can consult health-care professionals through virtual avatars, ensuring privacy and reducing the need for physical clinic visits.
- Medication Adherence: Medication adherence is tracked and incentivized within the metaverse, helping patients manage their treatment regimens effectively.
- Peer Support: Virtual support groups are hosted, connecting people living with HIV for emotional support and information sharing.

Collaborative Research and Development

The metaverse facilitates global collaboration among HIV/AIDS researchers, accelerating progress toward better treatments and a potential cure.

- Virtual Research Labs: Researchers worldwide have access to a virtual research laboratory, enabling them to simulate experiments, analyze data, and collaborate on HIV/AIDS research.
- Real-Time Data Sharing: The metaverse-based research hubs allow for real-time data sharing, expediting the evaluation of experimental therapies and vaccines.
- Simulated Clinical Trials: Virtual clinical trials within the metaverse aid in testing new treatments, providing insights into their efficacy and side effects.

Patient Support and Mental Health

The metaverse provides a safe space for individuals living with HIV/AIDS to access mental health support and connect with others facing similar challenges.

- Virtual Support Groups: Support groups, led by trained mental health professionals, offer a space for users to discuss their experiences, share coping strategies, and receive emotional support.
- Stigma Reduction: Education within the metaverse promotes stigma reduction, fostering a supportive and inclusive community for those affected by HIV/AIDS.

7.2.3 Conclusion

This case study illustrates how the metaverse can revolutionize HIV/AIDS management by addressing educational, clinical, research, and mental health needs. By leveraging the immersive and accessible capabilities of the metaverse, health-care providers can enhance disease prevention, treatment, and support services, ultimately improving the quality of life for individuals living with HIV/AIDS. As technology continues to evolve, the metaverse presents an exciting frontier for innovative health-care solutions.

8 Future Scope

The future scope for the metaverse in disease prevention and treatment is vast and transformative. It promises highly personalized preventive health care, featuring AI-driven algorithms for tailored health assessments and lifestyle recommendations [49]. Virtual health coaches and specialized disease-specific virtual clinics within the metaverse will provide continuous support and care [38]. Advanced technologies will facilitate remote surgeries, pain management, and rehabilitation, while also accelerating drug development and testing through virtual simulations [40]. Global collaboration among health-care professionals and researchers will lead to more effective preventive strategies and treatment innovations [41]. Additionally, the metaverse will empower patients to engage actively in their health care, bridge accessibility gaps, and revolutionize medical education and training. However, it also presents challenges related to data security and ethical considerations, which must be addressed as this technology evolves.

Moreover, AR and wearable devices will enable noninvasive diagnostics and real-time health monitoring [47]. Mental health services and wellness programs will expand within the metaverse, addressing the growing mental health crisis [4]. As the role of the metaverse in health care grows, regulations and ethical guidelines for data usage, AI, and virtual health-care practices will need development and enforcement [13]. Ultimately, the integration of the metaverse with the Internet of Things (IoT) will allow continuous monitoring of health parameters, further enhancing disease prevention and treatment [49].

9 Conclusion

In conclusion, the emergence of the metaverse as a transformative force in disease prevention and treatment offers a tantalizing glimpse into the future of health care. The amalgamation of augmented and virtual realities promises to revolutionize medical education, making it more engaging and accessible than ever before. Furthermore, the ability of the metaverse to facilitate real-time data sharing and global collaboration is a game-changer in the context of pandemic preparedness, enabling rapid responses and information dissemination on a scale previously unimaginable.

Nonetheless, it is paramount to acknowledge the challenges that accompany this groundbreaking integration. Ethical dilemmas, privacy concerns, and the potential for bias must be addressed comprehensively. The safeguarding of patient data and the establishment of robust regulatory frameworks are essential steps in harnessing the full potential of the metaverse, without compromising individual rights and safety.

As we venture into this new frontier of health care, it is a delicate balancing act between embracing innovation and safeguarding the principles of patient care and ethical practice. With careful consideration, responsible implementation, and a commitment to transparency, the metaverse holds the promise of not only transforming the way we prevent and treat diseases but also ensuring that health care remains patient-centric, equitable, and inclusive in this digital age.

References

1. Mitra, A., Roy, U., & Tripathy, B. K. (2022). IoMT in healthcare industry – Concepts and applications. In B. K. Tripathy, P. Lingras, A. K. Kar, & C. L. Chowdhary (Eds.), *Next generation healthcare informatics, studies in computational intelligence* (Vol. 1039). Springer. https://doi.org/10.1007/978-981-19-2416-3_8
2. Tripathy, B. K., Chiranjilal, L. C., Kar, A. K., & Lingras, P. (2022). *Next generation healthcare informatics* (Springer AISC series). Springer.
3. Mystakidis, S. (2022). Metaverse. *Encyclopedia, 2*(1), 486–497.
4. Mejia, J. M. R., & Rawat, D. B. (2022, July). Recent advances in a medical domain metaverse: Status, challenges, and perspective. In *2022 thirteenth international conference on ubiquitous and future networks (ICUFN)* (pp. 357–362). IEEE.
5. Thomason, J. (2021). Metahealth-how will the metaverse change health care? *Journal of Metaverse, 1*(1), 13–16.
6. Mohanty, R. K., & Tripathy, B. K. (2022). Decision-making in healthcare Nanoinformatics. In B. K. Tripathy, P. Lingras, A. K. Kar, & C. L. Chowdhary (Eds.), *Next generation healthcare informatics, studies in computational intelligence* (Vol. 1039). Springer. https://doi.org/10.1007/978-981-19-2416-3_6
7. Jain, A., Goel, I., Maheshwari, S., & Tripathy, B. K. (2022). Contemporary technologies to combat pandemics and epidemics. In B. K. Tripathy, P. Lingras, A. K. Kar, & C. L. Chowdhary (Eds.), *Next generation healthcare informatics. Studies in computational intelligence* (Vol. 1039). Springer. https://doi.org/10.1007/978-981-19-2416-3_11
8. Tan, T. F., Li, Y., Lim, J. S., Gunasekeran, D. V., Teo, Z. L., Ng, W. Y., & Ting, D. S. (2022). Metaverse and virtual health care in ophthalmology: Opportunities and challenges. *The Asia-Pacific Journal of Ophthalmology, 11*(3), 237–246.
9. Brownstein, J. S., Freifeld, C. C., & Madoff, L. C. (2009). Digital disease detection – Harnessing the web for public health surveillance. *The New England Journal of Medicine, 360*(21), 2153.
10. Randazzo, G., Reitano, G., Carletti, F., Iafrate, M., Betto, G., Novara, G., et al. (2023). Urology: A trip into metaverse. *World Journal of Urology*, 1–11.
11. Gruson, D., Greaves, R., Dabla, P., Bernardini, S., Gouget, B., & Öz, T. K. (2023). A new door to a different world: Opportunities from the metaverse and the raise of meta-medical laboratories. *Clinical Chemistry and Laboratory Medicine (CCLM).*
12. Fernandez, C. B., & Hui, P. (2022, July). Life, the metaverse and everything: An overview of privacy, ethics, and governance in metaverse. In *2022 IEEE 42nd international conference on distributed computing systems workshops (ICDCSW)* (pp. 272–277). IEEE.
13. Kshetri, N. (2022). Policy, ethical, social, and environmental considerations of Web3 and the metaverse. *IT Professional, 24*(3), 4–8.
14. Wang, G., Badal, A., Jia, X., Maltz, J. S., Mueller, K., Myers, K. J., et al. (2022). Development of metaverse for intelligent healthcare. *Nature Machine Intelligence, 4*(11), 922–929.
15. Solaiman, B. (2023). Telehealth in the metaverse: Legal & ethical challenges for cross-border care in virtual worlds. *Journal of Law, Medicine & Ethics, 51*(2), 287–300.
16. Kerdvibulvech, C. (2022, June). Exploring the impacts of COVID-19 on digital and metaverse games. In *International conference on human-computer interaction* (pp. 561–565). Springer.
17. Jiaxin, L., & Gongjing, G. (2022, June). Socializing in the metaverse: The innovation and challenge of interpersonal communication. In *2022 8th international conference on humanities and social science research (ICHSSR 2022)* (pp. 2128–2131). Atlantis Press.
18. Contreras, G. S., González, A. H., Fernández, M. I. S., Martínez, C. B., Cepa, J., & Escobar, Z. (2022). The importance of the application of the metaverse in education. *Modern Applied Science, 16*(3), 1–34.
19. Kliestik, T., Novak, A., & Lăzăroiu, G. (2022). Live shopping in the metaverse: Visual and spatial analytics, cognitive artificial intelligence techniques and algorithms, and immersive digital simulations. *Linguistic and Philosophical Investigations, 21*, 187–202.

20. Dionisio, J. D. N., Iii, W. G. B., & Gilbert, R. (2013). 3D virtual worlds and the metaverse: Current status and future possibilities. *ACM Computing Surveys (CSUR), 45*(3), 1–38.
21. Kye, B., Han, N., Kim, E., Park, Y., & Jo, S. (2021). Educational applications of metaverse: Possibilities and limitations. *Journal of Educational Evaluation for Health Professions, 18*, 32. Balica, R. Ş., Majerová, J., & Cuţitoi, A. C. (2022). Metaverse applications, technologies, and infrastructure: Predictive algorithms, real-time customer data analytics, and virtual navigation tools. *Linguistic and Philosophical Investigations*, 21, 219–235.
22. Leenes, R. (2007). Privacy in the metaverse: Regulating a complex social construct in a virtual world. In *IFIP international Summer School on the future of identity in the information society* (pp. 95–112). Springer US.
23. Yeung, A. W. K., Tosevska, A., Klager, E., Eibensteiner, F., Laxar, D., Stoyanov, J., & Willschke, H. (2021). Virtual and augmented reality applications in medicine: Analysis of the scientific literature. *Journal of Medical Internet Research, 23*(2), e25499.
24. Zeng, Y., Zeng, L., Zhang, C., & Cheng, A. S. (2022). The metaverse in cancer care: Applications and challenges. *Asia-Pacific Journal of Oncology Nursing, 9*(12).
25. Liu, Z., Ren, L., Xiao, C., Zhang, K., & Demian, P. (2022). Virtual reality aided therapy towards health 4.0: A two-decade bibliometric analysis. *International Journal of Environmental Research and Public Health, 19*(3), 1525.
26. Al-Jaroodi, J., Mohamed, N., & Abukhousa, E. (2020). Health 4.0: On the way to realizing the healthcare of the future. *IEEE Access, 8*, 211189–211210.
27. Mesko, B. (2022). The promise of the metaverse in cardiovascular health. *European Heart Journal, 43*(28), 2647–2649. https://doi.org/10.1093/eurheartj/ehac231
28. Skalidis, I., Muller, O., & Fournier, S. (2022). CardioVerse: The cardiovascular medicine in the era of metaverse. *Trends in Cardiovascular Medicine.*
29. King, C. E., & Sarrafzadeh, M. (2018). A survey of smartwatches in remote health monitoring. *Journal of Healthcare Informatics Research, 2*, 1–24.
30. Tripathy, B. K., Parimala, B., & Thippa Reddy, G. (2021). Prediction of diseases using innovative classification and regression models. In S. S. Roy et al. (Eds.), *Data analytics in biomedical engineering and healthcare* (pp. 179–203). Academic Press. https://doi.org/10.1016/B978-0-12-819314-3.00012-4
31. Jat, A. S., & Grønli, T. M. (2022, June). Smart watch for smart health monitoring: A literature review. In *International work-conference on bioinformatics and biomedical engineering* (pp. 256–268). Springer.
32. Debon, R., Coleone, J. D., Bellei, E. A., & De Marchi, A. C. B. (2019). Mobile health applications for chronic diseases: A systematic review of features for lifestyle improvement. *Diabetes & Metabolic Syndrome: Clinical Research & Reviews, 13*(4), 2507–2512.
33. Amagai, S., Pila, S., Kaat, A. J., Nowinski, C. J., & Gershon, R. C. (2022). Challenges in participant engagement and retention using mobile health apps: Literature review. *Journal of Medical Internet Research, 24*(4), e35120.
34. Isakadze, N., & Martin, S. S. (2020). How useful is the smartwatch ECG? *Trends in Cardiovascular Medicine, 30*(7), 442–448.
35. Chapman, J. R., Wang, J. C., & Wiechert, K. (2022). Into the spine metaverse: Reflections on a future metaspine (uni-)verse. *Global Spine Journal, 12*(4), 545–547.
36. Zhang, Y., Xing, Y., Li, C., Hua, Y., Hu, J., Wang, Y., et al. (2022). Mirror therapy for unilateral neglect after stroke: A systematic review. *European Journal of Neurology, 29*(1), 358–371.
37. Schuelke, S., Aurit, S., Connot, N., & Denney, S. (2019). Virtual nursing: The new reality in quality care. *Nursing Administration Quarterly, 43*(4), 322–328.
38. Wiederhold, B. K. (2022). Metaverse games: Game changer for healthcare? *Cyberpsychology, Behavior, and Social Networking, 25*(5), 267–269.
39. Usmani, S. S., Sharath, M., & Mehendale, M. (2022). Future of mental health in the metaverse. *General Psychiatry, 35*(4).
40. Ensor, J. R., & Carraro, G. U. (1998). Peloton: A distributed simulation for the world wide web. *Simulation Series, 30*, 159–166.

41. Carraro, G. U., Cortes, M., Edmark, J. T., & Ensor, J. R. (1998, February). The peloton bicycling simulator. In *Proceedings of the third symposium on virtual reality modeling language* (pp. 63–70).
42. Petrigna, L., & Musumeci, G. (2022). The metaverse: A new challenge for the healthcare system: A scoping review. *Journal of Functional Morphology and Kinesiology, 7*(3), 63.
43. Zhang, C., Feng, S., He, R., Fang, Y., & Zhang, S. (2022). Gastroenterology in the Metaverse: The dawn of a new era? *Frontiers in Medicine, 9*, 904566.
44. Suh, I., McKinney, T., & Siu, K. C. (2023, April). Current perspective of metaverse application in medical education, research and patient care. In *Virtual worlds* (Vol. 2, No. 2, pp. 115–128). MDPI.
45. Çerçi, P., & Kendirlinan, R. (2022). Can metaverse provide any new developments in the field of allergy and immunology? *International Archives of Allergy and Immunology, 183*(10), 1060–1061.
46. Thomason, J. (2022). Metaverse, token economies, and non-communicable diseases. *Global Health Journal, 6*(3), 164–167.
47. Ali, S., Abdullah, Armand, T. P. T., Athar, A., Hussain, A., Ali, M., et al. (2023). Metaverse in healthcare integrated with explainable AI and blockchain: Enabling immersiveness, ensuring trust, and providing patient data security. *Sensors, 23*(2), 565.
48. Chengoden, R., Victor, N., Huynh-The, T., Yenduri, G., Jhaveri, R. H., Alazab, M., et al. (2023). *Metaverse for healthcare: A survey on potential applications, challenges and future directions*. IEEE Access.
49. Yang, D., Zhou, J., Song, Y., Sun, M., & Bai, C. (2022). Metaverse in medicine. *Clinical eHealth, 5*, 39–43.
50. Sun, M., Xie, L., Liu, Y., Li, K., Jiang, B., Lu, Y., et al. (2022). The metaverse in current digital medicine. *Clinical eHealth.*
51. Lee, S. H., Lee, Y. E., & Lee, S. W. (2022, February). Toward imagined speech based smart communication system: Potential applications on metaverse conditions. In *2022 10th international winter conference on brain-computer interface (BCI)* (pp. 1–4). IEEE.
52. Tang, F., Chen, X., Zhao, M., & Kato, N. (2022). The roadmap of communication and networking in 6G for the metaverse. *IEEE Wireless Communications*.
53. Okegbile, S. D., Cai, J., Yi, C., & Niyato, D. (2022). Human digital twin for personalized healthcare: Vision, architecture and future directions. *IEEE Network.*

Role of Metaverse in Pioneering Healthcare 4.0

Nagendra Singh Yadav and Vishal Goar

1 Unveiling the Metaverse: A Virtual Utopia in Healthcare

The metaverse is a collective virtual shared space created by the convergence of physical and virtual reality. It goes beyond traditional VR experiences, aiming to provide users with immersive, interactive, and persistent digital environments. In the metaverse, users can engage with one another and digital objects in real time, fostering a sense of presence and interaction that mimics the physical world. This concept has gained traction in various industries, including entertainment, education, and now healthcare [1].

The word "metaverse" was mentioned for the first time by Neal Stephenson back in 1992, and one of the science novels "Snow Crash" is about the mesmerizing and another VR (virtual reality). The metaverse is based on the internet's 3-dimensional virtual world, where the user can execute their daily actions with the help of avatars reflecting their imaginary selves in a real virtual world [2]. In other words, this very virtual world becomes their real world as another life in which the digital themselves can take part in social activities but can also have an economic life.

To understand the structure and technology transforming the metaverse, they can be segmented into four categories as mentioned below:

- *AR (Augmented Reality)*—It is a digital graphic that surrounds in real-time an existing real world. This consists of lenses, glasses, or smart devices. The idea of the metaverse is to apply further information to real-life surroundings [3]. Some of these implementations exist today as 3D aminations in medicine and Pokemon Go.
- *Lifelogging*—This is an enlargement of the internal world. Smart devices that are distinguished from augmented reality have been acquired to record day-to-day

N. S. Yadav (✉) · V. Goar
Engineering College Bikaner, Bikaner, Rajasthan, India

C. L. Chowdhary (ed.), *The Metaverse for the Healthcare Industry*,
https://doi.org/10.1007/978-3-031-60073-9_10

lives on the web. Some of these implementations can be seen on social media platforms and health monitors.

- *Mirror World*—A mirror world is an imitation of the real world. How the object appears in the real world, related information, and structure are then sent to virtual space, which enables the performance of actions using web or mobile applications. Some of these implementations can be seen in Google's popular products, i.e., Google Maps and Earth.
- *VR (Virtual Reality)*—It consists of 3D virtual reality with avatars enabled by the internet and prompt tool of communication that simulate the internal world. The personalization can be applied to the avatars, but the physical and social attributes differ from reality. The avatars can connect with other objects to complete their objectives, i.e., consultation room and virtual hospital.

The metaverse can be seen as a location in which the real world is expanded, integrated, and reproduced alongside virtual reality, and hence another world is created [4]. It is critical to understand that the metaverse will be the place to generate the digital world and where objects can spend part of their daily lives. These factors should be considered, especially after the COVID-19 pandemic, which accelerated the development of the metaverse. The pandemic restricted physical life interaction along with other daily activities, i.e., education and medical care. This integration with the metaverse is enabled by emerging technologies that allow individuals to be a part of 24 h a day, irrespective of their locations. These physical devices, i.e., smartwatches or smartphones, are allowing healthcare education along with the self-management of chronic illnesses or home care [5].

From diversified industries to tech businesses, all are investing in the metaverse. The healthcare domain has started to interact with the metaverse to unlock the potential of the virtual world to prevent and treat patients with clinical conditions through research, education, or training [6].

The healthcare sector tops the chart when it comes to identifying the sectors that can take advantage of the power of technology. The relationship between them is fairly new, but the success of these two domains is aimed toward timely diagnosis, better care, and an enhanced experience for the patients and they need to manage or maintain the data tons of it. It's not an unknown fact that the metaverse is already revamping the healthcare domain, and this happened during the era of COVID-19, when the evolution of the metaverse was accelerated by the pandemic. Later on, the metaverse became a necessity for the existence of virtual and physical worlds, all because of the social distancing norms introduced by a pandemic.

The metaverse has already made an impact on medical training in which VR (virtual reality) is adopted to train an individual in simulated surroundings to reduce the learning and development costs [7]. On top of it, health 2.0 and the metaverse will play a crucial role in preventing and treating diseases. The physicians can meet with patients in a "3D meta hospital" with the help of services offered by telemedicine, mobile phone-based applications and wearable sensors [8]. The metaverse has already started contributing toward the technologies related to surgery, where augmented reality can enable surgeons to carry out surgeries and provide hassle-free access to patient data using mappings of 3D virtual models onto the bodies of patients.

With the estimation of a larger market size, the metaverse is taking over at a phenomenal pace. The metaverse includes the convergence of three technology trends—AI (artificial intelligence), AR (augmented reality) and VR (virtual reality). When combined, they can open several new methods for delivering treatments at lower costs and improving results for patients in the healthcare.

In the metaverse, boundaries melted away and reality took on a new dimension. The metaverse wasn't just about the physical and the digital; it was a realm where both coexisted seamlessly. This innovative blend of technology and human experience held the potential to revolutionize healthcare in ways never before imagined.

2 Applications in Healthcare 4.0

The integration of the metaverse into Healthcare 4.0 introduces numerous groundbreaking applications that have the potential to enhance patient care, medical training, research, and more [9]. Telemedicine, for instance, can be elevated to new heights by enabling doctors to interact with patients in a lifelike virtual environment, overcoming geographical barriers, and fostering a more personal connection. Medical professionals could perform remote surgeries with precision by virtually manipulating medical instruments [10].

Moreover, medical training and education can be transformed through the metaverse-based simulations. Aspiring doctors could engage in realistic surgical procedures, diagnosis scenarios, and patient interactions in a safe and controlled environment [11]. This hands-on experience would not only expedite learning but also enhance practical skill development.

Collaborative research and development can also benefit from the metaverse. Experts from around the world can gather virtually to collaborate on projects, share data, and conduct experiments in simulated environments. This cross-border collaboration could accelerate medical advancements and enable faster drug discovery and treatment development.

3 Characteristics of the Metaverse

The metaverse is characterized by several fundamental features:

- *Immersive Environment*—The metaverse provides a seamless and immersive digital space where users can interact with objects and people as if they were present in the physical world.

- *Persistent World*—Unlike traditional video games or virtual experiences, the metaverse exists continuously and independently of individual users. Changes made by one user may impact the experience of others.
- *Interconnectivity*—Different virtual worlds, applications, and experiences within the metaverse are interconnected, allowing users to move between them effortlessly.
- *User-Created Content*—The metaverse empowers users to create and contribute their content, such as virtual assets, environments, and experiences.
- *Social Interaction*—Communication and social interaction are core components of the metaverse. Users can communicate with each other using voice, text, or avatars.
- *Economy and Commerce*—Within the metaverse, virtual assets can be bought, sold, and traded. A virtual economy can emerge, where users can earn and spend digital currency.

4 Channels Fueling the Use of Metaverse in Healthcare

4.1 Telemedicine

The use of telemedicine has gained a lot of grips during the COVID-19 pandemic as it can deliver healthcare services remotely to patients. The metaverse will act as a supplement for telemedicine, where a patient can visit a virtual office to meet their physician in a 3D clinic, irrespective of each other's location.

This is estimated to enhance the user's experience using teleconsultation services remarkably. The use of virtual reality in the metaverse for healthcare services can unlock the next level of experience by enabling the sense of being present at a place unlike the other environments, i.e., social media or website. This will not limit the patients to being treated by only specific specialists at their physical locations. This is more significant in places where poor supply exists for medical personnel, and for patients who are based in remote areas, those patients would have to go long miles to visit or consult with the doctors.

The metaverse can be highly impactful in therapy. The patients can walk through the scenarios that cause them anxiety to them in a protected environment where each aspect of the interaction is closely observed and controlled [12]. For example. Gamechange, which is a virtual reality system created by Dr. Daniel Freeman and his team at the University of Oxford, utilizes the use of a virtual reality-enabled system to heal psychosis using DTx (digital therapeutics), which is a medical technology [13].

At the heart of the metaverse's influence on healthcare lies its transformative impact on patient care. Telemedicine transcended its traditional confines, evolving into a rich, immersive experience. Doctors and patients, no longer separated by geographical distances, interacted in lifelike virtual environments. The metaverse enabled physicians to conduct thorough examinations, diagnose ailments, and even perform surgeries remotely. This not only expedited healthcare delivery but also fostered a more personal doctor-patient connection, which was often lost in conventional telemedicine [14].

4.2 *Blockchain*

Blockchain is a very crucial part of the metaverse, considering the healthcare domain, as it can enable the decentralized communities to be managed with the help of smart contracts, and the ownership of the environment is digitally managed along with digital items. The secured management of precious health data is the best use case in the healthcare domain.

As of today, the way data is transferred among many companies is not efficient and transparent to the owners of actual data, as health records are managed on a centralized system, which is likely vulnerable to being stolen and sold on the dark web. It's a very time-consuming and frustrating process, even for those who have valid access to it, such as professionals treating patients (Fig. 1).

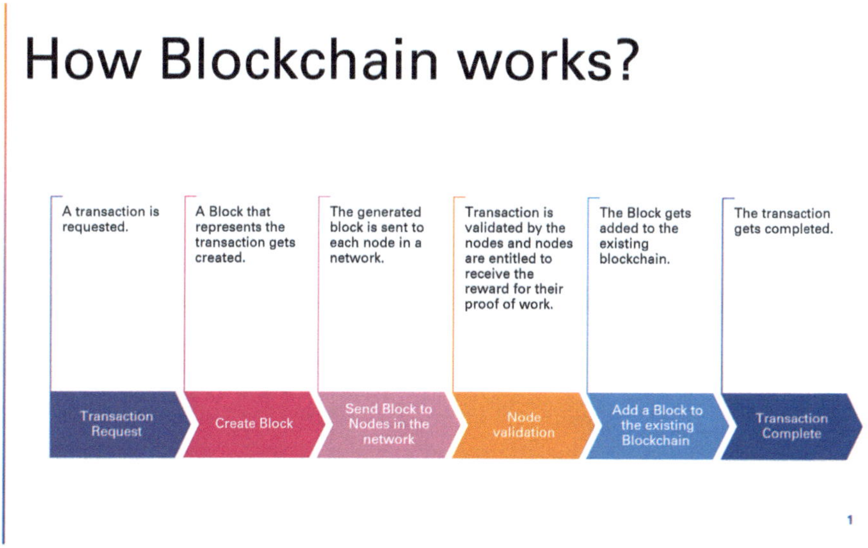

Fig. 1 How blockchain works?

4.3 Digital Twins

The digital twins refer to a virtual model or simulation of objects and procedures that are generated with the help of real-life data to understand their real-life counterparts. The digital twin of the patient can be the patient itself.

Digital twins can be considered healthcare services online with expertise in occupational health that are used as "test subjects/dummies" for an individual to predict the results. Starting from when the person will recover from surgery or how he will react to the medications. This will progress as our capacity to map and understand individual genomes increases.

Consider a virtual method to reflect each known medication for the individual's disease that can be tested. This will enable better treatment for individuals and determine which one works for them. This can observe the virtual entity, notify the doctors if the medical state ends up developing a side effect, and take preventive action. Several large MedTech organizations, i.e., Siemens Healthineers and GE Healthcare, are currently working on digital twins. These organizations will need crucial assets, i.e., large amounts of patient data, to achieve their goals (Fig. 2).

4.4 Education in a Virtual Operating Theater: Training Enhanced

Medical education faced a paradigm shift in the metaverse. Aspiring doctors found themselves in virtual operating theaters, dissecting digital cadavers, and performing simulated surgeries. These interactive experiences honed skills and

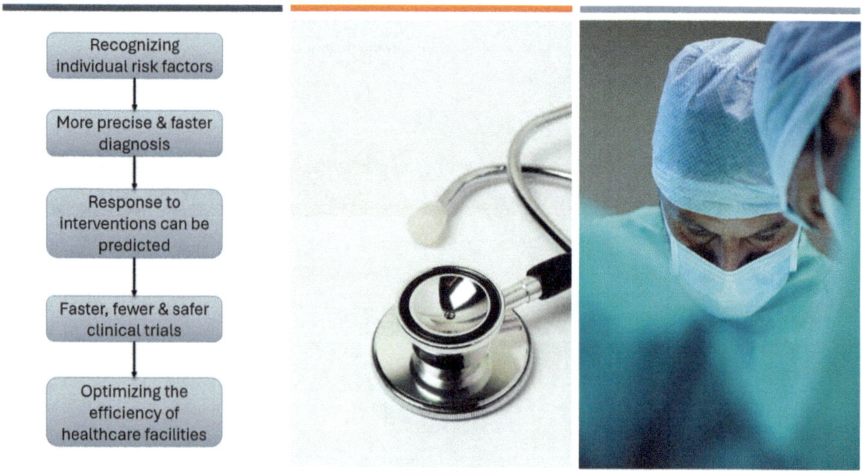

Fig. 2 Applications of digital twins in healthcare

boosted confidence, preparing future physicians for real-world challenges. Anatomy lessons transcended the pages of textbooks, and medical students could explore the human body from the inside out. Diagnosis scenarios turned into immersive puzzles, where the right solution was a matter of life and death. Medical training was elevated to an unprecedented level of realism and efficacy.

4.5 *Laboratories Without Borders: Collaborative Research Redefined*

The metaverse facilitated a borderless collaboration among researchers, scientists, and medical experts. Digitally constructed laboratories became the crucibles of innovation, where data flowed seamlessly, transcending geographical limitations. Experts from diverse corners of the globe converged virtually to exchange ideas, analyze complex medical data, and conduct experiments in virtual environments. The metaverse accelerated the pace of discovery, enabling faster drug development and breakthroughs in treatment methods. Collaborative research leaped forward, unfettered by physical constraints.

5 Why Metaverse for Healthcare?

The opportunity for healthcare lies in three low-risk accelerators each of which comes with a high-value driver created to enable the metaverse for the healthcare journey [15] (Fig. 3).

5.1 *Accelerates Learning*

It improves knowledge and learning using the experiment-based education system and training to improve the retention and interconnection between the development and knowledge of skills that are valuable to society [16].

- *Simulation of Real Life*—The metaverse simulates a real-life situation in an immersive environment. The doctors can prepare for an operation with a surgical monitor before the actual surgery [17]. As medical students, they can enter the virtual reflection of a human body into a full-scale virtual view.
- *Training*—This is a very natural aspect of the metaverse. The new nurses can enter the virtual room of patients and practice the standard of setting up the patient's monitor. Other healthcare professionals can acquire the knowledge and get to know several other medical equipment.

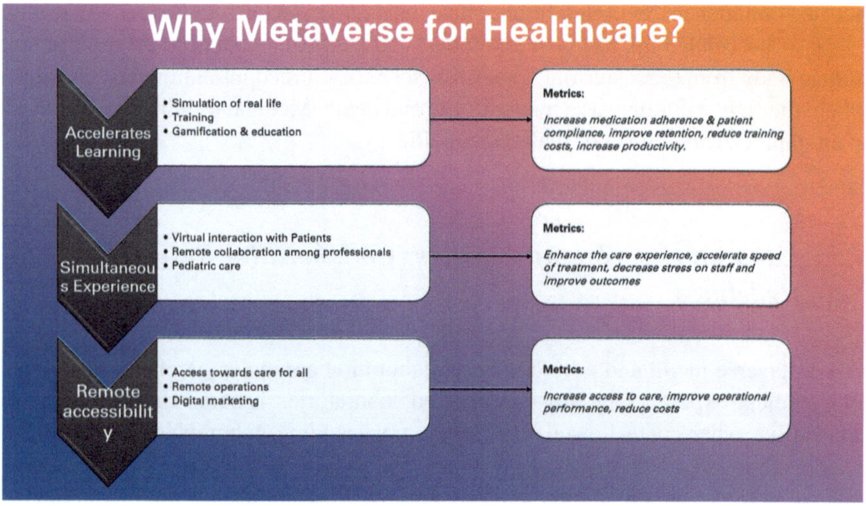

Fig. 3 Why Metaverse for Healthcare

- *Gamification and Education*—This can turn the process of acquiring knowledge into interesting exercises in the metaverse [18]. The patients can start practicing how to start using nebulizers the right way for their child, and all of this is done virtually. Other patients can start viewing the multi-dimensional view of blocked arteries and start scoring points as they learn about the symptoms and signs of the same [19].

5.2 *Simultaneous Experience*

The metaverse generates an immersive environment for collaboration, enabling patients and service providers to improve the care experience and engagement over time.

- *Virtual Interaction with Patients*—The patients can virtually interact with providers & their families as patients are the authentication mark for the metaverse. The exercises for a relaxed and safe setting can be demonstrated by a physical therapist. Patients with similar experiences can interact with each other virtually.
- *Remote Collaboration Among Professionals*—Remote collaboration among professionals utilizes extended reality and virtual space to streamline the exchange of information between different hospitals and service providers to facilitate consultations on complex cases or across the caring teams to facilitate the process of discharge.

- *Pediatric Care*—This is the best-suited place for the metaverse as teenagers and children have been growing up with enhanced reality technologies. The enhanced reality technologies are a welcome distraction for pediatric patients who are receiving chemotherapy treatment in their next cycle of treatment [20].

5.3 Remote Accessibility

This is possible due to the secure network of healthcare professionals who can now provide better care access to a diversified population.

- *Access Toward Care for All*—This adds a whole new meaning to the metaverse. As an individual, one can take part in hybrid clinical trials, both virtually and in person, to take advantage of the lifesaving treatments.
- *Remote Operations*—Remote operations are very valuable as the metaverse enables a set of people to interact from any location, enabling the opportunity for humans in the loop to facilitate the work from remote locations and manage the medical equipment with precision from a safe distance.
- *Digital Marketing*—Digital marketing in the metaverse is far more responsive. The organizations offering healthcare services can invite the patients to try the exercise equipment virtually at their wellness centers or ask any physician to explore genetic testing in their practice.

6 Case Studies: Metaverse in Healthcare Domain

6.1 Dassault Collaborates with Research Organizations to Produce 3D Simulated Radiotherapy Room

In June 2022, the collaborative efforts of Dassault Systèmes, the Hartmann Radiotherapy Institute, and the Rafael Institute gave birth to a groundbreaking initiative known as Project VORTHEx. This venture unveiled the world's inaugural fully immersive 3D simulation of a radiotherapy room. Pioneering in its approach, the project aimed to revolutionize patient experiences during treatment by incorporating virtual reality (VR) technology. Despite the commendable strides made in the efficiency and precision of radiotherapy over the past years, the conventional radiotherapy treatment room often poses a less-than-pleasant environment for patients.

The primary goal of the VORTHEx initiative is to elevate the overall well-being of patients by alleviating discomfort, reducing anxiety, and fostering a deeper comprehension of their treatment processes. As the actual treatment commences, individuals who have undergone the simulation will find themselves more at ease in the treatment room, where a dynamic and rotating apparatus is the sole company they encounter.

The digital replica of a room at the H. Hartmann Institute of Radiotherapy and Radiosurgery mirrors the environment of the VORTHEx project. This virtual space, crafted with precision, is a product of Dassault's 3DExperience Lab and 3DExcite solutions, offering state-of-the-art VR equipment and an immersive encounter.

While the inclusion of a robotic system in a radiotherapy treatment room is undeniably groundbreaking, it introduces a potentially intimidating element to the treatment process, particularly for patients undergoing this innovative approach for the first time. The simulated environment serves to replicate not only the technical intricacies and procedural elements of the treatment but also meticulously reconstructs the treatment room, the robotic arm, the patient's orientation, and the various conditions and procedural steps through an immersive 3D simulation.

The immersive encounter comes with the support of a dedicated healthcare team member who is readily available to address any queries about the scenario. These organizations are gearing up to initiate clinical trials aimed at evaluating the effectiveness and influence of the virtual reality educational program across the entirety of a patient's experience.

In the realm of the metaverse, we witness an innovative application of technology where companies leverage virtual collaborations to enhance both patient education and treatment outcomes. Within this digital landscape, the potential for 3D simulations to revolutionize education on a diverse range of treatments becomes apparent, ushering in a new era of immersive and effective learning experiences.

7 Future of Metaverse in Healthcare

7.1 Ease Things for Patients

The clinics will have the ability to offer further integrated treatment services and bundles, which are lacking in the current healthcare system, with the evolution of core technology in the metaverse. These technology-oriented solutions are improving the results and experiences of patients. The simplest of the procedures, i.e., blood draws, can take advantage of it, i.e., a technology-based solution that forms a map of veins on the skin of the patient.

Another med-tech giant recently acquired an AI-enabled surgical simulation platform called "Digital Surgery," which utilizes Microsoft's HoloLens to connect the real world with the virtual world. These significant investments in a med-tech domain are enabling organizations to unlock the potential of the metaverse.

7.2 *Enable Association Between the Professionals of the Healthcare Domain*

The capacity to share information promptly among healthcare professionals will enable quick identification of the cause of illness. Observing the patient's actions in the metaverse can enable the easy tracking of variables, i.e., compliance, which acts as an aid in diagnosis and illness treatment.

"Veyond Metaverse" is enabling healthcare professionals across the world to collaborate for planning, education, and training, as well as for medical operations. It utilizes inventive technology consisting of cloud and real-time communication to "enable doctors to upgrade or upskill their skill set with high accuracy to make sure everyone receives the best available healthcare services all the time & wherever."

There is a probability that the metaverse, combined with healthcare, will revolutionize the MedTech domain for over a few years. There are still several hurdles on the roadmap to make the metaverse fully functional in the healthcare domain, which includes smart technology mostly for the elderly population. Healthcare services-oriented companies are required to create a new business model that is integrated with the health insurance of patients, compensation, and prescriptions in a virtual world.

8 Metaverse Platform for Healthcare

The metaverse is developed to serve as a forever decentralized, collaborative, and interoperate offering and business model that will enable organizations to extend their operations digitally. A generic metaverse foundation for healthcare and medical services can consist of seven different layers, as mentioned in Fig. 4, from bottom to top, not being strict and likely to change based on several matrices, i.e., application, services offered, scalability, and requirements.

- *Infrastructure*—From the bottom, the infrastructure layer reflects all technologies required for infrastructure support and to develop the immersive, fully functional, and interoperable metaverse. Wireless communication and networking using 6G, 5G, or WIFI, the architecture of cloud storage systems, VR devices, and GPUs (graphics processing units) are required alongside several critical technology collections to develop a healthcare metaverse. This can enable uninterrupted connections with decentralized healthcare & medical centers. As of today, the metaverse stands for the foundation of high-performance computers that are lined with medical circuits, components of communication, health, medical hardware, and a mix of reality hardware.
- *Human Interface*—This layer reflects the devices that allow doctors or patients to feel the actual immersive experience in virtual life. This layer consists of devices, i.e., VR headsets, haptic-enabled gloves, smart glasses, and human

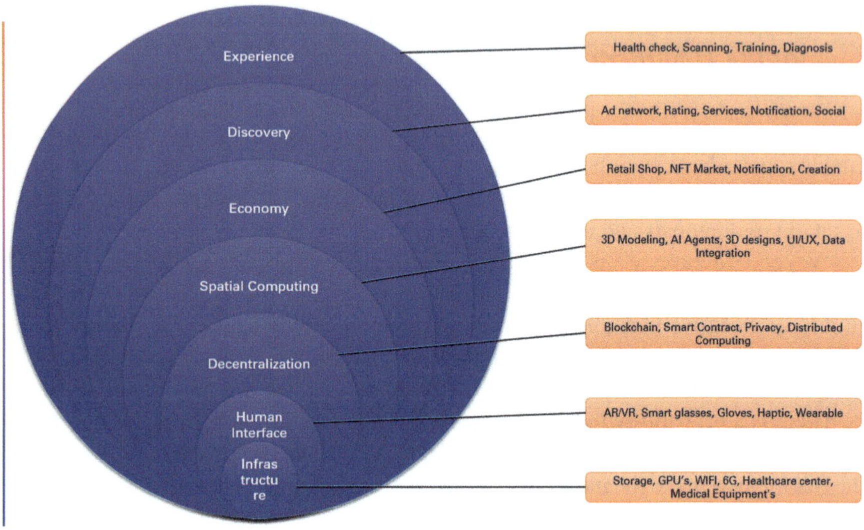

Fig. 4 Metaverse for healthcare platform

brain-computer inference systems. Using the technology of haptics, users can use electronic gadgets in mid-air without touching the screen or buttons, i.e., pick a 3D lung object to rotate and zoom in for analysis.

- *Decentralization*—The metaverse should be decentralized in the healthcare domain. It is required to be governed by one entity, and no one owns it, but it is a service available to everyone at any point of time. Decentralization consists of blockchain, which is a self-known digital identity method, smart contract, open access platforms to help facilitate the growth of distributed computing incrementally over time, and microservices of healthcare in scalable environments serving several crowds of patients and communities of medical experts. The host of healthcare metaverse projects, which are decentralized in nature, can make use of blockchain to serve the patient owner's private data and shared clinical experience in a traceable and transparent way to carry out the interaction and transaction.
- *Spatial Computing*—It refers to the combination of the real and virtual worlds. Spatial computing blurs the line between the ideal and actual worlds. Considering the domain of healthcare services, spatial computing is the sum of material, library, and collection of AI tools that are essential to developing the immersive 3D experience for real-life healthcare and wellness applications and medical services. Now because of the metaverse, medical students have the opportunity to put their skills into practice without risking anything with the help of virtual surgical training in the metaverse. A few 3D design engines, i.e., unreal engines, aid in 3D modeling and rendering with the help of GPUs to display the animation and geometry. Spatial computing aids in linking the diversified healthcare and

medical data from several hardware devices and sources to serve the end goal of visualization and animation with the help of VR devices.

- *Economy*—This layer is accountable for economic establishment and development inside the metaverse. Patients, doctors, and institutions of healthcare and medical groups can run their businesses in several distinctive ways. Here, patients can grant permission to service providers so that they can start using their private data for research initiatives and other non-commercial usage. The service providers can start rewarding patients for their participation using assets or virtual goods. There are a few economic schemes offered by medical and healthcare organizations, i.e., medical training, remote collaboration of diagnosis and treatment plans, and trading of health stuff and medical equipment. These can be placed in a retail shop of virtual world. This has huge potential for expansion economically by developing the virtual space not only for patients/doctors but also for content creators and designers so that they can interact in the metaverse.
- *Discovery*—Discovery can be seen as the promotion of an ecosystem consisting of the placement of stores, ratings, and system recommendations from users and service providers. This layer transfers the learning of experiments, which can be obtained as the end result of the push and pull of information consistently. In the metaverse-oriented healthcare and medical fields, pull refers to the inbound system where patients actively search for useful information and experiences, i.e., symptoms of a disease. Push, in particular, refers to more outbound and incorporates notice processes related to what kind of experience is waiting for patients in the metaverse. A larger set of modules are deployed in the metaverse generally to generate profits, consisting of a search engine, content that is driven by the community and outbound with display promotions, email, and other social handles.
- *Experience*—This interface consists of what the majority of businesses and individuals must be focused on. All the users, i.e., patients, and clinic employees, have several interactions during activities with each other and with virtual objects using the setting that are digitally driven with the help of digital content, i.e., declaration of symptoms of diseases, health checks, collaboration on diagnosis remotely, training, and medical education. The metaverse is way more than just some 3D reflection of reality, and it was built for immersive virtualization of physical space or products altogether to generate the seamless virtual but real ecosystem with built-in applications and offerings as services, i.e., the interactive VR surgery application can help the doctors discover the anatomy of interest and use the information that is valuable by learning it from an AI model to improve the medical image quality in real-time.

9 Prevention and Treatment Using Metaverse

The metaverse can be equipped for diagnostic and surgical processes and rehabilitation for anxiety, pain, depression, and several other disorders with considerable satisfying results [21, 22]. Considering cancer care This artificial intelligence technology can be a method to not only prevent it but also identify, treat, and rehabilitate the corresponding patients [23].

The concept of Healthcare 4.0 revolves around smart machines that can have access to large sets of data, enabling them to make decisions with minimal human interactions. It consists of a wider range of technological possibilities that can act as a foundation for new developments coming up in the healthcare domain. A widely popular and adopted concept is health 4.0, as it connects innovative technology such as virtual reality. It can not only enable us to observe the population but can also raise awareness amongst the people using community activities.

The first phase of Healthcare 4.0 has seen peak usage of the Internet of Medical Things along with the medical cyber systems, health cloud, machine learning, etc. This has significantly enhanced the cost-effectiveness, quality, and dependability of medical services.

The second phase of Healthcare 4.0 introduces the concepts of augmented reality and virtual reality. These digital technologies can be considered an alternative to the model of healthcare delivery where avatars can be allowed personalized care with the help of consultations [24]. The physicians can meet with the patients using the metaverse in a 3D clinic that utilizes the telemedicine service, and home devices, i.e., wearable sensors and mobile applications, can be used to observe the health status remotely.

Several distinguished devices can be equipped to observe the health condition remotely at home, as real life is connected with virtual life. The observation of the clinical aspect is critical, and as a result, the person's health who is located remotely can be easily monitored using 12 lead electrocardiograms for the heart, blood pressure equipment to check the cardiovascular system, and blood glucose calculator mainly for people having diabetes. Heart frequency monitors are widely used when it comes to the measuring or evaluating physical performance.

Smartwatches have been adopted worldwide lately and integrate the frequency of the heart with blood saturation and accelerometers. It also uses the data of the GPS (Global Positioning System) so that health status and physical performance can be captured and chronic diseases can be managed [25]. Smartwatches are frequently integrated with smartphones, and these smartphones are integrated with communities where individuals can differentiate their data from others and acknowledge challenges. There is a huge potential for smartwatches to promote health programs. Proactive and concurrent monitoring is possible as a part of the online world, which increases the possibility of signing up for fitness initiatives and opting for a healthy lifestyle [26]. The smartwatch can be hardware to keep individuals active in the world of the metaverse. The observation of health aspects 24 h a day can enable quick prevention in problematic situations, i.e., atrial fibrillation, enabling the health service provider to enhance their security measures for prevention. Other than proactive monitoring, another crucial factor to look for is virtual or artificial intelligence avatars in the metaverse, or perhaps an assistant who can share personal feedback and use the interference to promote a change in behavior. This can be achieved using avatars provided by new technology that can react realistically to their speech, body language, and expressions. Virtual reality can be opted for to build the pre-operational plans by evaluating the scenarios in 3D and collecting the feedback of other experts integrated with the internet. It can also be connected with several therapies, considering how effective it is for several medical situations that come with the pros of cost, compliance, and accessibility. Virtual reality can be used as a technique for rehabilitation, i.e., mirror therapy, which is a method to create a visual illusion so that the impaired limb (after stroke) is operating correctly to re-educate the motion of cognitive designs [27].

The last factor to keep in mind is the probability of creating avatars, which can be a "virtual caretaker or nurse" to proactively monitor the patients and care for or interact with them, explaining what is going on around them and how it works. This will not only monitor them, but in real-time, quality surveillance will ensure patient safety, the physician's activity, and discharge or admitting activities can be monitored as well. Although the metaverse can act as a transitional method before the real-life experience, healthcare professionals who are with the patients each step of the way in specific environments improve the effectiveness of treatments. Virtual models for care with psychological support group initiatives can be the right intervention. For chronic illness, i.e., diabetes, and mental health issues, remote virtual nursing with robotic users can be a bit of aid [28]. The metaverse with an anonymous virtual room will be a more comfortable place to talk about things or issues with professionals for people going through mental health issues [29]. Below is the figure reflecting an alternate method for the relationship between doctor and patient (Fig. 5).

The promotion of health can be carried out in teaching rooms, just the way students are being educated. Health promotion initiatives refer to enabling individuals to have their own space for training. Virtual rooms can be seen as places where individuals can meet each other and train together. Similarly, Peloton which is a virtual space for bicycling, which is existing and widely adopted. This virtual sports simulator utilizes virtual reality, and lately, it has come with interactive video, enabling groups of individuals to compete or workout together with the help of virtual space.

10 Benefits and Advantages of Metaverse

The metaverse's integration into Healthcare 4.0 brings forth a multitude of benefits. Firstly, it enhances accessibility to healthcare services, particularly for individuals in remote or underserved areas. Patients can consult specialists and receive medical guidance without the need for travel, reducing both costs and time constraints.

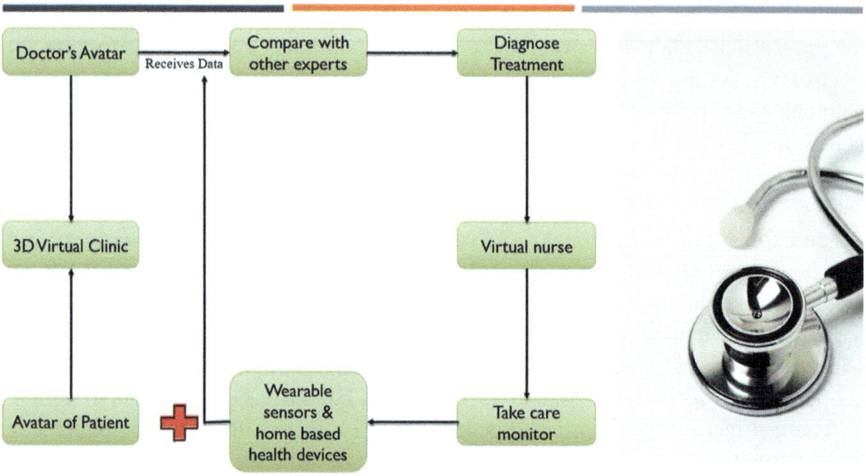

Fig. 5 probable relationship virtual model of doctor and patient

Secondly, the metaverse improves medical training and education by providing a risk-free platform for learning and practice. Medical professionals can refine their skills through realistic simulations, leading to better-prepared doctors and ultimately improving patient outcomes.

Thirdly, collaborative research becomes more efficient and dynamic within the metaverse. Scientists and researchers can interact, analyze data, and conduct experiments in immersive digital laboratories, accelerating the pace of discovery.

11 Ethical Considerations

While the metaverse offers transformative potential, it also presents several challenges and ethical considerations. Privacy and security are paramount concerns, as personal health data could be vulnerable to breaches and misuse in virtual environments. Striking a balance between convenience and data protection becomes crucial. Safeguarding sensitive medical information within the metaverse demanded novel approaches to encryption and authentication. Ensuring equitable access to the metaverse-driven healthcare was another hurdle, as marginalized populations could be left behind due to a lack of digital resources and skills [30].

Additionally, the digital divide may exclude certain demographics from fully benefiting from the metaverse-based healthcare. Access to high-speed internet, advanced devices, and digital literacy skills are prerequisites for participation, potentially leaving marginalized groups behind.

Ethical issues regarding the authenticity of virtual medical procedures also arise. Ensuring that virtual surgeries and treatments are as effective and safe as their physical counterparts requires stringent validation processes. Striking the balance between embracing innovation and upholding patient safety was paramount.

12 Limitations of the Metaverse

The key limitations of the metaverse are focused on the management of data, privacy risks, cyber-attacks, and probable restrictions when it comes to access, i.e., internet connectivity issues, and for individuals with low vision. The metaverse can be prone to possible sophisticated crimes, i.e., personal data theft (Table 1).

The initial aspect to focus on is the problem related to the management of data and its storage. There is a huge commercial interest, and individuals could have very restricted power to control their data, specifically with whom it should be shared and what those conditions will be. Therefore, it becomes the priority to solve the issues related to the security and privacy of data, along with legislative and regulation issues. There are always concerns related to ethics, security, and privacy as healthcare adopts the online model of operation, and that's why security enhancement for data security is essential, along with central regulatory oversight. This is a way to grant controlled access and organize data on complex networks such as blockchain. Blockchain can help enable the security of healthcare data sharing and storage. Blockchain is decentralized, transparent, traceable, and private, which makes it more reliable for trusting data. Furthermore, blockchain can be linked with artificial intelligence, which can aid in cardiovascular medicine by personalizing it for increased data readymade for AI development purposes, sharing an algorithm for generalization, and segmenting databases by decentralizing them for innovative solutions to generate improved results. Blockchain can aid in encrypting the data of patients, and therefore it can enforce compliance with standard medical records, keeping in a way that becomes a standard practice across healthcare professionals. The application of cardiovascular medicine with blockchain is still in the early phases of development, as concerns exist regarding its development. This way, healthcare services can keep track of medical history, and the doctors can access it only if they have the digital token shared by the patients, thereby ensuring that the patient's data stays confidential.

The second factor to focus on is the in-person interaction. It becomes much easier to check in with patients in person, by using a call or perhaps a social mode of communication, than compared to a far-fetched science idea. The metaverse is estimated to be proactively used for nursing and medical education. Though the metaverse can improve knowledge around nursing education, it is not as impactful as the rest of other modes of education considering domain skills, confidence, and performance time. Social engagement in the metaverse appears to be weaker than that of real-world interactions, as it is greatly expensive [31].

The last factor to focus on is the loss of freedom in the coming years. That's how the reality must be, and that's the actual pro of the metaverse. The key issue is identifying who should administer the metaverse: (a) is it the general public

Table 1 Challenges and future direction

Hurdles	Description	Probable solution	Future direction
Risks related to Cybersecurity	Data captured digitally from many devices are prone to attacks from hackers In several ways of information sharing	1. The software and components of gadgets utilized In the system should be able to identify the attacks 2. Communication rules should be enforced between the existing hardware in the network of the metaverse 3. Trust no one policy must he adopted unless the source is verified	1. Healthcare companies should have a security layer as a strict protocol 2. Lightweight Blockchain technology can be adopted with techniques of cryptography and consensus algorithms to secure the data of users
Risks related to Privacy	1. Securely saving the identity of the virtual patient 2. Adopting emerging technologies to create a virtual environment in the healthcare field. i.e. AI & IOT can expose sensitive data of users to the outside world and thus privacy breach occurs	1. Implementing encryption at the application layer can help to ensure the privacy of users data in a virtual environment 2. Technologies related to the enhancement of privacy should be adopted i.e. (PETs) which can be used to hide the sensitive data captured from sensors and later this masked data can be shared with cloud services	Techniques related to Federated learning should be adopted to enhance the confidentiality of patients data
Communication hurdles	1. It is required to setup reliable communication between heterogeneous devices in the Metaverse such that there are no delays or loss of data 2. A High-speed communication channel is required for Metaverse to facilitate the data transfer	1. Auction-based deep reinforcement learning can be created to enhance the efficiency of communication 2. Incentive-based techniques can be implemented in blockchain technology	Service models or 6G networks can be adopted to facilitate the hustle-free service using metaverse in healthcare
Computing and prediction hurdles	Huge computation capabilities are required even tough AI solutions for metaverse sharpen the QOS	1. Optimized and efficient AI models can be designed 2. AI can be deployed at Edge	1. lightweight AI models can result in improved prediction by reducing the computing 2. Explainable AI (XAI) can be adopted to enhance the prediction by efficiently understanding AI models

or (b) it multi-millionaire organizations that are keen on developing it over time? The metaverse might exist with the public to reflect the reality along with the private organizations. This way, the government has to start working on investing in alternate worlds that can ensure public space, education programs, and events. Public and private organizations must ensure the safety of personal data through consultations.

13 Conclusion: Healing in a New Reality

The metaverse will revamp the landscape of the healthcare domain by utilizing the new evolving technologies, i.e., AI, AR, blockchain, digital twinning, and VR. The metaverse can never replace real-world interaction using eye contact and in-person communication, as facial expressions and gestures are required in the healthcare domain.

There will be some legal implications for introducing the metaverse in the healthcare domain. The first is how healthcare will be accessible in the metaverse or how to ensure the regulation of applications that are utilized to deliver those services. The U.S. Food and Drug Administration has been working to share advice on the development of digital health and several of those technologies, which can be termed medical devices. The next challenge will be the protection of data. The organizations offering services in the metaverse will have the ability to collect a large amount of data. "The Health Insurance Portability and Accountability Act" of the USA protects the data of the patients and ensures that patients' data only stays within the offices of doctors. The question of intellectual property will continue to grow complicated, which can include patents, trademarks and copyrights all due to the decentralized metaverse, i.e., the patents for design will play a critical aspect as they are required to adopt the existing laws since the metaverse is all about visualization. Several considerations will show up when it comes to the "New Technology File System" to ensure how the copyrights can be determined for images, video, and artwork in the digital assets and to safeguard the interests of associate trademarks.

The metaverse is poised to redefine healthcare in the era of Healthcare 4.0. Its potential to enhance telemedicine, medical training, research, and collaboration can revolutionize the way healthcare services are delivered and experienced. However, addressing challenges related to privacy, access, and authenticity is crucial to harnessing its full potential. By carefully navigating these challenges, the healthcare industry can leverage the metaverse to usher in a new era of patient-centric, efficient, and innovative healthcare solutions.

The utilization of the metaverse in healthcare is growing at a phenomenal pace, and it will continue to evolve the existing performance of healthcare services. It is very important that the existing infrastructure of the system can sustain the growth, and several other domains like the law will continue to shape around the same. The metaverse can opt for a method to enhance the quality of the healthcare system by introducing interventions and treatments, providing education for individuals around the globe with standard training, and aiding the research for the development of a world database. The young generation can also start practicing sports and learn something new by spending some time in the metaverse.

Healthcare 4.0's integration of the metaverse promised a new era of patient-centric, efficient, and innovative solutions. However, this journey was not without its trials. The metaverse's role in healthcare 4.0 stood as a testament to human ingenuity, reminding us that even in the boundless realm of virtuality, the quest for a healthier future remained ever-grounded in the well-being of humanity.

References

1. Chen, L., & Wang, J. (2023). Virtual reality applications in Healthcare 4.0: A metaverse perspective. *International Journal of Medical Informatics, 147*, 1–10.
2. Lee, S., & Kim, Y. (2023). Integrating augmented reality and virtual reality in Healthcare 4.0: The role of metaverse. *Journal of Medical Systems, 47*(6), 1–11.
3. Johnson, M., & Roberts, D. (2021). Augmented reality for surgical training in Healthcare 4.0: A metaverse approach. *Journal of Surgical Education, 78*(3), 789–798.
4. Williams, L., & Davis, R. (2022). Virtual reality in medical imaging: Enhancing diagnostic accuracy in Healthcare 4.0. *Journal of Medical Imaging and Radiology, 15*(4), 210–220.
5. Martinez, C., & Gonzalez, E. (2022). The role of augmented reality in medical education within the context of Healthcare 4.0. *Medical Education, 27*(1), 1–11.
6. Brown, E., & Wilson, T. (2022). Metaverse-driven medical education in the context of Healthcare 4.0. Medical. *Science Educator, 32*(2), 567–576.
7. Lee, D., & Kim, Y. (2021). The metaverse in medical training and simulation for Healthcare 4.0. *Medical Education, 26*(1), 1–10.
8. Williams, E., & Davis, K. (2021). Using virtual reality to improve patient Engagement in Healthcare 4.0: A metaverse exploration. *Patient Education and Counseling, 104*(4), 789–798.
9. Kim, L., & Park, M. (2021). Enhancing medical training and education with augmented reality in Healthcare 4.0: The metaverse perspective. *Medical Teacher, 43*(9), 912–920.
10. Lee, H., & Kim, J. (2023). Metaverse-enhanced remote patient monitoring in Healthcare 4.0: A feasibility study. *Journal of Telemedicine and Telecare, 31*(6), 320–330.
11. Patel, R., & Gupta, M. (2022). Augmented reality navigation for surgical procedures in Healthcare 4.0: A metaverse perspective. *Journal of Surgical Research, 205*, 180–189.
12. Smith, P., & Johnson, R. (2023). Virtual reality exposure therapy in mental health treatment: A metaverse approach in Healthcare 4.0. *Journal of Anxiety Disorders, 47*, 1–11.
13. Gamechangevr Homepage. (n.d.). https://gamechangevr.com/. Accessed 08 Sep 2023.
14. Patel, R., & Gupta, M. (2021). Leveraging metaverse technologies for enhanced patient engagement in Healthcare 4.0. *Health Informatics Journal, 27*(2), 1–12.
15. Jackson, M., & Clark, R. (2023). Advancing telemedicine through the metaverse: Opportunities and challenges in Healthcare 4.0. *Telemedicine and e-Health, 29*(4), 285–293.
16. Smith, A. B., & Johnson, C. D. (2022). Exploring the potential of the metaverse in transforming healthcare delivery. *Journal of Healthcare Technology, 18*(3), 120–135.
17. Patel, J., & Gupta, A. (2021). Applications of augmented reality in surgical procedures within Healthcare 4.0: A metaverse perspective. *Surgical Innovation, 28*(5), 456–465.
18. Garcia, A., & Lopez, M. (2023). Gamification in metaverse-enabled Healthcare 4.0: Engaging patients for better health outcomes. *Games for Health Journal, 12*(2), 87–98.
19. Brown, J., & Wilson, K. (2022). Gamified rehabilitation exercises in metaverse environments for Healthcare 4.0. *Games and Health Journal, 11*(5), 301–310.

20. Chen, W., & Zhang, Q. (2023). Virtual reality pain distraction in pediatric Healthcare 4.0: Exploring metaverse applications. *Journal of Pediatric Nursing, 58*, 45–54.
21. Wong, K., & Tan, L. (2022). Enhancing rehabilitation services in Healthcare 4.0 using metaverse technologies. *Journal of Health Communication, 19*(5), 678–689.
22. Brown, M., & Wilson, R. (2023). Virtual reality for health behavior change in Healthcare 4.0: A metaverse exploration. *Health Education & Behavior, 50*(2), 124–135.
23. Patel, S., & Smith, K. (2021). Virtual reality pain management applications in Healthcare 4.0: A metaverse perspective. *Pain Management, 9*(3), 267–278.
24. Martinez, G., & Lopez, H. (2023). Metaverse-enhanced telehealth services in Healthcare 4.0: A case study on remote consultations. *Telemedicine and e-Health, 29*(6), 421–430.
25. Patel, N., & Gupta, S. (2023). Metaverse applications for remote monitoring of chronic conditions in Healthcare 4.0. *International Journal of Medical Informatics, 149*, 1–9.
26. Garcia, P., & Martinez, J. (2021). The role of virtual worlds in remote patient monitoring in Healthcare 4.0. *Journal of Telemedicine and Telecare, 27*(8), 432–441.
27. Wang, Q., & Li, M. (2022). The potential of virtual reality-based rehabilitation in Healthcare 4.0: A metaverse approach. *Disability and Rehabilitation, 37*(10), 879–888.
28. Rodriguez, A., & Martinez, B. (2022). Metaverse-based health support groups: Fostering peer-to-peer connections in Healthcare 4.0. *Journal of Community Psychology, 50*(3), 301–312.
29. Kim, S., & Park, H. (2023). Metaverse-based mental health interventions in the era of Healthcare 4.0. *Cyberpsychology, Behavior, and Social Networking, 26*(1), 56–64.
30. Kim, N., & Lee, S. (2022). Enhancing patient empowerment through metaverse-driven Healthcare 4.0: A user experience study. *International Journal of Human-Computer Interaction, 38*(7), 589–600.
31. Taylor, B., & White, G. (2021). Exploring social interaction in Healthcare 4.0 metaverse environments: Implications for patient support. *Health Communication, 26*(8), 610–621.

A Revolution in Health Care Using the Metaverse for the Elderly

Zahra Alidousti Shahraki and Mohsen Aghabozorgi Nafchi

1 Challenges of the Metaverse

The metaverse is a new technology based on virtual reality, which is based on people's imagination. Virtual reality can display all-natural events in the form of mental imagery. On the other hand, transforming imagination in mind-space into natural reality can have tremendous effects on human life using the metaverse. The metaverse's initial idea was taken from science-fiction stories, and attempts have been made to transform this idea into platforms. Online gaming platforms are an example of the metaverse technology that can be placed among different age groups. These online game platforms are based on social and political policies and beliefs in different countries. Therefore, it can be said that the metaverse technology can have different applications according to the needs of each society. The most important challenge in the discussion of the metaverse is examining the needs of the elderly.

A criticism of virtual reality technology is that it creates crises in both life and society. The implementation of mental imagery along with the benefits of presenting ideas may cause confusion and division among people. The wrong policies and decisions that come to people's minds should pass through people's logical points of view using correct thinking. If incorrect decisions are implemented without a logical analysis of people, they can cause different crises in different areas of life. These challenges must be investigated to develop practical and useful technologies. The intelligentization of applications based on virtual reality requires the ability to make decisions and analyze people's feelings. In this case, the metaverse revolution can compete with humans. We hope that in the near future, it will be possible to

Z. A. Shahraki (✉)
Department of Computer Engineering, University of Isfahan, Isfahan, Iran

M. A. Nafchi
Department of Computer Science and Engineering, Shiraz University, Shiraz, Iran

C. L. Chowdhary (ed.), *The Metaverse for the Healthcare Industry*,
https://doi.org/10.1007/978-3-031-60073-9_11

establish emotional, logical, and intelligent bilateral cooperation between humans and virtual reality. Examining the challenges in designing smart applications based on the metaverse is an important issue that has been discussed in different sections of this chapter. The implementation of ideas presented in the metaverse, based on applications for different age groups, can greatly improve quality of life. The effort was made to help increase their health level and quality of life by examining the various applications of virtual reality in the lives of the elderly.

2 The Metaverse-Based Virtual Hospitals for Health Care

The health of people of different age groups is a challenging issue that has always been considered by doctors and medical communities. According to repeated reports from the World Health Organization, some daily deaths are due to non-compliance of people in the field of health. The care of people of different age groups by medical centers and self-care should be monitored by medical centers. Because it is not possible to control and monitor the health of all people in person, the metaverse technology can play a good role in this regard. Self-care through the metaverse-based applications can lead to significant transformations in the health-care industry. Smart applications that use virtual reality to establish treatment and improve conditions for people can be welcomed by different age groups. Owing to their old age and lack of control over their physical conditions, the elderly can optimally use the metaverse technology. This special group can be under the control of medical centers during the day and receive special treatment in case of changes in the immune system, blood pressure, blood sugar, and other factors.

Virtual hospitals [1] can help control patients under different conditions and times. A virtual hospital can help them to be under the control of doctors at any time of the day and night with online visits and examinations of patients. One of the most important aspects of a doctor's examination is to recognize the facial expressions of the patients; therefore, taking a selfie of the patients can help in the diagnosis and treatment of the patients in the virtual world. The metaverse technology can help in processing images of patients and diagnosing their disease. Taking selfies is a way to communicate in today's world, creating interactions among people. Diagnosing the disease from processed images of the face can determine the patient's state, feelings, and amount of pain due to the disease. Along with the great benefits of taking selfies, other challenges must also be considered. A patient's sense of security when using social networks and interactions is an important factor that challenges the use of virtual reality systems in treatment. The preservation of patient privacy and information when communicating with doctors should be the most important part of the design of the metaverse-based treatment care systems. Therefore, the design of a virtual hospital based on the metaverse can transform the online interaction of patients and doctors into virtual reality. The use of algorithms based on data mining and blockchain helps maintain the security of patient information, and a virtual hospital system based on a safe metaverse is available to all people.

According to research in [2], the use of the metaverse virtual interactive systems reduces feelings of loneliness and depression in the elderly. This result can be used in the process of treating the elderly in virtual hospitals in the metaverse. Providing a special virtual environment for the elderly in a virtual hospital allows them to interact with each other, and the feelings of sympathy between them reduce their depression and loneliness. In addition, the trend of the metaverse social interactions among the elderly has caused virtual communities to be created under treatment. This community is treated at low cost. However, doctors visit and treat patients online because they spend less time and energy. Among the tiring aspects for doctors is the one-on-one interaction with patients, which sometimes leads to repeated visits and safety recommendations. Therefore, a metaverse virtual hospital can save doctors' time and energy, and increase their work efficiency.

One of the challenges is the training of nurses in emotional management in virtual reality [3]. Nurses play an important role in strengthening morale and raising positive energy in patients, especially the elderly who are hopeless. Therefore, virtual reality can provide an opportunity for nurses to practice more to control their emotions. However, this poses a significant challenge. The main goal of interactions between patients and nurses is physical and mental health. The patients require support from experienced nurses. Therefore, the virtual reality environment should not be an opportunity for nurses and doctors to learn through experience; on the other hand, the health of patients may be endangered due to the inexperience of nurses. If patients, especially the elderly under care, feel uncomfortable during the treatment period, the treatment staff will experience problems during their treatment period. It is also possible that some patients experience acute mental health problems. In a more general way, it should be emphasized that virtual reality is not a so-called laboratory environment for patients, where their health becomes someone else's toy.

Covid-19 has many weaknesses, owing to its unpredictability. One of these weaknesses is the inconsistency among doctors, patients, and nurses [4]. However, owing to long-term quarantine, the opportunity to learn in various fields, especially health, has been damaged. Useful experiences can be gained from these unpredictable events. For example, the design of intelligent platforms can reduce the complications caused by epidemics of unknown viruses and other factors that affect the health of society in an uncontrollable manner. The design of these platforms helps to prevent abnormalities in the medical health system. Using the metaverse technology and creating a 3D virtual reality keep people's communication safe in all conditions and improve the quality of health in society. The tele-observation (tele-obs) tool [5] has been effective in controlling patients in emergency departments. During the Covid-19 pandemic, this tool was able to have a very good effect in preventing patients from becoming infected in emergency departments. With this smart technology, patients' length of stay, hospitalization, and treatment costs have been investigated. This method can help to treat patients faster, reduce treatment costs, and save patients' places in hospitals by controlling patients remotely.

To create a hospital at home, a set of data is collected, including patients' information about age, sex, type of illness, medical history, and other factors that

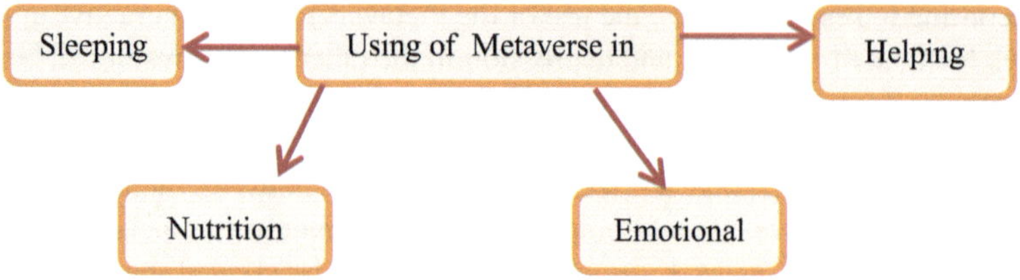

Fig. 1 Using of the metaverse in relation to health

help the patient diagnose the type of illness [6]. This information can be stored in a database, and data analysis of patients under different conditions can be performed using data mining algorithms. Machine learning patterns can predict the critical conditions of new patients and help create mobile hospitals in their homes. Based on the experiences created in communities regarding Covid-19, each community must design a smart hospital according to its own conditions. Widespread diseases with unknown symptoms are expected to occur in the future. Therefore, the world of the metaverse must have the ability to control and take necessary measures for society's health. The metaverse technology will create an all-encompassing power in the world and an intelligent global health organization in the whole world that will manage the health of people in different sectors. In a word, it is necessary to say that a virtual hospital based on virtual reality can control patients' conditions remotely and play an effective role in predicting patients' conditions using machine learning. Based on the history of the patients, the number of drugs that the patients take, the necessary data, and new information that can predict changes in disease conditions in patients with different symptoms can be extracted. Predicting patients' conditions using deep learning helps an intelligent system based on the metaverse achieve better control over the patients' treatment system (Fig. 1).

3 Using ChatGPT in the Metaverse and Its Impact on Health

ChatGPT [7] is the latest and most challenging smart technology of the twentieth century and was released worldwide in November 2022. This artificial intelligence chatbot could become the most powerful intelligent tool in less than 2 months and could be a great revolution in artificial intelligence. Tutorials in the chatbot library using deep learning algorithms were able to understand the concepts of questions in different fields and establish a very good interactive relationship with humans. One of the most challenging effects of this chatbot is its ability to answer questions related to human understanding and imagination. Thus far, the ChatGPT has been able to answer meaningful questions with a very low error rate. One of the limitations that has been raised about this robot thus far is incorrect answers to questions, which seems to be due to a misunderstanding of the concepts as well as the lack of updating of its information [8]. This robot was trained using data from 2021 and earlier, and new events and concepts after 2022 are unknown. Therefore, it should be trained daily on new science topics and concepts using machine learning algorithms so that it can perform successfully during the test.

The ChatGPT is a generation of language models that can understand languages and concepts from languages. This application is a stronger version of natural language processing, which performs numerous processes on data with a lower percentage of errors. One of the wonders of this emerging application is the processing of thousands of billion pieces of data. The cost of training data is extremely high and requires a powerful processor for analysis. The algorithm used in ChatGPT has a complex structure that can be described as multi-dimensionally collected data that runs at a high speed. Therefore, the analysis of these data requires a powerful graphics processor unit (GPU).

ChatGPT has a significant impact on the medical industry and human health. Communicating with different age groups, understanding the type of their disease, and prescribing medicine to them can make people no longer need doctors. Of course, the important point is that with the daily development of science, the intelligent robot should also update its information; if there are new unknown diseases, the doctor should prescribe medicines that are suitable for the type of new disease. This means that the robot can never be without the need for humans, and cannot continue its work independently. Artificial intelligence, with its great developing power, cannot be without the presence of scientists. Data scientists should keep the ChatGPT chat data updated daily, and data analysts should check different sciences and ensure the correctness of the training algorithms in the correct analysis of topics. Therefore, smart robots with the ability to diagnose and analyze questions in various sciences still need to be verified and approved by data scientists.

In medicine and health science, this robot should be able to treat patients with a small percentage error; hence, it requires a large amount of data. Big data algorithms should be able to perform data mining at high speeds and should inform patients about the results of the disease. Using smart algorithms based on the metaverse on big data can create a safe space for storing and exploring data. A cloud using blockchain algorithms can maintain the privacy of data and make it possible for GPT chatbots to perform training on big data. This can reduce the percentage of errors and patient care by using intelligent robots with higher accuracy. ChatGPT has been able to understand the concepts well and answer questions that were asked of it. The training given to this application has made it stay in mind based on questions that are frequently asked. This point can be useful for questions and answers that the elderly ask during the treatment period. Some elderly people suffer from forgetfulness or mental confusion due to mental disorders caused by their old age, in which case, the ChatGPT algorithm can remind them of the necessary points during the treatment period. On the other hand, the ChatGPT algorithm recognizes concepts well from the tone of voice, can analyze natural signal processing, and provides the correct answer to the questions of the elderly. Other services that can be added to ChatGPT include strong ones that make this application work strongly in the field of health.

The use of the metaverse-based chatbots can be a powerful tool for virtual reality. The combination of these two powerful technologies in the health industry can have many similarities to human behavior. Doctors can trust this technology and leave difficult medical operations, postoperative care, and care of special patients, such as the elderly and the physically and mentally disabled, to these ChatGPT robots based on virtual reality. Reaching this stage requires passing different challenges and tests to ensure the health of the patients throughout their treatment.

In [9], the opinions of Twitter users regarding this robot were reviewed. Based on the analysis of user comments, it seems that the majority believe that ChatGPT can answer questions about all topics. Accordingly, this robot can have a significant impact on virtual reality. The metaverse technology can create wonderful virtual reality based on the analysis of patients' questions, which provides the ability to communicate strongly with humans and understand human concepts well. Based on this, it is possible to implement the ChatGPT application based on neuroscience to create the ability to analyze voice and answer questions using the voice of the ChatGPT robot via signal processing. Such a revolution in the application of ChatGPT and the ability to communicate through conversation based on an understanding of human concepts can bring a real robot-like human into the medical industry. It is not surprising that a chatbot playing the role of a skilled doctor can fully treat patients. Analyzing patients' disease conditions accurately based on their facial expressions, voices, and images allows this robot to prescribe the necessary drugs to patients. Communicating and talking with this robot in the role of a doctor can have a positive effect on the mental state of patients, especially the elderly, who need more mental care. In summary, the ChatGPT can play a significant role in the health and care of patients, especially the elderly, in the metaverse industry. The role of this robot in communicating with the elderly can be of great help in improving their conditions.

In [10], ChatGPT was examined using a reinforcement learning algorithm. This learning technique allows the robot to gain new experience during its activity and shows better output results. Just as doctors can provide better treatment for other patients based on the experiences they gain during the treatment of patients, artificial intelligence applications that are programmed based on reinforcement learning techniques can also evaluate and analyze the data obtained at the output. Again, reinforcement learning helps the application to show better results with a lower error percentage in the output. In the metaverse industry, reinforcement learning algorithms can help introduce better treatment conditions for patients. Statistical analysis of patients' conditions using the metaverse-based applications designed with artificial intelligence reinforcement learning algorithms, such as age, disease history, sex of patients who need special care, and other effective conditions during the treatment period, helps identify patients according to their stored experiences. In the database of the application, a more accurate prescription for their disease will be dealt with, and they will experience a better treatment period.

4 The Metaverse in Social Networking Platforms

With the expansion of various social networking platforms, direct communication between people has significantly decreased. Based on existing observations, this range will soon increase in the coming years and cover various fields of communication such as business, health, medical care, and other factors in human life. If the metaverse environment is implemented on social networks, it will cause people to spend more time online. The metaverse allows social networks to operate in a virtual reality environment. Indeed, without the metaverse, the world of virtual communication would still have a sense of being virtual, and communicating with feelings and emotional reactions would not create a strong and friendly relationship among users. The metaverse resolves this deficiency and creates emotions in the virtual world. As we have seen in recent years since 2021, the social networking platforms Instagram and Facebook were able to name Meta their logos. This shows that these social networks (Instagram and Facebook) were able to use the idea of being the metaverse to expand their platforms. This causes many users to register on these platforms over a short period. The idea of being the metaverse in the communication of users on social networks will strengthen the mental conditions of users. The feeling of empathy and mutual understanding in the virtual communication managed by the metaverse leads to satisfaction of the emotional needs of users. The metaverse attempts to ensure users' physical health by establishing strong communication in a social network environment. Examining the challenges in the communication process on social networks using the metaverse should be considered, and the factors that cause damage to users' virtual reality communication should be limited.

With the combination of the metaverse, blockchain, artificial intelligence, digital currencies, and IoT, a wonderful combination of virtual reality can be displayed. The use of this combination in social media enables the design of a super-intelligent platform that can create strong and close connections among users on social networks. Thus, the feeling of being far from one another in social interactions can be reduced to its lowest level. It is interesting that the new tools that are added to meta-platforms, such as Instagram and WhatsApp, make distance communication more attractive. Face and voice change filters, gifts, animations used in user stories, and especially the new tool for translating the text and photos of stories and comments into the desired language have made this platform very popular among users worldwide. These tools have transformed the platform into virtual reality and have increased the possibility of its productivity to a high extent.

Since the elderly are one of the most popular age groups on these platforms under Meta Company, the metaverse has been able to create virtual reality for this age group as well. Based on the observations that we have during our daily lives with elderly age groups, the tendency to use virtual networks is increasing. Thus, the metaverse can design special tools for seniors to use on networking platforms. The use of these tools makes the establishment of social relationships among the elderly increase in social networks under the metaverse, and as a result, strengthens their motivation and increases their mood. It seems that if it is possible to design a metaverse platform suitable for the elderly for medical and health care, their despair and hopelessness during their treatment period can be reduced, and empathy and sympathy can increase. Social networks for the elderly can be designed according to their needs and user-friendly methods can be used to provide services on these platforms.

Indeed, one of the challenges faced by the elderly when using social networking platforms is the negative feeling toward its user-friendliness. It takes a long time for most seniors to connect well to these platforms. A good feature that should be used in the design of these platforms is the use of user interface experience methods. These methods make social network platforms tend toward virtual reality. Elderly people with a weak spirit in communicating with social networks can open up a new world of communication using these methods. The metaverse world for the elderly makes them feel happy when communicating. Virtual reality can strengthen spiritual and emotional needs. Seniors who talk to each other on social networking platforms based on the metaverse can create a wide range of communication. The most important goal of these platforms is to reduce the feeling of people being far from each other and to create two-way or multiperson communication in less time and at a higher speed. Traditional ways of communicating with each other using these platforms have been reduced, enabling people anywhere in the world to communicate with each other. Based on this, the emergence of the metaverse was able to provide an additional feeling for long-distance communication, which led to the improvement of the physical and mental health of people (especially the elderly).

In [2], the conditions of the elderly living in rehabilitation centers were studied. Some of these seniors have used virtual reality systems to interact, and the results have shown that the level of loneliness, isolation, and depression in this group of seniors has decreased significantly. By examining this challenge, it appears that long-term planning should be designed to improve the quality of life of the elderly. The Corona era has been a turning point in the lives of all people worldwide, with their own special conditions. This pandemic brought the world to the brink of major changes in communication. Elderly people were among a special age group that was generally affected by this epidemic owing to their physical problems. A model for designing social platforms for the elderly was proposed [2], in which the spiritual needs of the elderly, social needs, and needs of society were determined separately, and the level of communication between these needs was determined to be 90. The obtained model is a complete graph that includes a set of types of communication, the conditions of the elderly, and their needs in terms of virtual communication. In this system, communicating with the audio and video system of the elderly can provide human-computer interaction. Using input sensors, it is possible to analyze different hand movement gestures and recognize the needs of the elderly based on the type of hand movement. The use of cloud services allows the elderly to communicate with each other based on hand movements, tone of voice, and emotional changes by processing audio and video signals. Examination of the results obtained from the use of this platform showed that the quality of life of the elderly increased with the use of VR systems based on virtual reality.

However, virtual reality can also help patients with cognitive disorders [31]. Physical, emotional, cognitive, and social disorders are important in establishing a balance in people's lives, which can be aided by using artificial intelligence and virtual reality. In solving physical disorders, the level of pain and the strength and ability of people to move should be examined, as well as the level of concentration, the ability to control anger and rage, and the ability to interact with people with cognitive disorders should be considered. The levels of happiness, peace, and prevention of depression, isolation, and lack of self-confidence in the elderly are also included in the emotional disorders section, in which virtual reality can help improve the level of well-being of the elderly by eliminating these disorders [31].

5 Sleeping by the Metaverse

Based on the theories that exist so far about the metaverse and metaphysical space, another challenging issue is the effect of the metaverse on improving the quality of sleep of people, especially those who suffer from sleep disorders. Sufficient sleep is an important physical and mental health concern. If people have enough sleep for an average of 8 hours during the day, they can experience a healthy quality of life physically and mentally. Based on this, the metaverse can optimize sleep. The metaverse-based applications can help people to experience deeper sleep. In fact, virtual reality can help people fall asleep with the vision of their dreams. Whatever they are interested in, think, visualize, and continue visualizing during sleep. Interestingly, the metaverse can also play a role in people's dreams. By penetrating the mental system and understanding his interest in his past experiences or future dreams, he can make him pay as much as he is interested in seeing and re-experiencing his past events and reviewing his favorite memories during his sleep hours. This action can be exciting for the elderly population. This is because they had more experiences of pleasant and bitter events during their lifetime. Their experience can fill the metaverse design model with more data. The random selection of each event that they like to reenact in their dreams requires a camera and headphones that can convert virtual experiences into virtual reality.

As of the last days of 2022, ChatGPT was able to create a great revolution in communication. The metaverse can also affect people's sleep with the ChatGPT! It would be interesting if every person consulted ChatGPT based on his interest in a part of his life that happened in the past or part of his dreams that he would like to happen in the future! The concept of ChatGPT with a metaverse-based application is a dream of virtual reality. The decision about the dream in which each person is interested can be a surprise for the world. Suppose I want to objectively observe what happened to me in the last 10 years! Viewing my past memories in a virtual reality space is so enjoyable that it cannot be compared to anything else. Therefore, by reading my mental space through ChatGPT, which is connected to the world of the metaverse, I can live my past life again in a limited time while sleeping. Living with people who no longer have us is a wonderful transcendental space that can make humanity wonder. With the help of the metaverse, artificial intelligence applications can create such events.

6 Security in the Use of the Metaverse

In [15], various factors that influence the metaverse in human life were investigated. Based on the obtained studies, factors such as culture play an important role in the speed of technological growth in society. Some societies do not believe in the metaverse or the role of virtual reality in life because of the traditional view of life. This causes society to slow down in the direction of modernity. In my opinion, beliefs and religious issues are also important factors in the impact of the metaverse on human life. In reality, the subject of the metaverse is beyond the problem of solid physics and requires a wide view of the human imagination and mind. The power of people's imaginations makes them believe in their interests. With the high level of believability of people toward virtual reality, their use of the metaverse patterns is also higher. Therefore, the metaverse revolution cannot be easily introduced into the lives of people in different societies. First, there should be cultural formation regarding modern technological issues, and then we should accept that virtual reality can also improve health.

There are various challenges to the metaverse medical laboratories that should be carefully investigated [15]. Despite the large amount of data obtained from laboratory results, the laboratory community needs a metaverse space to organize the data. The challenge that will arise in medical laboratories based on the metaverse is the security and privacy of data. Cryptographic algorithms should be able to cover bugs in the metaverse space and eliminate the adverse effects caused by the metaverse using new techniques. One of the driving factors in updating the metaverse technology is cultural change and user expectations from the medical laboratory environment. Therefore, management and evaluation of the economy and trade play a prominent role in the treatment of laboratory patients. Accordingly, the inflation and economic growth rates should be considered in any situation. Therefore, users can use the metaverse patterns in laboratory space. The metaverses can have a positive effect by reducing laboratory costs. Changing the type of communication of users and their level of communication with the treatment staff by the metaverse can help patients safely obtain better treatment. This ease of imagining has a direct impact on the process of improving health. Therefore, people should be provided with a sense of security when using virtual reality technology. The use of 6G era networks with their high-security policy [16] preserves the privacy of users when using the metaverse. The design of cryptographic algorithms in the metaverse-based systems on a new-generation network can increase the access level of users in smart applications based on the metaverse.

7 Emotional Intelligence in the Metaverse

Linguistic intelligence also plays an important role in designing the metaverse-based applications for the elderly [10]. As in the real world, verbal communication has a great effect on emotional relationships between people; in the metaverse world, it can also create effective communication. In the health industry, effective verbal communication between patients and doctors creates healthy emotional relationships. This relationship directly affects the healing process in patients. As patients are psychologically positive, their life expectancy plays a positive role in the treatment process [11]. Based on these studies, managing patients' feelings and emotions will control their body hormone levels, which will improve their health. The interaction between the human brain and computer can also be managed by doctors [12]. Owing to their old age, the elderly have different conditions in their emotional behaviors and interactions with others. Examining their physical and mental condition during treatment can help them manage their emotions and physical changes. If the elderly can always be monitored by virtual reality applications, their physical and mental changes can be predicted using deep learning algorithms. Forecasting these conditions will have a positive effect on lifestyle control and increase the life expectancy of the elderly.

One of the interesting things that can be done to improve patients' condition is their treatment by controlling their physical and mental conditions using an intelligent ChatGPT robot. This robot can be used in the role of a consulting doctor, who is set with the doctor's voice. This interaction is very effective for the elderly, who need a sympathizer to prevent isolation and depression. In addition, the interaction of the elderly with a robot that plays the role of another person can satisfy the needs of the elderly under care to establish social interactions. Understanding the emotions of the elderly in different situations during the day using this humanoid robot has taken a very effective step in the social revolution. It appears that the human brain was replaced by a chat robot. A robot that can work like a human in virtual reality and make decisions will help doctors and medical centers to make difficult decisions. In addition, the production of soothing sounds and music according to the mental needs of the elderly using an intelligent robot can also help improve the conditions of the elderly. According to psychologists, thinking about the fact that one can create something in the world through thought and imagination is somewhat true. Thinking about positive and negative thoughts that will attract them in life has been a challenging issue for researchers with religious beliefs, and how the universe can turn people's thoughts into truth has always been a controversial issue. It is interesting that today, chatbot, which is derived from the science of the metaverse, has been able to turn imagination into pure truth. Today, with smart robots, it is possible to turn a situation into reality by thinking about patients' health, thinking positively or negatively about the current situation, and thinking about the future. Elderly people can improve their mental and physical health many times with happy ideas about their stable lives. By understanding the mental concepts of the elderly, the metaverse-based applications turn their desired conditions into reality and turn the life built into the minds of the elderly into reality. The use of multidimensional cameras can help the elderly spend long hours of the day and night in another life from a different angle of view. These multi-dimensional cameras transform the elderly into different minds, bodies, and thoughts, which cause extraordinary mental changes. The metaverse can make people no longer need one another, either physically or mentally. In addition, the metaverse can ensure the health of patients, especially the elderly, who no longer need the actual presence of doctors to some extent. With all the brilliant results that this robot has in understanding emotions and interacting with the brain of the elderly, it will have errors that do not make humans redundant with the existence of a real doctor. It can be said that this robot will create a significant revolution in the metaverse industry. Again, humans are purest creations that meet the needs of their fellow humans.

8 The Metaverse in the Health Care of the Disabled People

Various physical conditions should be considered when examining the health and care challenges of the elderly. Indeed, the presence of disabled people in society is not rare, and steps should be taken to ensure the well-being and health of this group of people. Disabled people face problems in work and education [13], and when these problems are not solved, they become elderly people with low IQs and low efficiency in society. In every society, it is not possible to provide an ideal life for different age groups with different conditions, and we must anticipate the conditions of people with disabilities in their old age. Examining the physical and mental condition of disabled and mentally retarded elderly people is a challenging issue that can be predicted using machine learning. Artificial intelligence applications using the metaverse technology can provide ideal conditions for the elderly with disabilities. For example, in artificial intelligence applications, by analyzing the existing data obtained from the records of the elderly's illness, mental and physical needs, and life expectancy based on the processing of the image of the elderly's face, it is possible to predict the current conditions for the elderly. Elderly people with physical and mental disabilities can communicate their needs through observation. In this situation, the metaverse can act as a tool to meet their needs.

Designing personal robots for each elderly person with disabilities can be helpful for correctly understanding their thoughts and feelings. In other words, every personal robot uses the metaverse technology to understand the needs of every elderly person and predict their physical and mental needs according to their specific conditions. Teaching fun, educational, and fun activities to the elderly is helpful in keeping their mind dynamic and spirit alive. In the metaverse industry, the processing of neural signals by neuroscience algorithms should be performed properly in order to correctly understand the sensory perceptions of the elderly. In addition to machine learning, the metaverse industry plays an important role in saving time. Customer services for the elderly also play a positive role in welfare. Accurate diagnosis of the needs of the elderly in the shortest possible time can reduce fatigue and boredom and, on the other hand, bring vitality and happiness to the elderly. Such actions increase the life expectancy of the elderly (disabled and disabled).

Thus, the ChatGPT technology can be very useful for communicating with elderly people with disabilities. In particular, elderly people who are unable to communicate and talk because of speech disorders and cannot express the meaning of their speech well can use the ChatGPT to help them express their meaning. By analyzing their speech based on their condition, this application can predict their needs and help them. ChatGPT can be an effective companion for elderly people with disabilities. A correct understanding of the disorders of the disabled elderly and efforts to meet their needs owing to their defects are the most important reasons for supporting chatbots for disabled people. For example, elderly people with a speech disorder may not pronounce words correctly or may repeat them frequently; in this case, the chatbot will quickly understand their meaning and act to help. This action makes it possible to eliminate repetitive speech and reduce repetitive tasks, making the elderly more tired. All these efforts are aimed at predicting conditions using machine learning to create more welfare for people according to their specific physical and mental conditions and needs.

9 Healthy Nutrition with the Metaversal Techniques

Scientifically, it has been proven that healthy nutrition has a significant impact on the health of the human body and the soul. A healthy diet increases the life expectancy and reduces the risk of death. Currently, various factors in the machine world have caused weight gain and improper nutrition, which have resulted in heart attacks and kidney problems. This issue is particularly important for the elderly population. Because the elderly group should receive special care and attention from doctors due to their old age, unhealthy nutrition in this age group poses more risks to their health. You can look at the current world with all the harm it causes to people's physical and mental health, from a different perspective. Artificial intelligence systems can control people's nutrition, and in cases of improper consumption of nutrition, necessary warnings can be given to people. The design of artificial intelligence applications can check people's conditions and suggest a correct diet for people based on their physical and mental characteristics, disease records, gender, age, and use of different drugs.

Machine-learning applications can help predict people's desires for various foods. These applications allow every person to manage their nutrition properly. Therefore, it is important to pay attention to feeding elderly people using intelligent robots. Older adults are more susceptible to Alzheimer's than younger adults. Therefore, nutritional control plays an important role in maintaining health and longevity. Analyzing the condition of the elderly during the day and night based on their cognitive behaviors will help determine the level of changes in their hormones. By predicting changes in hormone levels, it is possible to suggest proper nutrition for the elderly population.

Notably, some people's food preferences are due to a false need for unhealthy food. Therefore, false food trends can be reduced in people with a metaverse revolution. Currently, nutritional psychologists offer this technique for appetite control. Mindfulness regarding food cravings is an important issue that can be addressed using the metaverse. Thinking about unhealthy food desires can fill the mind with false desires within a short period. When a person's mind is filled with false needs, their desire to eat decreases. Nutritional psychologists believe that a man is made of his own mind, and if one can eat mindfully about various issues, especially nutrition, bulimia can be eliminated.

Opinions have been expressed regarding the impact of the metaverse in transforming traditional medical processes. This is the effect of virtual reality on the treatment of patients with mental disorders [14]. According to the suggestions presented in [14], the metaverse can provide virtual training to doctors in geographically deprived areas and virtually perform surgeries without advanced facilities. This technology improves the speed of surgery and saves time for both the doctors and patients. Managing the condition of the elderly (such as controlling blood pressure, blood sugar, heart failure, and kidney failure) during surgery ensures their health during the surgical period.

Among the surgeries that are very common today are the slimming surgeries. Different people, due to improper nutrition and lack of knowledge of food consumption, become overweight, which causes physical and mental harm. Decreased self-confidence and feeling uncomfortable with oneself are examples of mental disorders in overweight individuals. Efforts to improve the physical and mental health of patients undergoing beauty and slimming procedures can be checked by the metaverse. Virtual reality applications can help people suffering from mental and physical disorders due to improper nutrition to treat themselves. Virtual designs of the physical and mental conditions of people in a healthy state make them feel pleasant and take necessary measures to improve their health. Everyone has a dream that makes them take big steps toward truly achieving their goal. Virtual reality cameras can be of great help to people so that they can see their thoughts and imaginations in the future and live in their ideal world for a while. These thoughts made participants feel satisfied and pleasant. Designing practical applications based on virtual reality for the elderly who are overweight owing to their inability to move can also have tremendous effects. By observing their physical and mental conditions using the metaverse cameras, the elderly can gain vitality and hope for life. Trying to feel physical satisfaction and fitness is an important issue that is always a concern. Humans are unconsciously interested in being beautiful and are seen as beautiful. Fitness is one of the most beautiful conditions for people of all age groups, which creates a pleasant feeling and confidence in people.

10 Quantum Medicine in the Metaverse

A quantum world is a space consisting of quantum bits that transmit data at high speed. In this space, communication is performed with a high security and speed. However, the metaverse world, which is a seemingly imaginary space, can contain quantum data and create an environment that goes beyond reality. In this regard, health can be guaranteed with a higher percentage of confidence. Examining the conditions of each person's disease, which are extracted based on the analysis of the data obtained from communication between people, can help improve people's health performance. A quantum world based on the metaverse will take a big step in the medical industry and greatly improve people's mental and physical health. Diagnosing the health of each person in the shortest possible time using quantum speed can help prevent disease occurrence.

In the metaverse world, people are not limited by time and space. In fact, people and their relationships are placed in the temporal dimension. This virtual world was neither physical nor digital. As presented in [32], this is a figital world, and human dynamics are defined in this fig space. In a physical space, the feelings, situations, relationships, and everything that make up the soul and body are physical and tangible. The figital world is a quantum space without the ability to touch objects physically. Human relationships, emotions, and their reactions to situations are displayed in quantum dimensions. Quantum figital space is part of the metaverse world that defines human dynamics in this virtual world based on quantum space. According to theory [32], a combination of place and space can define the dynamics of humans in a digital environment. This definition can affect the mental maps. Geographical physical maps become mental maps, and every person can obtain accurate ideas of geographical situations using the metaverse mentality. If we consider a human being as a physical being that has been transformed into the metaverse space, then different aspects of each human's reactions can be converted based on the metaverse space and place. The relationship space, mental space for thinking, relative space, and absolute space are four important parts of human nature displayed in quantum space [32]. It is scary and may be vague if we think that extraterrestrial beings will be born on the planet in the near future as humans with the metaverse nature. If these beings grow in quantum space with quantum mentality, they will not have any nature from the physical dimension, and this challenge is unbelievable for humanity, which has grown with physical nature! However, with the multiple speeds of technology and the metaverse world that we are currently facing, this issue will probably arise in the near future and will create a fundamental change in humanity. The birth of humans with quantum and metaphysical spaces will be a great revolution in the metaverse era, which can also affect the next generation.

The impact of quantum on human life and even on people who may have the metaverse nature in different dimensions of their lives can have a great impact on their health. The use of quantum computing models allows for faster diagnosis in treatment, improves the performance of patients throughout their lifetime, and

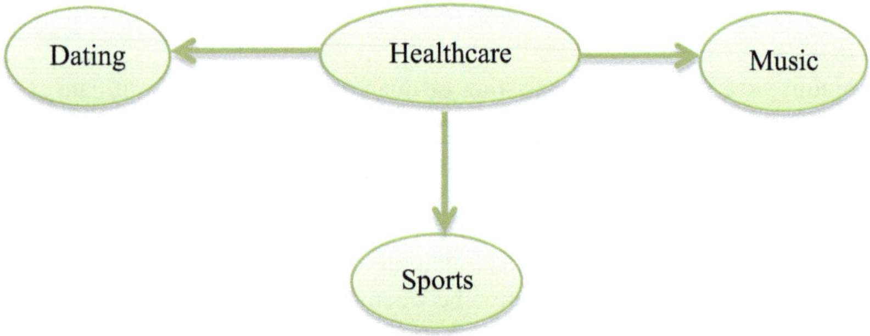

Fig. 2 Improving the lifestyle using the metaverse

can reduce the costs of treating patients [33]. Indeed, daily medical care and improvement of people's health rely on modern technologies. The use of quantum structures in human health can play a significant role in improving health. The idea of combining the metaverse and quantum structures is closely related. The transformation of the physical conditions related to people's health into a quantum environment creates a new space for the treatment and health of people. It is interesting to refer to medical care studies using quantum methods of quantum medicine as a big step in providing services to medical and special care centers. The implementation of quantum algorithms in health care requires the analysis of large amounts of data that include information about people's health levels. The study of the different structures of people's lives and the diseases they face is included in a large database. This database can be a good source for data analysis based on the structure of the quantum algorithms. If the database can be converted into a metaverse space based on quantum patterns, computing time and data storage space will be saved. Quantum space can store data in the metaverse space with different dimensions and obtain good results in the fastest processing time (Fig. 2).

11 Sports in the Metaversial Lifestyle

The metaverse systems on the web can also help people's health through sports movements. In [17], a system that can use multidimensional smart cameras to check the physical movements of the body during exercise, and if the movements change correctly or incorrectly, be warned. Designing sports applications based on the metaverse can motivate older adults to exercise. Physical sports activities with the help of virtual reality cameras under the metaverse help the elderly see the positive effects of sports movements on their physical and mental health and encourage them to exercise at home. Determining the amount of calories consumed in sports and the amount of metabolism of the elderly according to their physical activity in the metaverse-based applications can also put the elderly in a good mental condition. The power of imagination to achieve physical health through sports exercises improves people's health.

It is interesting to note that unveiling the Nikeland sports game as a Nike sports brand in the metaverse has created high interaction in the virtual and real world for users [18]. Nikeland sports, based on the metaverse, proved that age and emotions go beyond sports. In other words, the results obtained from the metaverse sports brand research have shown that sports concepts and the metaverse technology are not far from each other and can be viewed from an evolutionary perspective. In fact, the metaverse view of sports can multiply the pleasure of doing sports and help people who do not show much interest in sports find a positive way of thinking about sports. Designing different sports brands based on the metaverse can create healthy competition. These designs create smart applications with different features in the field of sports that can attract a large audience. Designers use different ideas of user friendliness to register a sports virtual reality system with different brands. This action is a big step toward encouraging different segments of the society to engage in sports. The elderly must be under special care when exercising due to special physical conditions and sometimes due to physical disability due to old age. Therefore, user interface design can be helpful in designing the metaverse-based smart applications for physical activity.

Initial projects using the metaverse in online games were presented for the first time in the design of the Active World and the Palace [21], and online game platforms were presented in the 3D world. Social interaction using social networks began during this period. The design of multidimensional online games based on the metaverse could make significant changes to the Internet game industry. The communication of users in the 3D space of online games causes changes in traditional games. Subsequently, famous games such as Habbo Hotel [22], World of Warcraft [23], Minecraft [22], Fortnite [24], VRChat [25, 26], and game creation Roblox [27–29] expanded social interactions and the 3D virtual world.

With AltspaceVR, designed by Microsoft in 2017, virtual images have become virtual reality [30]. In 2021, Facebook turned its social platform into a meta platform to establish close connections between social interactions in virtual space and the metaverse. These games can have positive effects on mental and physical health, creating social interactions among different age groups. Establishing team communication in online games creates a sense of calmness and healthy interaction in the elderly and eliminates their feelings of isolation. With the introduction of technology, some seniors are unable to communicate well with smart devices. Therefore, the design of intelligent systems for the elderly can eliminate the feeling of weakness, because artificial intelligence is not used.

Additionally, the use of the metaverse sports can be divided into four patterns [19]. Augmented reality, life, virtual world, and mirror world are models of the metaverse that can affect different aspects of people's lives. Virtual reality tennis, table tennis, screen baseball, online sports coaches, sports smart watches, dance training, and virtual yoga are all examples of the role of the metaverse in sports and physical activity systems. By using each of the metaverse models, the different effects of sports can be seen in life. Sports that are suitable for physical and mental activity use different tools to improve health and longevity. In this regard, the metaverse models suitable for the elderly should be used. Teaching virtual yoga and specific physical and mental activities for the elderly can be better than engaging in hard physical activities, such as baseball and football. Therefore, the design of virtual reality systems for the elderly, young people, and even children should be based on age and gender. An issue that should be considered in the health of the elderly during exercise is the control of their heart rate using smartwatches. Adjusting the blood pressure and blood sugar levels of the elderly is also effective in improving their immune system performance during physical and mental exercise. Therefore, the metaverse systems should intelligently control the condition of elderly individuals.

Examining the impact of different sports on people's bodies is an important issue that was further investigated after the coronavirus pandemic and the start of online sports. The popularity of online games has reached its maximum growth rate [20]. It seems that the Corona era was able to create a close relationship between real life and smart life. Examining the relationship between different sports and the metaverse makes it possible to design an intelligent system based on the metaverse, which is suitable for each sport. Traditional and modern sports require their own smart systems to help people exercise through virtual reality cameras. In the design of smart sports systems, the types of individual and team sports should be considered so that good possibilities can be considered in the design of sports systems based on the metaverse. Team sports create healthy competition between people and have positive effects compared to individual sports. Of course, it goes without saying that individual sports can also have positive effects according to the mood and mental condition of each person. Playing team sports is more effective for the elderly in strengthening their mental condition and preventing their isolation. The metaverse-based applications using virtual reality cameras can help senior team sports create a happy and stress-free environment. Based on this, the metaverse can have positive effects on sports for the elderly.

12 Dating Applications Using Metaverse in Health

Dating has always been an important part of people's interactions with their lives. Communicating, hurting, sympathizing, and talking are inseparable parts of every person's life, so that they can live without feeling isolated or lonely. Having a social life is an important definition for everyone along with their personal lives. Every person tries to have the best conversations and interactions with people around them. Now that the age of technology has opened wide ways of communication to people, dating culture has undergone changes. Connecting people is associated with both positive and negative challenges. Overall, however, the positive effect of dating was greater than its negative effect. Communication has become unlimited and everyone can find people who match their mood and personality through social networking and dating applications. Socializing and talking with people who have similar personalities and feelings toward each other is the most enjoyable part of conversation and provides an important part of people's need for conversation. The physical feeling of being together cannot be denied by all interactions that people can have in virtual dating. The physical absence of people is always visible in virtual conversations in dating networks. However, along with the positive aspects that this technology has had in life, negative aspects have also emerged. Virtual dating with the metaverse can provide a feeling of a person's physical existence to some extent. Virtual reality cameras can help anyone visualize another person according to their needs, based on their conversation needs. Virtual reality helps to make a virtual conversation not only completely virtual, but also without expressing feelings. Communicating feelings, including sadness, laughter, and happiness, through virtual reality can turn a conversation into a more intimate interaction. The metaverse managed to reduce the distance between the virtual conversations and the emotional world. The metaverse has created a turning point in the establishment of virtual dating. The metaverse was able to reduce communication distances in virtual conversations and reach an optimal level of people's need for interaction with the help of emotional communication.

13 The Effect of Metaverse on Educational Health Care

As it is known, the world has been affected by the coronavirus since 2019 and it has affected all the important parts of every person's life. The education system of universities and health centers, which cover an important part of the education and health system of society, was involved in many challenges during the coronavirus epidemic. Based on this evidence, during this period, educational centers continued their activities online. The use of different platforms in universities can significantly alter education. Although these changes were negative, they created a wide range of communication. Access to educational courses and concepts has also increased. In this situation, the metaverse was able to hold virtual training at a better level and with higher educational quality [34]. As scientific education in the field of health in universities plays an important role in the health and lives of people, it should be possible to provide good solutions to increase the educational quality of professors and students in special care courses. Educator applications that can use virtual reality to establish scientific communication between medical students and professors will increase the quality of education, and as a result, the health level of society will be guaranteed by increasing scientific health information.

14 The Metaversial Music in the Health of Humanity

Music has always been a food source for the human soul. Few people have reached peace of mind by listening to pleasant voices and soothing music. Music has always been suitable for all age groups, and anyone in any situation, such as happiness, sadness, stress, and excitement, can listen to music that suits their mood, reduces their stress and anger, or increases their happiness and excitement. The metaverse music can also be used to improve the quality of music. The metaverse can turn the music space into virtual reality [35] and bring a deep spiritual feeling to the text and sounds of music. Every person can have a better understanding of the sound and text of music by listening to the sound of music that has been brought closer to the space of reality by the metaverse. The metaverse music is also useful in music science. The design of musical notes based on the use of the metaverse can provide another model of music for the world [36]. This music can be designed for any age group, according to specific mental and physical conditions. The elderly can also order different models of music using virtual reality based on their special mood and use a certain style of music in different situations. Such actions can offer music in virtual reality, and everyone can order special notes based on their needs in any situation to feed their souls. Such a revolution in the music industry based on the metaverse can guarantee the health of the human soul.

15 Conclusions

The metaverse has been able to provide good power for artificial intelligence. The conversion of application systems in various fields that humans need to the power of the metaverse has made ways of communication, treatment, service, and treatment of humanity to be done more quickly and efficiently. However, challenges that arise with the expansion of the metaverse should be carefully examined. In any case, the growth of technology industries, along with its advantages, also has weaknesses, which certainly are not without merit in the use of the metaverse. The health-care industry in every country can use the metaverse-based applications to provide patients with better services. In this chapter, the role of the metaverse in various fields related to health care is discussed and investigated. Since the elderly are an important part of every society and are more exposed to physical and mental injuries due to their physical disability, the role of the metaverse in improving their quality of life and health was specifically investigated. In the near future, the metaverse will take over the world with the help of chat-GPT, positively and negatively affecting people's health. We should try to use this technology to achieve positive efficiency. We hope that this chapter will be an effective step toward increasing the efficiency of the metaverse and its impact on the medical industry.

References

1. Marzooqi, I., & AlMarzooqi, I. (2023). Virtual hospitals – A literature review. *ScienceOpen Preprints*.
2. Liang, H., Li, J., Wang, Y., Pan, J., Zhang, Y., & Dong, X. (2023). Metaverse virtual social center for the elderly communication during the social distancing. *Virtual Reality & Intelligent Hardware, 5*(1), 68–80.
3. Dubovi, I., & Itzhaki, M. (2023). Playing the role of a nurse in a virtual reality simulation: A safe environment for emotion management. *Nurse Educator, 48*(1), 13–18.
4. Jung, O. S., Graetz, I., Dorner, S. C., & Hayden, E. M. (2023). Implementing a COVID-19 virtual observation unit in emergency medicine: Frontline clinician and staff experiences. *Medical Care Research and Review, 80*(1), 79–91.
5. Abiri, A., Keadey, M., Hughes, G., Pitts, S. R., Moran, T. P., & Ross, M. A. (2023). The impact of virtual care in an emergency department observation unit. *Annals of Emergency Medicine, 81*(2), 222–233.
6. Tan, M. W. J., Arciga, M. G. A., Arba'in, J. B., Towle, R. M., Lim, S.-F., Tang, W. H., & Low, L. L. (2023). Outcomes of a "hospital at home" programme for the supervised home recovery of COVID-19 patients in Singapore. *Proceedings of Singapore Healthcare, 32*, 20101058231152049.
7. Roose, K. (2023) The brilliance and weirdness of ChatGPT. *NYTImes*. December 5, 2022 .
8. Lakshmanan, L. (2022, December 16). Why large language models like ChatGPT are bullshit artists. *becominghuman.ai*. Archived from the original on December 17, 2022. Retrieved January 15, 2023. The human raters are not experts in the topic, and so they tend to choose text that looks convincing. They'd pick up on many symptoms of hallucination, but not all. Accuracy errors that creep in are difficult to catch.
9. Taecharungroj, V. (2023). "What can ChatGPT do?" Analyzing early reactions to the innovative AI Chatbot on Twitter. *Big Data and Cognitive Computing, 7*(1), 35.
10. Wang, F.-Y., Miao, Q., Li, X., Wang, X., & Lin, Y. (2023). What does chatGPT say: The DAO from algorithmic intelligence to linguistic intelligence. *IEEE/CAA Journal of Automatica Sinica, 10*(3), 575–579.
11. Shahraki, Z. A., & Nafchi, M. A. (2023). The effect of emotional intelligence applications on the lifestyle of the elderly. In *Multidisciplinary applications of deep learning-based artificial emotional intelligence* (pp. 216–233). IGI Global.
12. Shahraki, Z. A., & Nafchi, M. A. (2023). The impact of brain–computer interface on lifestyle of elderly people. In *Brain-computer interface: Using deep learning applications* (pp. 77–100).
13. McGunnigle, C. (2022). *Disability and the academic job market*. Vernon Art and Science Incorporated.
14. Ahuja, A. S., Polascik, B. W., Doddapaneni, D., Byrnes, E. S., & Sridhar, J. (2023). The digital metaverse: Applications in artificial intelligence, medical education, and integrative health. *Integrative Medicine Research, 12*(1), 100917.
15. Gruson, D., Greaves, R., Dabla, P., Bernardini, S., Gouget, B., & Öz, T. K. (2023). A new door to a different world: Opportunities from the metaverse and the raise of meta-medical laboratories. *Clinical Chemistry and Laboratory Medicine (CCLM)*.
16. Nafchi, M. A., & Shahraki, Z. A. (2022). IT governance and enterprise security policy in the 6G era. In *Next-generation enterprise security and governance* (pp. 227–245). CRC Press.
17. Lee, J., Yoon, H.-K., & Kim, D. (2023). Design of metaverse-based physical fitness service for the enhancement of exercise capability for youth. *Mobile Information Systems, 2023*.
18. Demir, G., Argan, M., & Halime, D. İ. N. Ç. (2023). The age beyond sports: User experience in the world of metaverse. *Journal of Metaverse, 3*(1), 19–27.
19. Yu, J.-E. (2022). Exploration of educational possibilities by four metaverse types in physical education. *Technologies, 10*(5), 104.

20. Mohamad, M. D., & Asyraf. (2023). Sports in the metaverse. In *Metaverse applications for new business models and disruptive innovation* (pp. 150–168). IGI Global.
21. "Active Worlds for Windows (1995)". *MobyGames*. Archived from the original on November 11, 2021. Retrieved November 3, 2021.
22. Brown, D. (2021, August 30). What is the 'Metaverse'? Facebook says it's the future of the Internet. The Washington Post. Retrieved November 1, 2021.
23. Woods, B. (2022, May 7). In Microsoft's Activision deal, it's not just stock prices but a future world at stake. CNBC. Retrieved May 8, 2022.
24. Webster, A. (2021, March 18). Fortnite's experimental story is an attempt to create 'The entertainment experience of the future'. The Verge. Archived from the original on May 3, 2021. Retrieved May 3, 2021.
25. Crawford, A., & Smith, T. (2022, February 23). Metaverse app allows kids into virtual strip clubs. BBC News. Retrieved March 6, 2022.
26. Smith, Q. (2022, May 17). Making sense of VRChat, the 'Metaverse' people actually like (video). Design and art direction by Anni Sayers. People Make Games. Retrieved June 24, 2022 – via YouTube.
27. Wakefield, J. (2021, March 10). Roblox: How the children's game became a $30bn bet on the Metaverse. BBC News. Retrieved January 9, 2022.
28. Sidhwani, P. (2021, March 12). "The history of roblox: From 2004 until now. *TechStory*. Archived from the original on April 20, 2021. Retrieved November 3, 2021.
29. Nike gets ahead of the Metaverse and creates 'Nikeland', its own virtual world on Roblox. entrepreneur.com. Archived from the original on November 26, 2021. Retrieved November 26, 2021.
30. Langston, J. (2021, March 2). 'You can actually feel like you're in the same place': Microsoft Mesh powers shared experiences in mixed reality. *Innovation Stories*. Archived from the original on November 3, 2021. Retrieved November 3, 2021.
31. Chaze, F., Hayden, L., Azevedo, A., Kamath, A., Bucko, D., Kashlan, Y., Dube, M., et al. (2022). Virtual reality and well-being in older adults: Results from a pilot implementation of virtual reality in long-term care. *Journal of Rehabilitation and Assistive Technologies Engineering, 9*, 20556683211072384.
32. Sui, D., & Shaw S.-L. (2022). New human dynamics in the emerging metaverse: Towards a quantum phygital approach by integrating space and place (Vision Paper). In *15th international Conference on Spatial Information Theory (COSIT 2022)*. Schloss Dagstuhl-Leibniz-Zentrum für Informatik.
33. Channi, H. K., & Chowdhary, C. L. (2023). Role of quantum computing for healthcare. In *Handbook of research on quality and competitiveness in the healthcare services sector* (pp. 84–96). IGI Global.
34. Durak, G., & Cankaya, S. (2023). Metaverse technologies and applications in the future of online learning. In *Shaping the future of online learning: Education in the metaverse* (pp. 1–16). IGI Global.
35. Turchet, L. (2023). Musical metaverse: Vision, opportunities, and challenges. *Personal and Ubiquitous Computing*, 1–17.
36. Marlen, D. R., Nastiti, P., Primasari, C. H., Wibisono, Y. P., & Negara, J. G. P. (2023). Analysis of the effect of gamelan metaverse on acceptance of music education methods using technology acceptance model 2. *JISAMAR (Journal of Information System, Applied, Management, Accounting and Research), 7*(1), 22–34.

The Metaverse Game

C. Vanmathi, Harpreet Kaur Channi, Muhammad Fazal Ijaz, Ritik Srivastava, Sai Meghana Bommana, Lauryn Arora, and Chiranji Lal Chowdhary

1 Introduction

The metaverse games are immersive virtual experiences that enable players to partake in various activities within a persistent virtual world. This chapter delves into the multifaceted nature of these games, offering a unique blend of social interaction, exploration, and creativity. Players can personalize avatars, construct virtual homes, and engage in diverse activities and events [1].

A defining characteristic of the metaverse games is their open-world design, allowing players to navigate the virtual realm at their own pace, connect with others, and uncover new activities. This openness fosters emergent gameplay, empowering players to craft their narratives and experiences within this dynamic virtual space.

This chapter explores a spectrum of activities within the metaverse games, spanning combat, exploration, crafting, trading, and socializing. Some games even empower players to create their own games within the overarching game framework, utilizing tools and resources provided by developers [2].

Beyond entertainment, the metaverse games hold the potential to offer educational and career prospects. With increasing sophistication, these games demand skilled developers, designers, and content creators for their creation and maintenance. Furthermore, the virtual economies within these games' present opportu-

C. Vanmathi · R. Srivastava · S. M. Bommana · L. Arora · C. L. Chowdhary (✉)
School of Computer Science Engineering and Information Systems, Vellore Institute of Technology, Vellore, Tamil Nadu, India
e-mail: vanmathi.c@vit.ac.in; chiranji.lal@vit.ac.in

H. K. Channi
Electrical Engineering Department, Chandigarh University, Mohali, Punjab, India

M. F. Ijaz
School of IT and Engineering, Melbourne Institute of Technology, Melbourne, VIC, Australia
e-mail: Mfazal@mit.edu.au

C. L. Chowdhary (ed.), *The Metaverse for the Healthcare Industry*,
https://doi.org/10.1007/978-3-031-60073-9_12

nities for entrepreneurship and financial gains. In essence, the metaverse games usher in a new era of interactive entertainment, providing players with a distinctive and immersive virtual encounter that blurs the boundaries between fantasy and reality [3]. This chapter will delve deeper into these facets, providing an insightful exploration of the evolving landscape of the metaverse games.

2 Background

The notion of a metaverse has roots dating back decades, with initial manifestations found in science fiction literature and cinematic works. However, recent advancements in virtual reality and blockchain technology have propelled the creation of more engaging and interactive metaverse experiences. An early illustration is the emergence of Second Life, a virtual world introduced years ago, enabling users to craft avatars, acquire virtual properties, and engage in immersive interactions within a 3D environment [4]. At its zenith, Second Life boasted over a million active users, exemplifying the growing interest in such virtual spaces.

The integration of blockchain technology has further expanded the horizons of the metaverse experiences, exemplified by the advent of Decentraland in 2017. This decentralized virtual world empowers users to transact virtual real estate using cryptocurrencies, fostering interactions, activities, and events within its virtual landscape. Another noteworthy instance is the Sandbox, a decentralized gaming platform launched in 2019. Here, users can conceive, share, and monetize their gaming experiences, with blockchain facilitating ownership and trading of virtual assets [5].

Reflecting on earlier works in the metaverse gaming domain, Habitat stands out as one of the pioneers, developed in the mid-1980s by Lucasfilm Games (now LucasArts). Habitat, an online multiplayer game for the Commodore 64, allowed players to customize avatars, explore shared virtual realms, and partake in various activities. Similarly, WorldsAway, developed by Fujitsu in the early 1990s, presented an online chat platform featuring graphical avatars, real-time interaction, and immersive environments, laying the groundwork for future metaverse games [6].

The late 1990s and early 2000s witnessed the emergence of the notable metaverse games, including Second Life and There. Linden Lab's Second Life, launched in 2003, remains a prominent example, offering users the ability to shape avatars, own virtual land, and engage in persistent social interactions. There, developed by Makena Technologies in 2003, also emphasized social interaction and creativity. These early metaverse games not only showcased the potential of immersive virtual worlds for fostering social interaction and creativity but also served as foundational inspirations for contemporary metaverse gaming developments. Their enduring impact continues to influence the evolving landscape of the metaverse experiences [7].

The period from 2002 to 2023–2024 witnessed significant evolution in the realm of the metaverse gaming. Following the success of Second Life and There in the early 2000s, developers and innovators continued to push boundaries, introducing new technologies, gameplay mechanics, and social dynamics. This era marked a transition from early experiments to more sophisticated and diverse metaverse experiences [7].

In the mid-2000s, platforms like Second Life continued to thrive, attracting a dedicated user base. However, the landscape saw a diversification of offerings with the introduction of virtual worlds emphasizing specific aspects, such as social interaction, gaming, or immersive experiences. The gaming industry, in particular, saw the rise of massively multiplayer online role-playing games (MMORPGs) that incorporated the metaverse elements, providing expansive virtual worlds for players to explore and interact within [8].

The advent of advanced graphics, improved computing power, and enhanced internet connectivity contributed to more visually stunning and seamless virtual environments. This period also witnessed the integration of augmented reality (AR) and virtual reality (VR) technologies, further enhancing the immersive nature of the metaverse gaming experiences [9].

Blockchain technology continued to play a pivotal role not only in facilitating virtual asset ownership and trading but also in the emergence of blockchain-based games and decentralized economies within the metaverse environments. NFTs (non-fungible tokens) gained prominence as a means to represent ownership of unique in-game items, contributing to the development of virtual economies [10].

During this time, diverse genres of the metaverse games emerged, catering to a wide range of player preferences. Some games focused on narrative-driven experiences, while others emphasized competitive gameplay, creative building, or social interaction. User-generated content became a central theme, allowing players to contribute to the evolving narratives and landscapes within these virtual worlds [11].

The metaverse gaming industry also saw collaborations with real-world industries, such as education, health care, and business, exploring innovative ways to leverage virtual environments for various purposes.

As we approach 2023–2024, the metaverse gaming landscape continues to evolve, with ongoing advancements in technology, an expanding user base, and an increasing integration of virtual and real-world elements. The journey from the early 2000s to the present day represents a dynamic and transformative period in the development of the metaverse games, shaping the future of interactive entertainment and virtual experiences.

3 Preliminaries: Some of the Most Popular Metaverse Games

3.1 Dark Forest

Dark Forest is a blockchain game designed by MIT graduate Brian Gu, also known as Gubsheep. It stands out as the first decentralized incomplete-information game, blending cutting-edge cryptography with science fiction themes. The game challenges players to explore the potential applications of new technologies, offering a unique gaming experience. It fosters a transparent blockchain and enables the creation of autonomous decentralized digital worlds.

Dark Forest has been recognized as a prime example of a "new vision for the metaverse" in which blockchain technology serves as the foundation for transparent and decentralized social systems. By pushing the boundaries of blockchain technology, Dark Forest is not just revolutionizing the gaming industry but also redefining our understanding of social systems within the metaverse. It represents a significant step forward in the ongoing evolution of blockchain technology and its applications [12].

3.2 *Axie Infinity*

Axie Infinity is a metaverse game that incorporates advanced technologies such as blockchain, cryptocurrencies, NFTs, and AR to create a distinctive gaming experience. Utilizing Ethereum, Axie Infinity ensures safe, transparent, and tamper-proof transactions within the game, eliminating the need for intermediaries. The game employs cryptocurrencies, particularly Axie Infinity Shards (AXS), as a chief currency, allowing players to make in-game purchases and receive rewards. Players can earn AXS through battles, quests, and trading. Axie Infinity leverages NFTs to represent the unique characteristics of each Axie, making each in-game creature one-of-a-kind. The rarity of certain Axies contributes to a thriving marketplace on cryptocurrency platforms. The integration of AR technology enhances player immersion, allowing them to engage with their Axies in the real world by scanning QR codes with their smartphones.

Unique Gaming Environment: Axie Infinity's utilization of blockchain, cryptocurrencies, NFTs, and AR results in a decentralized gaming experience where players can earn real-world rewards while enjoying the game [13].

3.3 *Second Life*

Second Life is a highly customizable virtual world that has been a prominent player in the metaverse landscape since its development by Linden Lab in 2003. A unique feature is the ability for users to create and customize avatars, allowing for diverse appearances from realistic humans to fantasy creatures.

Users can purchase virtual land to create personalized spaces, contributing to the virtual real estate market and the in-game economy, facilitated by Linden Dollars. Second Life is known for its rich and diverse community, engaging in activities from socializing to gaming [7]. The platform encourages creativity, with users designing virtual clothing, buildings, and more.

Beyond gaming, Second Life has been used for educational and research purposes, simulating historical events, hosting virtual classrooms, and facilitating virtual meetings and conferences. Users have the potential to make real money by selling virtual creations in the marketplace or offering custom services to other players, adding an economic dimension to the virtual world.

These metaverse games showcase the diverse ways in which technology, creativity, and innovation intersect to create immersive and transformative virtual experiences. Each game contributes uniquely to the evolving metaverse landscape, pushing boundaries and redefining the possibilities within virtual worlds.

4 How Are Newer Metaverse Games Better?

How have contemporary metaverse games improved upon their predecessors? While the concept of the metaverse games has existed for decades, recent years have witnessed a noteworthy evolution in their design and implementation. Following are the key distinctions between older and newer metaverse games.

4.1 Technological Advancements

Early metaverse games were constrained by the technology of their time, such as text-based interfaces in games like Habitat and LambdaMOO from the 1980s and 1990s. Later games like Second Life and World of Warcraft (launched in 2003 and 2004, respectively) introduced 3D graphics but were limited by available hardware. Modern metaverse games leverage advances in virtual reality (VR) and augmented reality (AR) technology, providing more immersive and interactive gaming experiences.

4.2 Social Interaction Focus

Older metaverse games often centered around single-player experiences, offering limited social interaction. Modern counterparts, like Fortnite and Roblox, prioritize social experiences, emphasizing collaboration and community building. Players can team up to complete challenges or construct virtual structures, fostering a more communal gaming environment.

4.3 Openness and Extensibility

A distinctive feature of contemporary metaverse games is their openness. Unlike earlier closed systems, modern games are designed to be extensible and adaptable.

Developers can create apps and add-ons that seamlessly integrate within the game world, expanding functionality and unlocking new opportunities for players.

4.4 Scalability Improvements

Newer metaverse games exhibit enhanced scalability. Early games, such as Second Life, faced limitations in supporting concurrent players, often breaking down beyond a certain threshold. Modern games like Minecraft and Roblox utilize cloud computing and advanced technologies to accommodate millions of players, contributing to their widespread popularity.

4.5 Evolution of Business Models

Shifts in business models distinguish old and new metaverse games. Early games were typically standalone products purchased for a fixed duration. In contrast, contemporary metaverse games often adopt a free-to-play model, granting players free access to the game world while enabling the purchase of virtual items or upgrades using real-world currency. This model allows developers to generate ongoing revenue and establish a more sustainable business framework.

In summary, the continuous development of the metaverse games has led to substantial improvements in technology, social interaction, openness, scalability, and business models, collectively contributing to a more dynamic and engaging gaming experience.

5 Latest Developments in the Architecture of a General Metaverse Game

5.1 Client-Side Architecture

- Utilizing advanced rendering techniques, including real-time ray tracing and AI-based graphics enhancements, to deliver visually stunning and realistic game environments.
- Ensuring seamless experiences across diverse devices, encompassing desktop computers, mobile devices, and emerging technologies like extended reality (XR) headsets.

5.2 *Network Architecture*

- Implementing blockchain technology to enhance the security and transparency of in-game transactions, including virtual asset ownership and trading.
- Exploring decentralized networking solutions to optimize performance, scalability, and reliability, ensuring a smooth and immersive experience for users.

5.3 *Game Engine*

- Incorporating machine learning algorithms within the game engine to enhance AI behavior, providing dynamic and adaptive non-player characters (NPCs) for a more engaging gaming experience.
- Improving physics simulations for greater accuracy, realistic lighting, and shadows, ensuring a heightened level of immersion for users.

5.4 *Database*

- Leveraging blockchain for secure storage of virtual assets, ensuring transparency, ownership, and preventing fraudulent activities.
- Implementing distributed database systems for improved scalability, handling vast amounts of player data while maintaining performance and data integrity.

5.5 *Middleware*

- Exploring decentralized identity services to enhance user authentication, privacy, and reduce reliance on centralized servers for increased security.
- Adhering to industry standards for middleware services, fostering seamless integration with external services, and maintaining high levels of data security and privacy.

5.6 *Application Programming Interface (API)*

- Following OpenAPI standards to provide third-party developers with a well-documented, user-friendly, and feature-rich API for building applications that interact with the metaverse game.

- Exploring decentralized API gateways for increased reliability, reduced latency, and a resilient infrastructure to support third-party developers.

These architectural advancements signify ongoing efforts to enhance technology, security, and user experiences within the metaverse games, contributing to more immersive, scalable, and interconnected virtual worlds.

6 Components of a Metaverse Game (Table 1)

Before diving into the components of a metaverse game, it is essential to understand the multifaceted nature of these virtual environments. Metaverse games are not just

Table 1 Components of a metaverse game

Component	Description	References
Virtual world	The primary game environment, fully or partially 3D, with different regions for player exploration	[14]
Avatars	Player-controlled characters representing the player within the game, customizable in appearance and abilities	[15]
Social interaction	Tools and systems for player interaction, including chat systems, messaging, voice chat, and other social features	[16]
Economy	In-game currency or mechanisms for exchanging value, such as virtual goods, services, or real-world currency	[17]
Object creation	Tools for players to create and customize objects, including building or programming tools and 3D modeling software	[18]
Quests/challenges	Pre-determined or dynamically generated goals or challenges for players, providing rewards or benefits upon completion	[19]
Game mechanics	Underlying systems governing gameplay, including movement, combat, physics, and other mechanics	[20]
User-generated content	Ability for players to create, share, and distribute their content, including objects, levels, characters, and assets	[21]
Augmented reality	Integration of virtual objects or information into the real-world environment through mobile devices or wearable technology	[22]
Virtual reality	Immersive technologies allowing players to experience the game world in 3D, often through head-mounted displays and VR hardware	[23]
Blockchain technology	Use of blockchain and cryptocurrency technology to facilitate ownership, trade, and exchange of virtual assets within the game	[24]
Artificial intelligence	Use of intelligent agents or AI systems to provide dynamic, responsive, or personalized gameplay experiences	[25]

simple games but complex ecosystems that blend various technologies and interactive elements to create immersive, persistent virtual worlds. These components work together to enhance player engagement, foster social interactions, and support a vibrant economy. Below is an overview of the primary components that constitute a metaverse game, each playing a crucial role in shaping the overall player experience.

7 Core Concepts Involved in the Metaverse Games

7.1 Reinforcement Learning (RL)

As the metaverse games evolve, non-player characters (NPCs) require increased intelligence. Reinforcement Learning (RL) is pivotal in achieving this, enabling NPCs to make intelligent decisions. The metaverse games, mimicking the real world, feature complex environments with numerous NPCs. Implementing RL-based NPCs in such games involves addressing large-scale reinforcement learning tasks, particularly challenging due to the vast number of tasks requiring reward functions. However, the metaverse games often provide limited feedback to RL-based agents, posing difficulties in achieving success for complex tasks. To mitigate these challenges, incorporating a curiosity mechanism proves effective. This mechanism enables agents to learn intrinsic rewards based on curiosity, reducing the need for manually designing sparse reward functions.

7.2 Blockchain Technology

Blockchain, a decentralized digital ledger, ensures secure and transparent information storage. Unlike centralized databases, blockchain's distributed nature prevents data tampering. Originally designed for cryptocurrencies, blockchain has found applications in the metaverse games. Popular blockchain games, including Axie Infinity and Decentraland, utilize this technology for secure ownership, trade, and exchange of virtual assets. Blockchain in gaming extends to in-game currency transactions, preventing fraud and theft through encryption. Additionally, it authenticates users and uses digital signatures to ensure transaction authenticity, enhancing privacy and security in the metaverse gaming environments.

7.3 Cryptography

Cryptography plays a crucial role in ensuring the security and privacy of in-game transactions and interactions in the metaverse games. It involves using mathematical algorithms to secure communication against third-party interference. Cryptography applications include encrypting payment information to protect sensitive data and authenticating users to ensure authorized access. Digital signatures authenticate in-game transactions, assuring players of transaction legitimacy. Cryptography also addresses privacy concerns, encrypting messages and sensitive data to safeguard player privacy and restrict access to authorized parties.

7.4 Non-Fungible Tokens (NFTs)

NFTs, or non-fungible tokens, have gained popularity in the metaverse games as representations of and trading platforms for virtual assets. In the metaverse games, NFTs represent unique and valuable in-game items, providing players with true ownership. Built on blockchain technology, NFTs ensure security, verifiability, and authenticity of traded assets, preventing fraud. Beyond ownership, NFTs offer avenues for players to monetize in-game activities, creating new opportunities for income. NFTs also facilitate asset transfer between different games or platforms, allowing players to retain control over assets even when switching games or platforms.

7.5 Augmented Reality (AR)

AR enhances the immersive experience in the metaverse games by blending physical and virtual elements. In mobile games, AR uses smartphone cameras to overlay digital objects onto the real world, creating a unique sense of excitement and adventure. AR further fosters social interactions by allowing players to see virtual representations of friends' avatars in real-world surroundings, enhancing the sense of community. Customization is another AR advantage, enabling users to personalize their game experience by placing virtual objects in real-world surroundings. The interactive nature of AR, where real-world objects unlock virtual content, adds dynamism to the gaming experience, making it more engaging.

These core concepts collectively contribute to shaping the dynamic and evolving landscape of the metaverse games, providing players with new dimensions of engagement, ownership, security, and personalization. As the popularity of the metaverse games continues to grow, these concepts will likely play an even more pivotal role in shaping the future of gaming.

8 Drawbacks of the Metaverse Games

8.1 Technological Restrictions

The Metaverse games demand cutting-edge technology, putting a significant strain on computational power. Gamers with outdated or underpowered equipment may struggle to enjoy the game, leading to dissatisfaction and potential expulsion from the gaming community.

8.2 Network Restrictions

A stable and high-speed internet connection is crucial for the proper functioning of the metaverse games. Slow or unstable connections can result in latency, disconnections, and technical issues that degrade the overall gaming experience for players.

8.3 Risks Related to Security

The metaverse games based on blockchain and cryptocurrencies are susceptible to security risks and hacking attempts. The integrity of the game and its environment may be compromised, leading to the loss of valuable assets and confidential data. Hacking attempts, phishing assaults, and other strategies may be employed by malicious actors to steal players' assets or gain unauthorized access to their accounts. Centralized servers storing player data and insecure third-party marketplaces for in-game items pose additional risks, exposing players to potential data breaches, fraud, and scams.

8.4 Complexity

The metaverse games introduce a significant technical disadvantage due to their complexity. Integrating cutting-edge technologies such as blockchain, virtual and augmented reality, non-fungible tokens (NFTs), and cryptocurrencies can make these games challenging to develop and enjoy. Skilled developers are essential to create a stable and immersive gaming environment. The complexity of these games may also pose a barrier for new players, as understanding and navigating the game may be challenging without familiarity with the underlying technologies. This complexity could potentially limit the market appeal of the metaverse games.

9 Future Research Directions in the Metaverse Games

As the metaverse games continue to evolve, researchers and developers are exploring new avenues to enhance user experiences, address challenges, and unlock the full potential of this immersive gaming genre. Several exciting future research directions are emerging and are discussed below.

9.1 Advanced Artificial Intelligence (AI) Integration

Dynamic NPCs: Research could focus on refining reinforcement learning algorithms to create more intelligent and adaptive non-player characters (NPCs) within the metaverse games. Developing NPCs that exhibit advanced decision-making and adaptability in complex virtual environments remains a key challenge.

Curiosity Mechanism: Further exploration of the curiosity mechanism in reinforcement learning can be undertaken to enhance the learning process for AI agents, especially in scenarios where traditional reward structures are sparse.

9.2 Blockchain Innovations

Scalability and Efficiency: Research may target enhancing blockchain technology for the metaverse games, addressing scalability issues, and improving overall efficiency in handling large-scale virtual economies.

Interoperability: Research may explore ways to improve interoperability between different blockchain-based metaverse games, enabling seamless asset transfer and interactions across diverse virtual worlds.

9.3 Cryptography and Security

Privacy Solutions: Future research could focus on developing advanced cryptographic techniques to further safeguard user privacy in the metaverse games, especially in transactions and interactions involving sensitive information.

Anti-fraud Measures: Research may investigate innovative cryptographic solutions to prevent fraud, unauthorized access, and data manipulation, ensuring a secure and trustworthy gaming environment.

9.4 User Experience Enhancements

Cross-Platform Integration: Research may explore methods to enhance cross-platform integration, allowing users to seamlessly transition between different devices while maintaining a consistent and immersive gaming experience.

Innovative Interaction Models: Investigate novel interaction models, such as gesture-based controls, voice commands, and haptic feedback, to create more immersive and natural user interfaces within the metaverse.

9.5 Economic and Social Impacts

Virtual Economy Studies: Research may explore the economic dynamics of virtual worlds, including inflation, currency exchange, and the impact of player-driven economies on overall gameplay and user engagement.

Social Dynamics: Research may explore the social implications of the metaverse games, including the formation of virtual societies, governance structures, and the psychological impact of extended virtual interactions.

9.6 Educational Applications

Learning Environments: Research may investigate the potential of the metaverse games as educational tools, creating immersive learning environments for various subjects and age groups.

Skill Development: Research may focus on how the metaverse games can contribute to skill development, creativity, and problem-solving abilities in users.

9.7 Ethical Considerations

Ethics in Game Design: Delves into the ethical considerations surrounding the metaverse game design, including issues related to addiction, mental health, and the impact of virtual experiences on real-world behavior.

9.8 *Environmental Sustainability*

Energy Consumption: Research may focus on optimizing the energy consumption of the metaverse game platforms, exploring sustainable technologies to minimize the environmental impact of running large-scale virtual worlds.

9.9 *Inclusive Design*

Accessibility: Research may focus on ways to make the metaverse games more accessible to individuals with diverse abilities, ensuring that virtual worlds are inclusive and accommodating to a broad audience.

As the metaverse continues to expand and captivate audiences, ongoing research efforts will play a crucial role in shaping the future of the metaverse games, ensuring they remain innovative, enjoyable, and ethically sound.

10 Conclusion

In conclusion, the dynamic landscape of the metaverse games represents a frontier where technology, creativity, and user experiences converge to redefine the future of interactive entertainment. From the integration of cutting-edge technologies like AI, blockchain, and augmented reality to the intricate balance of economic ecosystems within virtual worlds, the metaverse games offer a glimpse into a realm where the boundaries between reality and fiction blur.

While the potential for unprecedented immersion and innovation is evident, challenges such as technological limitations, security risks, and the complexity of design must be navigated. Researchers, developers, and industry stakeholders are at the forefront of shaping this digital frontier, addressing these challenges, and unlocking new possibilities.

The metaverse is not merely a realm of entertainment but a canvas for interdisciplinary exploration, ranging from advanced AI architectures and cryptographic solutions to novel interaction models and educational applications. As the metaverse evolves, ethical considerations, environmental sustainability, and inclusive design become integral facets of its development, ensuring that this digital realm reflects the diversity and values of its users.

In this ongoing journey into the metaverse, collaboration and exploration will drive innovation. The convergence of technological prowess and human creativity promises a future where the metaverse games transcend boundaries, offering experiences that captivate, educate, and inspire. As we navigate this uncharted territory, the metaverse stands as a testament to the limitless possibilities that arise when imagination meets technology, forging a path toward a digital frontier that is both exciting and transformative.

References

1. Wang, G., Badal, A., Jia, X., Maltz, J. S., Mueller, K., Myers, K. J., Niu, C., Vannier, M., Yan, P., Yu, Z., & Zeng, R. (2022). Development of metaverse for intelligent healthcare. *Nature Machine Intelligence, 4*(11), 922–929.
2. Lee, C. W. (2022). Application of metaverse service to healthcare industry: A strategic perspective. *International Journal of Environmental Research and Public Health, 19*(20), 13038.
3. Bansal, G., Rajgopal, K., Chamola, V., Xiong, Z., & Niyato, D. (2022). Healthcare in metaverse: A survey on current metaverse applications in healthcare. *IEEE Access, 10*, 119914–119946.
4. Veerapen, M. (2013). Where do virtual worlds come from?: A genealogy of second life. *Games and Culture*, (2), 98–116.
5. Far, S. B., Rad, A. I., & Asaar, M. R. (2023). Blockchain and its derived technologies shape the future generation of digital businesses: A focus on decentralized finance and the metaverse. *Data Science and Management, 6*(3), 183–197.
6. Rauscher, A. (2019). From cineludic form to mise-en-game: The ludification of cinematic storyworlds in the star wars video games. *Franchise Era: Managing Media in the Digital Economy, 119.*
7. Santos, R. P. (2014). Second life physics: Virtual, real, or surreal? *arXiv* preprint arXiv:1405.6327. 2014 May 24.
8. Sun, S., Kim, J. H., Lee, K. M., & Nan, D. (2023). Exploring the association between the Proteus effect and intention to play massive multiplayer online role-playing games (MMORPGs). *Internet Research.*
9. Dincelli, E., & Yayla, A. (2022). Immersive virtual reality in the age of the Metaverse: A hybrid-narrative review based on the technology affordance perspective. *The Journal of Strategic Information Systems, 31*(2), 101717.
10. Christodoulou, K., Katelaris, L., Themistocleous, M., Christodoulou, P., & Iosif, E. (2022). NFTs and the metaverse revolution: Research perspectives and open challenges. *Blockchains and the Token Economy: Theory and Practice*, 139–178.
11. Dwivedi, Y. K., Hughes, L., Baabdullah, A. M., Ribeiro-Navarrete, S., Giannakis, M., Al-Debei, M. M., Dennehy, D., Metri, B., Buhalis, D., Cheung, C. M., & Conboy, K. (2022). Metaverse beyond the hype: Multidisciplinary perspectives on emerging challenges, opportunities, and agenda for research, practice and policy. *International Journal of Information Management*, (66), 102542.
12. Yao, N., Lin, Z., Wu, X., & Wang, L. (2022). Freedom and restraint in dark forest: A peek at the metaverse through a blockchain game. *IEEE Transactions on Computational Social Systems.*
13. Akkus, H. T., Gursoy, S., Dogan, M., & Demir, A. B. (2022). Metaverse and metaverse cryptocurrencies (meta coins): Bubbles or future? *Journal of Economics Finance and Accounting, 9*(1), 22–29.
14. Bhugaonkar, K., Bhugaonkar, R., & Masne, N. (2022). The trend of metaverse and augmented & virtual reality extending to the healthcare system. *Cureus, 14*(9).
15. Tan TF, Li Y, Lim JS, Gunasekeran DV, Teo ZL, Ng WY, Ting DS. Metaverse and virtual health care in ophthalmology: Opportunities and challenges The Asia-Pacific Journal of Ophthalmology 2022 11(3):237–46.'
16. Kerdvibulvech, C., & Chang, C. C.. (2022). A new study of integration between social robotic systems and the metaverse for dealing with healthcare in the post-COVID-19 situations. In *International conference on social robotics*, 2022 Dec 13 (pp. 392–401). Springer Nature.
17. Thomason, J. (2022). Metaverse, token economies, and non-communicable diseases. *Global Health Journal, 6*(3), 164–167.
18. Mourtzis, D. (2023). The metaverse in industry 5.0: A human-centric approach towards personalized value creation. *Encyclopedia, 3*(3), 1105–1120.

19. Dincelli, E., & Yayla, A. (2022). Immersive virtual reality in the age of the metaverse: A hybrid-narrative review based on the technology affordance perspective. *The Journal of Strategic Information Systems, 31*(2), 101717.
20. Yadav, C. (2023). Machine learning in the metaverse: Building intelligent virtual worlds. *Journal of Informatics Education and Research, 3*(2).
21. Kasapakis, V., & Gavalas, D. (2017). User-generated content in pervasive games. *Computers in Entertainment (CIE), 16*(1), 1–23.
22. Xu J. (2022). From augmented reality location-based games to the real-world metaverse. In *Extended abstracts of the 2022 annual symposium on computer-human interaction in play*, 2022 Nov 2 (pp. 364–366).
23. Nevelsteen, K. J. (2018). Virtual world, defined from a technological perspective and applied to video games, mixed reality, and the metaverse. *Computer Animation and Virtual Worlds, 29*(1), e1752.
24. Panda, S. K. (2023). Revolution of the metaverse and blockchain technology. *Metaverse and Immersive Technologies: An Introduction to Industrial, Business and Social Applications., 20*, 97–125.
25. Huynh-The, T., Pham, Q. V., Pham, X. Q., Nguyen, T. T., Han, Z., & Kim, D. S. (2023). Artificial intelligence for the metaverse: A survey. *Engineering Applications of Artificial Intelligence, 117*, 105581.

The Metaverse and Its Related Technologies in Telesurgery in Healthcare 5.0: A Case Study

Siva Rama Krishnan Somayaji

1 Introduction

1.1 Metaverse

The metaverse is a fictitious version of the Internet that is made possible using augmented reality (AR) and virtual reality (VR) headsets. It is a single, ubiquitous, and immersive virtual universe. Built on a foundation of blockchain technology, the metaverse [1] is a spatial computing platform that offers virtual experiences as an alternative to or a duplicate of the actual world, complete with all the essential elements of civilization, such as social interactions, currency, commerce, economy, and property ownership. A variety of three-dimensional worlds may be accessible by a headset, smartphone app, or website in the metaverse. People might engage and experience in real time over great distances with it. The result will be an extensive web application ecosystem. An almost infinite number of users can experience synchronously [2] and persistently a massively scaled and interoperable network of real-time rendered 3D virtual worlds with a sense of personal presence and continuity of data, including identity, history, entitlements, objects, communications, and payments.

As a rapidly developing paradigm for the future generation of the Internet, the metaverse seeks to create a completely immersive, hyperspatiotemporal, and self-sufficient virtual shared environment where people may interact, work, and play. The metaverse is transitioning from science fiction to an impending reality, propelled by recent developments in cutting-edge technology like blockchain,

S. R. K. Somayaji (✉)
School of Computer Science Engineering and Information Systems, VIT, Vellore, Tamil Nadu, India
e-mail: siva.s@vit.ac.in

C. L. Chowdhary (ed.), *The Metaverse for the Healthcare Industry*,
https://doi.org/10.1007/978-3-031-60073-9_13

artificial intelligence, and extended reality. By the Internet, the metaverse creates a virtual environment [3] where human emotions and movements are replicated. It encompasses the entire real-world and virtual world social and economic structures. In general, the technologies that businesses allude to when discussing "the metaverse" might include augmented reality, which blends elements of the digital and physical worlds, and virtual reality, which is defined by persistent virtual worlds that remain even when you are not playing. It is not necessary, though, for certain areas to just be accessible through VR or AR. Virtual worlds have begun calling themselves "the metaverse." Examples of these worlds include parts of Fortnite [4] that are accessible via PCs, game consoles, and even smartphones.

Notwithstanding the metaverse's encouraging signs, security and privacy concerns remain the main obstacles to its further growth. In the metaverse, a variety of security flaws [5] and privacy violations might occur from handling enormous data streams, ubiquitous user profiling, unfair AI algorithmic results, to the security of physical infrastructures and human bodies.

1.2 Telesurgery

Telesurgery, often known as remote surgery, is a newly developed surgical instrument that links patients and surgeons who are geographically separated by using wireless networking and robotic technology. The primary benefit of Telesurgery [6] is its capacity to get beyond the drawbacks of traditional surgery, which include extensive travel distances, financial expenditures, shortages of surgeons, and geographical barriers to quick, high-quality surgical care. By improving operation safety and offering technical correctness, this technology helps both patients and surgeons and delivers top-notch surgery to underprivileged medical settings, including remote communities, military bases, and spaceships. Surgeons at separate centers can receive simultaneous high-definition visual input [7] from today's 3D display systems, enabling real-time surgical cooperation between doctors at several hospitals.

Though Telesurgery came as a breakthrough especially during the COVID-19, there are several challenges. Concerns about patient privacy and safety, the high upfront and ongoing expenses of adoption, and ethical and legal issues are all considered. Privacy is very important, especially when sending sensitive photos of patient data over the Internet. But cyberattacks and erratic connections can make it more difficult to do Telesurgery in a way that is both morally and safely compliant. An unstable connection can also cause latency, increasing the possibility of errors occurring during surgery and lengthening the duration of the treatment (Fig. 1).

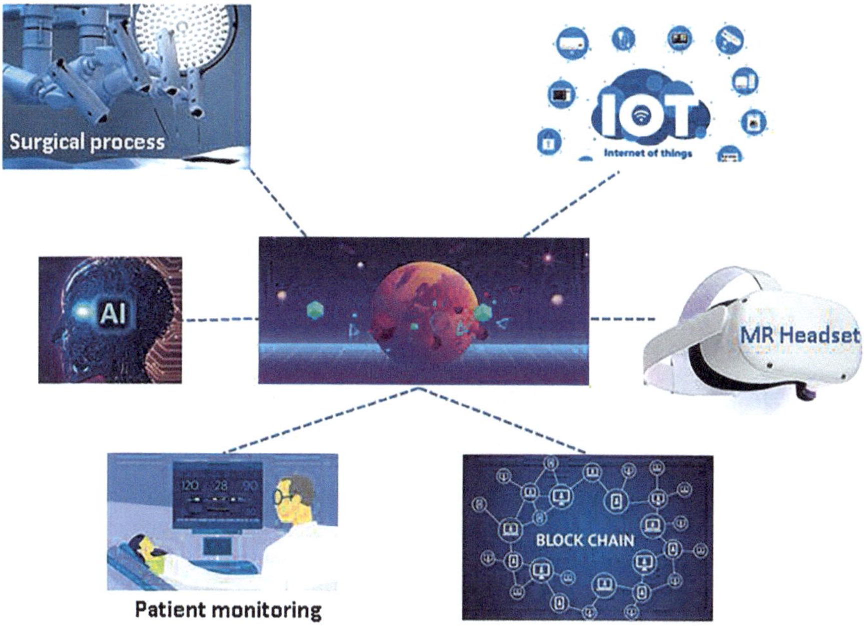

Fig. 1 The metaverse for Telesurgery

1.3 Industry 5.0

The Fifth Industrial Revolution, or Industry 5.0, is a new and developing stage of industrialization in which robots [8] with artificial intelligence (A.I.) and cutting-edge technology collaborate to improve workplace procedures. This is combined with a stronger emphasis on sustainability, resilience, and a more human-centric approach. People who collaborate with robots and intelligent machinery are referred to as Industry 5.0 workers. It is about using cutting-edge technology like big data and the Internet of Things (IoT) to enable robots to assist people in doing tasks more efficiently and quickly. It gives the efficiency [9] and automation cornerstones of Industry 4.0 a more intimate, human touch. Industry 5.0 aims to combine cognitive computing capabilities with human intellect and resourcefulness in collaborative operations as workplace devices become more intelligent and networked.

The primary benefit of Industry 5.0 is in the generation of higher-paying employment that provides customers with more personalization options and employees with more design flexibility. Human workers may devote more of their time to providing better, customized services and goods when industrial operations are delegated to automation, allowing automation to manage production processes frees up human laborers [10] to devote more of their time to providing better, customized services and goods. Industry 5.0 is a concept that transcends "industry." It holds true for any industry and any type of organization that comes to mind. Its usefulness is therefore far broader than Industry 4.0. Thus, we must adopt a wide and universal viewpoint that applies to all industries while debating the strategic implications of Industry 5.0. Industry 5.0 is built around three main pillars, as outlined by the European Commission in this infographic: human-centric, resilient, and sustainable. Adopting Industry 5.0 is costly as it calls for highly trained workers [11] and intelligent machinery to boost output and efficiency. Industry 5.0 has security challenges since building ecosystem trust is essential.

1.4 Blockchain

A blockchain is a distributed ledger or database that is shared by all nodes in a computer network. Though they have applications outside of cryptocurrencies, they are most recognized for playing a critical part in cryptocurrency systems that preserve a safe and decentralized record of transactions. Any sector may employ blockchain technology to make data immutable, or incapable of being changed. A blockchain is made up of programs known as scripts that carry out the operations that are typically performed in a database: entering, retrieving, and saving data, among other things. A distributed blockchain [12] requires many copies to be kept on numerous devices and must match in order for it to be considered legitimate. Transaction data is gathered by the blockchain and stored in blocks. When it is filled, an encryption technique is used to the data, resulting in the hash—a hexadecimal number—being generated. After that, the hash is encrypted along with the other data in the block and added to the next block header. As a result, a chain of linked blocks is produced. A blockchain enables data in a database to be dispersed over several network nodes, or computers or other devices running blockchain software, at different places. In addition to adding redundancy, this keeps the data accurate.

A smart contract is a collection of instructions [13] that are automatically performed and recorded on the blockchain to speed up transactions. In addition to many other things, a smart contract can specify parameters for the payment of trip insurance and corporate bond transfers. Every block has links to the ones that come before and after it. When an asset is transferred or ownership is changed, these pieces come together to form a chain of data. The blocks securely connect together to prevent any block from being edited or a block from being added between two existing blocks. They also certify the precise timing and order of transactions.

Blockchain-based tokenization of assets is known as non-fungible tokenization (NFT) [14]. They are given distinct identifiers and information to set them apart from other tokens. NFTs are produced using a procedure known as minting, in which a blockchain is used to record the NFT's data. In essence, the minting process comprises three steps: the creation of a new block, the validation of NFT data by a validator, and the closing of the block. Smart contracts that control the NFT's transferability and assign ownership are frequently incorporated during this minting procedure.

1.5 The Metaverse in Telesurgery

Healthcare 5.0, which offers emotional telemedicine, Telesurgery, wellness monitoring, virtual clinics, and individualized treatment, is the next evolution of smart healthcare. As a result, the metaverse presents itself as a useful instrument for utilizing digital connection to enhance healthcare in virtual settings. The metaverse's healthcare system offers interactive, immersive, and enjoyable healthcare services [15] that are tailored to each patient's requirements. The sophisticated technological innovations such as blockchain, telepresence, augmented reality, virtual reality, and artificial intelligence (AI) are all part of the metaverse and have a significant influence on healthcare. It is difficult to simulate a whole operating room in the actual world since the metaverse is a complex system that integrates several technologies. Furthermore, since Telesurgery requires extremely delicate and exact control, mistakes from a metaverse setting should be quite rare. The metaverse integrates a multitude [16] of cutting-edge technologies and has considerable promise for use in medical diagnosis, treatment, rehabilitation, and teaching, among other medical-related duties. However, there are also a lot of technological and application-level difficulties that the medical metaverse is now dealing with. The interactions between patients and doctors, patients and treatment resources, and other users are more frequent and complex in the medical process, which results in a massive amount of data being stored and transmitted in the metaverse. This is because the metaverse contains virtual models created by mapping specific real physical environments and reflects the complex interaction behaviors of users. Since the metaverse is heavily shared and medical procedures frequently entail private patient information, privacy and surveillance concerns arise with the acquired data containing users' personal information. The expense of these sophisticated technologies and the integrated technologies sometimes restrict the metaverse environment's wide range of applications since the metaverse combines several cutting-edge technologies to create whole systems.

2 Background

This section discusses the various technologies and method for deploying the metaverse in Telesurgery.

Digital transformation in the healthcare sector now includes digitalizing the social network through the use of metaverse technologies, in addition to virtual communication. Through the use of augmented reality (AR) and virtual reality (VR), the metaverse is a pervasive and immersive virtual environment. This study [17] is the first attempt to provide an extensive assessment covering seven areas (telemedicine, clinical care, education, mental health, physical fitness, veterinary, and pharmaceuticals) that looks at the most recent metaverse advancements in the healthcare business. The authors examine applications in the metaverse and go into great detail on the technological problems and solutions in each area that may be used to create a long-lasting, self-sufficient, and future-proof solution for healthcare systems in medicine. Lastly, the authors draw attention to the difficulties that need to be resolved before the healthcare sector can completely adopt the metaverse.

The metaverse is a platform for integrating the virtual and physical worlds. It allows people to interact with their avatars in a virtual reality, augmented reality, mixed reality, blockchain, digital twins, and artificial intelligence (AI) environment that is enhanced by virtually limitless data. Social media and entertainment platforms have lately given rise to the metaverse, but its application to healthcare might have a significant influence on clinical practice and public health. Ge Wang et al. [18] propose creation, testing, assessment, control, translation, and improvement of AI-based medicine, particularly medical imaging-guided diagnosis and treatment, can be aided by a metaverse of "medical technology and AI" (MeTAI). The authors talk about pertinent concerns with the MeTAI metaverse ecosystem, such as inequality, security, and privacy. Additionally, they pinpoint particular actions that should be taken in concert to develop the MeTAI metaverse in order to enhance patient happiness, cost-effectiveness, quality, and accessibility of healthcare.

A surgical metaverse—a virtual setting where procedures can be planned and carried out—may be created by combining artificial intelligence and extended reality (AI-XR) technology. In order to realize the full potential of an AI-XR surgical metaverse, a number of hurdles must be overcome, which is why this study [19] attempts to shed light on such applications. Additionally, the authors present a case study in which the execution of "an immersive surgical attack" on incision point localization is carried out in the context of preoperative planning within a surgical metaverse, underscoring the necessity of safe and reliable AI-XR surgical metaverses and illustrating the practical ramifications of security threats to the AI-XR surgical metaverses.

The arrival of the metaverse in medicine has been made possible by the recent integration of new virtual visualization modalities with artificial intelligence and high-speed Internet connections. Three-dimensional virtual models (3DVMs) of the patient's anatomy may be viewed and discussed using digital avatars in this fully virtualized setting. Enrico Checcucci et al. [20] offer a metaverse preoperative clinical case discussion prior to a minimally invasive partial nephrectomy for the first time. Before the surgery, the digital representations of the surgeons convened in a virtual room to discuss the surgical plan and clamping technique. The simulated surgical method is then followed while performing robotic or laparoscopic surgeries.

The advancement of augmented reality (AR) and virtual reality (VR) technologies has accelerated recently. But the medical community is starting to take notice of this technology more and more; both national and international surgical groups have acknowledged the advantages that VR and the metaverse will bring to surgical education and patient care. Kabir Matwala et al. [21] point out that throughout the next 20 years, VR-related technologies will become deeply ingrained in surgical procedures.

The review by the authors [22–25] discusses the combination of two crucial advancements in the field of minimally invasive robotic surgery, with a focus on hepatobiliary surgery: artificial intelligence (AI, which includes machine learning) and augmented reality (or rather, mixed reality (MR) visualizations). Some people refer to the combination of these methods as the "surgical metaverse." The possibility of this innovative idea to meet surgeons' practical need for simpler, more precise, and ultimately safer procedures is drawing attention. The existence of a "control tower," which makes it easier to display and analyze many digital data streams and is well suited for the robotic console, is essential for adopting these cutting-edge technologies. Therefore, expanding on the large surgical robot installation base may contribute to the development of an international ecosystem that encourages innovation and application. In addition, this line of thinking suggests that the ideal approach to achieve advancements in hepatobiliary surgery is to keep an eye on similar activities that take place throughout the surgical landscape.

Hamidu Hamisi Gobeka et al. [26] conducted an analytical comparison of 2D and 3D YouTube videos in terms of content and quality as supplementary teaching resources for phacoemulsification surgery. YouTube videos of 2D and side-by-side 3D phacoemulsification were obtained for this cross-sectional investigation by searching for "phacoemulsification," "phaco," and "cataract." The video power index, interaction index, and watching rate were used to calculate the popularity and interactivity of the videos. Videos were assessed by two senior ophthalmologists (SOs), two ophthalmology residents (ORs), and the global quality score (GQS) and usefulness rating systems.

The current pandemic has accelerated the use of telemedicine in cardiovascular health and spurred the development of innovative technical solutions like the metaverse, an innovative interactive blend of virtual and augmented reality. The word "cardioverse" refers to the metaverse's embrace by cardiovascular medicine [27], which encompasses all of its limitless potential as well as its difficulties and adds fresh perspectives to illness awareness, prevention, and diagnosis. It has several uses, including improving patient visits, supporting heart treatments, and changing the way medical education is delivered. While challenges are anticipated in a number of areas, including technological, legal, and regulatory, using non-fungible tokens as a security asset for patient data seems like a viable way forward.

Technology utilizing extended reality shows promise for having a significant influence on medical education in the future. This technology has an expanding portfolio of use cases that can be implemented at every level of medical education. Investigating and talking about these uses is important to securing the expansion and all-encompassing nature of our future medical education program. Integrative medicine [28] treats the whole person—mind and body—by combining various therapies and lifestyle modifications. Research keeps showing how integrated medicine improves morbidity outcomes and quality of life. Guided meditation, dietary counseling, yoga classes, and other mind–body treatments are just a few of the innovative integrative health techniques that the metaverse and expanded technologies may offer. Additionally, there is growing evidence that VR and AR can provide therapy for anxiety and post-traumatic stress disorder (PTSD) to people.

Novel 3-dimensional rendering techniques and other advances in computer sciences have made it feasible to create cloud-based virtual reality (VR) interfaces that allow peer-to-peer interaction in real time, even from faraway locations. The possible use of this technology to the teaching of microsurgery anatomy is discussed in this paper [29]. Several photogrammetry techniques were used to construct digital specimens, which were then put into a virtual laboratory simulating neuroanatomy dissection. A multiuser virtual anatomy laboratory experience was used to create a VR instructional application. Five visiting scholars from various countries who specialize in neurosurgery tested and evaluated the digital VR models as part of an internal validation process.

Eqram Rahman et al. [30] explore the fascinating connection between plastic surgery, aesthetic medicine, and the metaverse. The research focuses on how these domains interact to generate digital identities and how judgments about physical aesthetic modifications are influenced by digital avatars. The authors' consolidated six publications covering the metaverse, aesthetic plastic surgery, aesthetic and cosmetic medicine, and cosmetic dermatology were found through the search. These works serve as essential resources for understanding the development of aesthetic medicine and cosmetic surgery, comprehending the metaverse, exploring the intersection of these fields, discussing obstacles and moral conundrums, and identifying opportunities for the future.

Virtual reality may be a tremendous help for pain management and rehabilitation, lowering tension and anxiety and increasing therapy adherence. Virtual consultations can also improve access to care, cut down on distance and expenses. With its ability to transform intraoperative augmented reality and artificial intelligence as well as operation planning through 3D modeling and virtual surgeries, the metaverse offers the most promise in urologic surgery [31]. Residents may utilize this platform to learn in a safe setting at their own speed, and medical schools can use the metaverse to enhance their anatomy and surgery courses by offering an immersive learning environment. But using the metaverse in healthcare is not without its potential drawbacks and ethical dilemmas.

The metaverse can support the development of complicated clinical abilities and enhance the learning process in the field of medical education. The metaverse can assist medical professionals in performing orthopedic surgery [32] more precisely and securely. It can also enhance pain management, the use of rehabilitation procedures, and the encouragement of healthy lifestyles. Additionally, virtualization can enhance components of healthcare administration and information, improving organizational performance and process efficacy. This optimization may be especially important in departments where there is a lot of pressure from healthcare providers.

Physicians are thaumaturgical; they execute risky, complicated procedures to save lives. However, as physicians are also fallible human beings, mistakes can be made during such treatments that could lead to a mild complication or a deadly outcome. However, unlike people, robots are error-free. They are the ideal partner for jobs demanding extreme accuracy, such as challenging procedures. This study [33] will cover AR/VR-Assisted Robotic Surgery, its implications, the advantages of AR/VR in the medical field, and how they are radically transforming healthcare via surgery.

The most IoT devices are being used by the metaverse in their virtual workspace. In the blockchain-based metaverse [34], this data is utilized as traceable data and has a distinct identifying tag. Such data is increasingly being used as a useful resource for artificial intelligence in the metaverse. The use of these newest technologies will be accelerated. The metaverse combines blockchain technology and artificial intelligence to create a digital virtual world where you may securely and freely engage in social and economic activities that transcend the boundaries of the actual world.

With an immersive experience, the metaverse has the ability to effortlessly offer patients and medical professionals a wide range of health services. This article [35] suggests using blockchain technology with artificial intelligence in the metaverse to provide patients a more realistic, quicker, and safer experience while receiving healthcare online. The three environments that make up this system are the metaverse environment, the patient's environment, and the doctor's environment. Blockchain technology helps to create a metaverse environment where patients and clinicians communicate while protecting patient privacy, security, and safety. Avatars serve as the physicians', patients', and nurses' representations in the metaverse environment. These individuals join this environment through blockchain registration. Every consultation that takes place between the physician and the patient will be documented, and all of the data—pictures, audio, text, videos, clinical information, etc.—will be collected, sent, and kept on the blockchain.

By improving data security, patient empowerment, disaster victim identification, and the provision of dental treatments, blockchain technology and the metaverse have the potential to completely transform the fields of dentistry and healthcare. In this analysis, Ritik Kashwani [36] addresses the state of the art in dentistry now as well as its future, emphasizing the benefits and drawbacks of using blockchain technology to identify catastrophe victims. Applications of blockchain for Disaster Victim Identification (DVI) provide a humanitarian touch, assisting in providing comfort to bereaved families. Additionally, the ability of blockchain technology to create telemedicine platforms and virtual health clinics might alleviate healthcare gaps in underprivileged areas.

Lately, deep learning (DL) and advanced mathematical algorithms have become indispensable in the diagnosis of medical conditions. Furthermore, providing these services via a blockchain system improves transparency, safety, dependability, and data exchange tracking. It also results in cost savings because of increased productivity. Omid Moztarzadeh et al. [37] describe the design and implementation of a digital twin of cervical vertebral maturation (CVM), a crucial component in many types of dental surgery, within a blockchain-based metaverse platform. An automated diagnosis procedure for the forthcoming CVM pictures in the suggested platform has been developed using a DL technique. This technique makes use of MobileNetV2, a mobile architecture that enhances mobile models' performance across a range of benchmarks and workloads. Because of its low latency and cheap computational costs, the suggested method of digital twinning is easy to use, quick, and appropriate for medical professionals and the Internet of Medical Things (IoMT). This work makes a significant contribution by using DL-based computer vision as a real-time measuring technique, which eliminates the need for extra sensors in the suggested digital twin.

Because patients just need to provide their identity card to access a full medical record history, the introduction of electronic medical records, or EMRs, has made it easier to handle patient data. The medical industry has undergone a transformation thanks to digitalization, but there are two main issues with online records: security and trust. To protect and uphold total confidence with the data, an extra security framework is necessary because data saved on the Internet is not secure. This study [38] proposes a blockchain-based security architecture to protect EMR confidentiality. Using the patient's public key as a universal identification, this method is also utilized to securely access the patient's records in any hospital and to acquire the patient's medical record history much more rapidly, especially during crises.

Through the application of several relevant technologies, the metaverse seeks to provide consumers with 3D immersive and individualized experiences. How to safeguard the digital information and data of users in the metaverse is a natural concern, even with all of its advantages. Blockchain presents a possible answer in this area because of its unique decentralization, immutability, and transparency qualities. Huynh-The et al. [3] present a thorough overview of blockchain applications for the metaverse so that readers may have a deeper understanding of the technology's place in the metaverse. First, the authors provide an overview of blockchain technology and the metaverse, emphasizing the reasons for using it in the metaverse. Following that, the authors go into great detail on blockchain-based approaches for the metaverse from a technological standpoint, covering topics like data collection, storage, sharing, interoperability, and privacy protection. Additionally, they look at how blockchain affects important metaverse-enabling technologies like digital twins, big data, artificial intelligence, multisensory and immersive apps, and the Internet of Things.

The potential advantages of combining disruptive technologies have led to some significant advancement in the global economic expansion and healthcare revolution. Healthcare records require extra care and consideration when it comes to privacy, security, interoperability, and dependability. As a result, modern technologies are being used to enhance the sector's functions. Distributed database applications using blockchain are used to address privacy and complexity issues in a variety of industries, including healthcare. The COVID-19 pandemic has shown how crucial it is to set up strong, stable, and dependable patient and healthcare services. Digital solutions that use Blockchain [39] and artificial intelligence (AI) to guarantee supply chain integrity and data intelligence to operate more effectively and efficiently would be excellent for putting an end to this situation. Blockchain technologies improve the confidentiality, privacy, and immutability of medical information; however, AI-assisted diagnosis or detection is quicker, more precise, and safer than current methods.

3 Overall Challenges

The following are the challenges while deploying the metaverse in Telesurgery [15, 16, 40]:

- Huge amount of data: The interactions between patients and doctors, patients and treatment resources, and other users are more frequent and complex in the medical process, which results in a massive amount of data being stored and transmitted in the metaverse. This is because the metaverse contains virtual models created by mapping specific real physical environments and reflects the complex interaction behaviors of users.
- Device compatibility and interaction: The expanded reality technology—which now needs to be based on head-mounted devices like HoloLens, Pico, etc.—is the essential technology that powers the metaverse immersive experience. Head-mounted devices can occasionally restrict the operator's range of motion, and the patient's physical restrictions and the physician's range of motion during treatment frequently pose issues with head-mounted device use. There are certain difficulties in integrating computer vision with the metaverse. The computer vision-enabled metaverse could employ inaccurate projection techniques, leading to distorted surroundings within the metaverse.
- Connectivity issues: The largest barriers are technical ones, such as issues with digital devices, Internet access, hardware, and software, and usability of interfaces. There might be a delay in processing the data or visualizing the same in the headset due to network issues or weather conditions. Some rural areas may not have the sufficient bandwidth as a data carrier. This raises a major concern during the surgical process.
- Security concerns: Cybersecurity threats associated with metaverse applications in immersive 3D or 2D environments include patient data disclosure and hacking. Applications that enhance endpoint complexity and possible incoming portals for hacking, data instrumentation, and/or bad actor monitoring are those that need extra new networked hardware for clinical deployment. Because XR-related solutions have access to so much private patient data, there is a chance of a data breach in the metaverse. Any alteration or loss of this data will negatively impact patient privacy and healthcare, as well as the reputation of the treating physician.
- Huge cost: The XR devices are expensive, and the environment setup for Telesurgery with IoT interfacing involving body-aware sensors would be a complex task. Recruitment of experts to handle these devices and the maintenance of the hardware adds to the overhead cost.
- Live interaction and individual touch are lost: The distance between a patient and a doctor is widened by the current digital revolution of healthcare systems with telemedicine services and remote patient monitoring technologies. After obtaining the required patient history and current circumstances, or by examining digital health data without actually seeing the patients, doctors might recommend the remote treatment process. However, by offering practical and efficient interactive alternatives, the metaverse will provide patients and healthcare

practitioners an immersive virtual environment. A lack of face-to-face rapport and a unique bonding experience is felt by most patients as a result of the current digital style of therapy.

- Legal issues: The expanding practical uses of the metaverse in the healthcare industry, including several organizations like insurance companies, pharmaceutical firms, and healthcare providers to deliver effective patient care, might give rise to legal and regulatory challenges. The implementation of the metaverse might cause misunderstanding among different entities of the domain over intellectual property rights, trust issues, etc., because it lacks appropriate rules and procedures.

4 Case Studies

4.1 The Metaverse Potential for Life Sciences and Healthcare—TCS

Located at the intersection of innovative disruptive technologies like blockchain, Internet of Things (IoT), cloud, 5G, and AI-ML, among others, it is bringing about a new era of digital transformation and opening up new avenues for exploration. The life sciences and healthcare sector can benefit greatly from the metaverse's ability to create immersive, real-time, persistent, and decentralized virtual environments. It can assist in overcoming some of the most significant obstacles related to clinical trials, telemedicine, better illness diagnosis, patient outcomes, and medical education. The tech team in TCS [41] talks about future prospects, early adoption use cases to create commercial value, applications for the healthcare and life sciences sectors, and emergent metaverse trends.

The life sciences and healthcare sectors will benefit greatly from the metaverse's evolution and maturation as technology advances, and it will also help to solve some of the industry's upcoming problems. Although there are still some unclear areas, such as governance, additional regulatory guidance is anticipated. To stay ahead of the curve and ride the transition from the proto-metaverse to the more developed metaverse phase, life sciences and healthcare enterprises must collaborate with the appropriate players in the technological ecosystem.

4.2 The Metaverse of Healthcare Goes Beyond Virtual Reality—Boston Consulting Group

The majority of healthcare fields are already being impacted by the metaverse, despite the fact that it is still in its infancy. Technology is developing quickly, and its use is growing, indicating a major disruption in the works. Payers and providers must decide right now how they will react to these changes. Before defining their vision for how these next-generation technologies may help them and their patients, they need to have a thorough awareness of the variety of use cases that are currently available on the market as well as those that are being developed.

In November 2022, BCG conducted a study [42] with providers, payers, biopharma and medtech businesses to understand how established actors in the healthcare industry are addressing the metaverse. Most businesses, it turns out, are already experimenting with these technologies. Over one-third of payers and nearly three-quarters of healthcare providers said they have used XR, blockchain, or M-worlds in some capacity. Payers utilize blockchain more than other participants, at 25%, but they reported using XR less than other players, which makes sense given that most XR use cases now are provider oriented.

According to Boston study, the metaverse in healthcare appears to be evolving in three stages. Phase one, the first few years of testing, is coming to an end. Phase two, which will last for the next five years or more, will be characterized by the wider acceptance of existing use cases and the creation of new ones as technology develops. Phase three (the next ten years) will witness the creation of metaverse technologies in several healthcare domains and the development of increasingly sophisticated use cases.

4.3 Healthcare Metaverse: How Will It Change the Sector?—Relevant Software

The next great thing on the Internet that will disrupt every business, notably intelligent healthcare, is the metaverse, which is predicted to reach a valuation of 800 billion dollars by 2024. Surprisingly positive about the metaverse is the healthcare industry, which is frequently perceived as conservative. Improved Availability of Medical Services Relevant Software [43] renders healthcare IT consulting services, utilizing their in-depth knowledge of related technologies—like blockchain, artificial intelligence and machine learning, VR and AR tools, and 3D technology—to create cutting-edge applications.

4.4 The Convergence of Emerging Technologies Is Transforming Digital Healthcare—Accenture's Digital Health Technology Vision 2022 Report

The "metaverse continuum" is a spectrum of digitally enhanced worlds, realities, and business models that, according to the report "Accenture Digital Health Technology Vision 2022," will transform almost every aspect of life and business in the next ten years and beyond, including the healthcare sector. Accenture has announced the creation of the Accenture Metaverse Continuum business group, which brings together industry-leading capabilities in digital commerce, artificial intelligence, computer vision, blockchain, extended reality, and customer experience with metaverse expertise to assist healthcare organizations in designing, implementing, and speeding up their metaverse journeys.

Rich Birhanzel, Accenture's worldwide industrial health director, stated [44]: "The metaverse may appear futuristic, yet it's already beginning to take shape. We are looking forward to the opportunities it will provide to enhance patient engagement with healthcare organizations, patient data management, and patient assistance throughout their wellness and health journeys. The next generation of healthcare will be shaped by healthcare organizations that begin strategically investing now to establish a high-performing digital technology foundation. These organizations will put people at the center of their work and create greater access, better experiences, more trust, and improved outcomes."

According to the research, healthcare companies are also preparing for more technology advancements. For instance, over 80% of executives in the healthcare industry stated that during the previous three years, the number of edge and Internet of Things (IoT) devices installed in their companies had grown dramatically or enormously. Furthermore, almost all 96% believe that the long-term viability of their company will depend on the application of next-generation computing to issues that current computers are unable to resolve.

Senior managing director of Accenture Health Kaveh Safavi, M.D., J.D., stated: "Investing in a digital technology foundation for healthcare has allowed leading healthcare enterprises to make good progress." The Internet of location and the Internet of ownership in healthcare are available to us in the metaverse, which is the next frontier. Surgical teams, for instance, can learn new techniques without physically being in the same operating room. Alternatively, being able to safely allow a caregiver access to your medical records while on the go without needing to verify your address or get a doctor's approval.

4.5 Metaverse in the Healthcare Sector: Utilizations, Benefits, Difficulties, and More—Intelivita Private Limited

In order to establish a dynamic and integrated virtual healthcare ecosystem, the metaverse in healthcare makes use of technologies like virtual reality (VR), augmented reality (AR), mixed reality (MR), and sophisticated digital platforms. Through the use of virtual clinics and home consultations with medical specialists, people in this metaverse may get the care they need without being limited by distance or time constraints.

With the help of the metaverse's virtual medical simulations, medical education has never been more effective or immersive. Medical practitioners and students can participate in realistic scenarios through these simulations without endangering patient safety. Users may manage patient care in a risk-free setting, practice surgical methods, and diagnose medical diseases using virtual reality.

Whether during routine check-ups, operations, or even hospital stays, anxiety is often a part of the healthcare experience. A potent answer to this problem is provided by the metaverse. By exposing patients to calming virtual settings [45], tension and anxiety are reduced, making the encounter more pleasant and less intimidating. Patients can select from a range of tranquil settings, such as placid woodlands or beaches. These virtual getaways provide a digital haven away from the sometimes eerie hospital environments.

In virtual laboratories, researchers from all around the world may collaborate and exchange ideas. This cooperative setting fosters efficiency and creativity, which speeds up medical advancements. Regardless matter where they are in the world, scientists can collaborate easily to address some of the most urgent problems in healthcare. Better patient care is the result of quicker medical discoveries and breakthroughs made possible by this integrated approach to research.

4.6 Examining the Possibilities, Costs, and Procedures for Developing Metaverse in Healthcare—Appinventiv

Physical barriers have vanished with the development of telemedicine as it has integrated into the metaverse. The majority of patients and caregivers eventually used telehealth to supplement in-person consultations or visits with healthcare providers once it gained popularity during the epidemic. By taking care of urgent medical demands and guaranteeing the provision of healthcare services, integrating the metaverse opens up a world of opportunities. Patients may obtain medical professionals from the comfort of their virtual surroundings, enjoying accessibility and ease. Furthermore, the metaverse greatly facilitates multidisciplinary care by providing precise diagnosis and customized treatment regimens.

The first factor influencing the price of metaverse development services is your choice of development partner. For metaverse healthcare app development services [46], pick a company that employs a group of skilled, knowledgeable developers.

5 Conclusion and Future Directions

The metaverse in healthcare has many dimensions of use cases. One of the major scenarios of metaverse deployment is Telesurgery using smart body-aware sensors. This could enable the remote monitoring and control of patients in surgical process with an aid of robotics especially in situations where the surgeons are immediately required for a specialized operation. Though there are various complications in setting up the technological environment, it can be a life saver in several cases.

This chapter highlighted the technologies involved in the metaverse for Telesurgery and existing applications for diagnosis. The future directions would involve usage of quantum computing for quick processing of patient data, thus reducing the time and the overhead cost in the computational process.

References

1. Spiceworks AI. Retrieved October 10, 2022, from https://www.spiceworks.com/tech/artificial-intelligence/articles/what-is-metaverse/#:~:text=The%20Metaverse%20is%20a%20spatial,a%20bedrock%20of%20blockchain%20technology
2. Builtin media-gaming. Retrieved October 6, 2022, from https://builtin.com/media-gaming/what-is-metaverse
3. Gadekallu, T. R., Huynh-The, T., Wang, W., Yenduri, G., Ranaweera, P., Pham, Q. V., da Costa, D. B., & Liyanage, M. (2023). Blockchain for the metaverse: a review. *Future Generation Computer Systems, 143*, 401–419.
4. Builtin media-gaming. Retrieved June 15, 2023, from https://www.wired.com/story/what-is-the-metaverse/
5. Wang, Y., Su, Z., Zhang, N., Xing, R., Liu, D., Luan, T. H., & Shen, X. (2022). A survey on metaverse: fundamentals, security, and privacy. *IEEE Communications Surveys and Tutorials, 25*(1), 319–352.
6. News medical life sciences. Retrieved June 15, 2023, from https://www.news-medical.net/health/What-is-Remote-SurgeryTelesurgery.aspx
7. National library of medicine. Retrieved May 31, 2018, from https://www.ncbi.nlm.nih.gov/pmc/articles/PMC6067812/
8. twi-global industry-5-0. Retrieved November 5, 2023, from https://www.twi-global.com/technical-knowledge/faqs/industry-5-0
9. MasterControl GxP Lifeline. Retrieved July 30, 2020, from https://www.mastercontrol.com/gxp-lifeline/3-things-you-need-to-know-about-industry-5.0/#:~:text=The%20term%20Industry%205.0%20refers,pillars%20of%20automation%20and%20efficiency
10. Forbes Industry 5.0. Retrieved May 24, 2022, from https://www.forbes.com/sites/jeroenkraaijenbrink/2022/05/24/what-is-industry-50
11. Maddikunta, P. K. R., Pham, Q. V., Prabadevi, B., Deepa, N., Dev, K., Gadekallu, T. R., Ruby, R, & Liyanage, M. (2022). Industry 5.0: a survey on enabling technologies and potential applications. *Journal of Industrial Information Integration, 26*, 100257.
12. Investopedia Blockchain. Retrieved December 15, 2023, from https://www.investopedia.com/terms/b/blockchain.asp
13. IBM Blockchain. Retrieved January 14, 2020, from https://www.ibm.com/topics/blockchain
14. Investopedia NFT. Retrieved April 6, 2023, from https://www.investopedia.com/non-fungible-tokens-nft-5115211
15. Chengoden, R., Victor, N., Huynh-The, T., Yenduri, G., Jhaveri, R. H., Alazab, M., Bhattacharya, S., Hegde, P., Maddikunta, P. K. R., & Gadekallu, T. R. (2023). Metaverse for healthcare: A survey on potential applications, challenges and future directions. *IEEE Access, 11*, 12765–12795.
16. Shao, L., Tang, W. E. I., Zhang, Z., & Chen, X. (2023). Medical metaverse: technologies, applications, challenges and future. *Journal of Mechanics in Medicine and Biology, 23*(2), 2350028.
17. Bansal, G., Rajgopal, K., Chamola, V., Xiong, Z., & Niyato, D. (2022). Healthcare in metaverse: A survey on current metaverse applications in healthcare. *IEEE Access, 10*, 119914–119946.

18. Wang, G., Badal, A., Jia, X., Maltz, J. S., Mueller, K., Myers, K. J., Niu, C., Vannier, M., Yan, P., Yu, Z., & Zeng, R. (2022). Development of metaverse for intelligent healthcare. *Nature Machine Intelligence, 4*(11), 922–929.
19. Qayyum, A., Bilal, M., Hadi, M., Capik, P., Caputo, M., Vohra, H., Al-Fuqaha, A., & Qadir, J. (2023). Can we revitalize interventional healthcare with AI-XR surgical metaverses? arXiv e-prints, arXiv-2304.
20. Checcucci, E., Amparore, D., Volpi, G., De Cillis, S., Piramide, F., Verri, P., Piana, A., Sica, M., Gatti, C., Alessio, P., & Quarà, A. (2023). *Metaverse surgical planning with three-dimensional virtual models for minimally invasive partial nephrectomy, European urology*. Elsevier.
21. Matwala, K., Shakir, T., Bhan, C., & Chand, M. (2023). *The surgical metaverse, Cirugía Española*. Elsevier.
22. Van Leeuwen, F. W., & van der Hage, J. A. (2023). Where robotic surgery meets the metaverse. *Cancers, 14*(24), 6161.
23. Giannone, F., Felli, E., Cherkaoui, Z., Mascagni, P., & Pessaux, P. (2021). Augmented reality and image-guided robotic liver surgery. *Cancers, 13*, 6268.
24. Wendler, T., van Leeuwen, F. W. B., Navab, N., & van Oosterom, M. N. (2021). How molecular imaging will enable robotic precision surgery: The role of artificial intelligence, augmented reality, and navigation. *European Journal of Nuclear Medicine and Molecular Imaging, 48*(13), 4201–4224.
25. Garavand, A., & Aslani, N. (2022). Metaverse phenomenon and its impact on health: A scoping review. *Informatics in Medicine Unlocked, 32*, 101029.
26. Gobeka, H. H., Gülyeşil, F. F., Yozgat, Z., & Sabaner, M. C. (2021). Quality assessment and comparison of two-and three-dimensional YouTube videos as additional educational tools for cataract surgery:“METAVERSE”. *Irish Journal of Medical Science, 192*(5), 2427–2433.
27. Skalidis, I., Muller, O., & Fournier, S. (2022). CardioVerse: The cardiovascular medicine in the era of Metaverse. *Trends in Cardiovascular Medicine, 33*(8), 471–476.
28. Ahuja, A. S., Polascik, B. W., Doddapaneni, D., Byrnes, E. S., & Sridhar, J. (2023). The digital metaverse: Applications in artificial intelligence, medical education, and integrative health. *Integrative Medicine Research, 12*(1), 100917.
29. Gonzalez-Romo, N. I., Mignucci-Jiménez, G., Hanalioglu, S., Gurses, M. E., Bahadir, S., Xu, Y., Koskay, G., Lawton, M. T., & Preul, M. C. (2023). Virtual neurosurgery anatomy laboratory: A collaborative and remote education experience in the metaverse. *Surgical Neurology International, 14*, 1–10.
30. Rahman, E., Rao, P., Sayed, K., Webb, W. R., Philipp-Dormston, W. G., Carruthers, J. D., & Carruthers, A. (2023). Sculpting digital identities: The interplay of aesthetic medicine, plastic surgery, and the metaverse. *European Journal of Plastic Surgery, 46*, 845–854.
31. Randazzo, G., Reitano, G., Carletti, F., Iafrate, M., Betto, G., Novara, G., Dal Moro, F., & Zattoni, F. (2023). Urology: A trip into metaverse. *World Journal of Urology, 41*(10), 2647–2657.
32. Román-Belmonte, J. M., Rodríguez-Merchán, E. C., & De la Corte-Rodríguez, H. (2023). Metaverse applied to musculoskeletal pathology: Orthoverse and Rehabverse. *Postgraduate Medicine, 135*(5), 1–9.
33. Das, S., & Vyas, S. (2022). The utilization of AR/VR in robotic surgery: A study. In *Proceedings of the 4th International Conference on Information Management and Machine Intelligence* (pp. 1–8). ACM.
34. Mozumder, M. A. I., Sheeraz, M. M., Athar, A., Aich, S., & Kim, H. C. (2022). Overview: Technology roadmap of the future trend of metaverse based on IoT, blockchain, AI technique, and medical domain metaverse activity. In *2022 24th International Conference on Advanced Communication Technology (ICACT)* (pp. 256–261). IEEE.
35. Ali, S., Abdullah, Armand, T. P. T., Athar, A., Hussain, A., Ali, M., Yaseen, M., Joo, M.-I., & Kim, H.-C. (2023). Metaverse in healthcare integrated with explainable AI and blockchain: enabling immersiveness, ensuring trust, and providing patient data security. *Sensors, 23*(2), 565.

36. Kashwani, R., & Sawhney, H. (2023). Dentistry and metaverse: A deep dive into potential of blockchain, NFTs, and crypto in healthcare. *International Dental Journal of Students' Research, 11*(3), 94–98.
37. Moztarzadeh, O., Jamshidi, M., Sargolzaei, S., Keikhaee, F., Jamshidi, A., Shadroo, S., & Hauer, L. (2023). Metaverse and medical diagnosis: A blockchain-based digital twinning approach based on MobileNetV2 algorithm for cervical vertebral maturation. *Diagnostics, 13*(8), 1485.
38. Krishnan, S. S. R., Manoj, M. K., Gadekallu, T. R., Kumar, N., Maddikunta, P. K. R., Bhattacharya, S., Suh, D. Y., & Piran, M. J. (2020). A blockchain-based credibility scoring framework for electronic medical records. In *2020 IEEE Globecom Workshops* (pp. 1–6). IEEE.
39. Uma, S. (2023). Blockchain and AI: disruptive digital technologies in designing the potential growth of healthcare industries. In *AI and Blockchain in Healthcare* (pp. 137–150). Singapore.
40. Tan, T. F., Li, Y., Lim, J. S., Gunasekeran, D. V., Teo, Z. L., Ng, W. Y., & Ting, D. S. (2022). Metaverse and virtual health care in ophthalmology: Opportunities and challenges. *The Asia-Pacific Journal of Ophthalmology, 11*(3), 237–246.
41. TCS Life sciences. Retrieved December 24, 2022, from https://www.tcs.com/what-we-do/industries/life-sciences/white-paper
42. BCG Healthcare. Retrieved January 19, 2023, from https://www.bcg.com/publications/2023/reaping-the-benefits-of-the-healthcare-metaverse
43. Relevant Metaverse. Retrieved August 4, 2023, from https://relevant.software/blog/metaverse-in-healthcare/
44. Accenture Newsroom. Retrieved June 21, 2022, from https://newsroom.accenture.com/news/2022/accenture-report
45. Intelivita Metaverse healthcare. Retrieved October 11, 2023, from https://www.intelivita.com/blog/metaverse-in-healthcare/
46. Appinventiv Metaverse healthcare. Retrieved November 23, 2022, from https://appinventiv.com/blog/metaverse-in-healthcare/

Challenges, Ethics, and Limitations of the Metaverse for the Health-Care Industry

Chiranji Lal Chowdhary and Abhishek Ranjan

1 Introduction

The convergence of the metaverse and health care promises revolutionary transformations in patient care, medical training, and collaborative research. However, as we embark on this journey, it is crucial to examine the challenges that may impede progress, the ethical concerns that demand our attention, and the inherent limitations that may shape the trajectory of the metaverse adoption in health care [1].

1.1 Challenges in Implementing the Metaverse in Health Care

The incorporation of the metaverse into health-care systems is not without its challenges. These hurdles span various domains, from technological intricacies to user adoption concerns and regulatory landscapes. In this section, we delve into the specific challenges encountered in seamlessly integrating the metaverse into the health-care industry [2].

Technological Challenges The successful amalgamation of the metaverse with health care is contingent on overcoming several technological challenges [3].

C. L. Chowdhary (✉)
School of Computer Science Engineering and Information Systems, Vellore Institute of Technology, Vellore, Tamil Nadu, India
e-mail: chiranji.lal@vit.ac.in

A. Ranjan
Faculty of Engineering and Technology, Botho University, Accra, Ghana
e-mail: Abhishek.ranjan@bothouniversity.ac.bw

C. L. Chowdhary (ed.), *The Metaverse for the Healthcare Industry*,
https://doi.org/10.1007/978-3-031-60073-9_14

(a) Interoperability issues:

One of the primary technological obstacles lies in ensuring seamless interoperability between diverse systems and platforms within the metaverse and existing health-care infrastructures. Achieving compatibility is crucial to facilitate the smooth exchange of information and functionality across virtual and real-world environments.

(b) Data security and privacy concerns.

As health care inherently involves sensitive patient data, ensuring robust data security and privacy protection mechanisms is paramount. The metaverse introduces novel dimensions to data management, necessitating a careful balance between accessibility for health-care professionals and the safeguarding of patients' confidential information.

(c) Bandwidth and connectivity constraints.

The immersive nature of the metaverse demands substantial bandwidth and stable connectivity. Overcoming bandwidth limitations and ensuring reliable connections are essential to prevent disruptions in virtual health-care interactions. Addressing these constraints becomes pivotal in guaranteeing a seamless and effective integration of the metaverse into health-care practices.

User Adoption Challenges The successful implementation of the metaverse in health care relies heavily on the acceptance and active participation of both health-care professionals and patients [4]. This subsection explores the multifaceted challenges associated with user adoption.

(a) Resistance to change among health-care professionals:

Health-care professionals, accustomed to traditional practices, may exhibit resistance to adopting metaverse technologies. Overcoming this resistance requires targeted educational programs, demonstrating the advantages and efficiency gains offered by virtual health-care platforms. Encouraging a shift in mindset is crucial for the successful integration of the metaverse into medical workflows.

(b) Patient acceptance and engagement:

For the metaverse to truly enhance health-care experiences, patient acceptance and engagement are pivotal. Ensuring that patients are comfortable with virtual medical interactions and actively participate in their health care through these platforms involves addressing concerns related to trust, usability, and the overall patient experience.

(c) Accessibility for diverse populations:

(d) The metaverse should cater to diverse populations, considering factors such as age, socioeconomic status, and technological literacy. Making virtual health care accessible to all requires a focus on inclusivity, user-friendly interfaces, and strategies that bridge the digital divide. Overcoming accessibility challenges ensures equitable health-care delivery through the metaverse technologies.

Regulatory and Legal Challenges Navigating the regulatory and legal landscape is a critical aspect of integrating the metaverse into the health-care industry. This subsection delves into the challenges posed by existing regulations and legal considerations [5].

(a) Compliance with existing health-care regulations:
Adherence to established health-care regulations is essential for the metaverse technologies to gain acceptance and trust. Ensuring that virtual health-care platforms comply with existing standards and guidelines guarantees the ethical and legal use of these technologies within the health-care sector.

(b) Liability issues in virtual medical environments:
Virtual medical interactions raise unique liability concerns. Determining responsibility in case of errors or adverse events within virtual environments requires careful consideration and legal frameworks. Addressing liability issues is crucial for fostering confidence in the safety and reliability of the metaverse-enabled health-care services.

(c) Intellectual property concerns in virtual health-care spaces:
The creation and utilization of virtual health-care environments give rise to novel intellectual property challenges. Protecting innovations, designs, and content within these virtual spaces necessitates a nuanced understanding of intellectual property laws. Establishing clear guidelines and regulations mitigates disputes and ensures a fair and ethical landscape for innovation in virtual health care.

1.2 Ethics in the Metaverse–Health-Care Nexus

Ethical considerations are central to the successful and responsible implementation of the metaverse in health care. This section examines ethical challenges and principles that arise in the intersection of the metaverse and health care [6].

Privacy and Confidentiality Privacy and confidentiality are paramount in health care, and their preservation in virtual environments is critical for the ethical use of the metaverse [7].

(a) Protection of patient data in virtual environments:
Maintaining the confidentiality and security of patient data is a foundational ethical requirement. Robust encryption, secure storage, and strict access controls must be implemented to safeguard patient information within the virtual realm. Ethical considerations demand the establishment of practices that mirror or exceed traditional health-care privacy standards.

(b) Informed consent in virtual medical interactions:
In virtual medical interactions, ensuring informed consent is a nuanced challenge. Transparent communication about the nature of virtual health care, potential risks, and the use of patient data is essential. Establishing protocols for

obtaining informed consent in virtual environments upholds ethical standards and respects patients' autonomy.

Equity and Accessibility Ethical considerations extend to addressing disparities and ensuring accessibility for all, irrespective of individual circumstances [8].

(a) Addressing disparities in access to virtual health care:
Ethical metaverse integration demands a commitment to addressing disparities in access. Initiatives should focus on reducing barriers related to technology, connectivity, and education to ensure that virtual health care is accessible to diverse populations, regardless of socioeconomic or geographical factors.
(b) Ensuring inclusivity for individuals with disabilities:
Virtual health-care platforms must be designed with inclusivity in mind, catering to the needs of individuals with disabilities. Ethical practices involve prioritizing accessibility features, such as adaptive technologies and user interfaces, to ensure that virtual health-care services are inclusive and equally accessible to all.

Ethical Use of AI and Virtual Agents The ethical deployment of AI and virtual agents in health care within the metaverse requires careful consideration and oversight [9].

(a) Ensuring fairness and transparency in AI algorithms:
Ethical AI algorithms in virtual health care must prioritize fairness and transparency. Algorithms should be designed to avoid bias, and mechanisms for transparency in their decision-making processes should be implemented. Ethical considerations emphasize the importance of fairness in health-care outcomes, regardless of the virtual or real-world setting.
(b) Mitigating biases in virtual medical consultations:
Virtual medical consultations facilitated by AI agents must be vigilant against biases that could impact health-care decisions. Ethical practices involve continuous monitoring, auditing, and refinement of AI algorithms to minimize biases and ensure that virtual medical consultations are impartial and equitable.

1.3 Limitations of the Metaverse Integration in Health Care

Understanding and acknowledging the limitations inherent in the metaverse's integration into health care is crucial for realistic expectations and effective utilization [10].

Technological Limitations Technological advancements are ongoing, but acknowledging current limitations and potential future advancements is essential.

(a) Current capabilities and potential advancements:
While the metaverse holds promise, it's crucial to recognize its current capabilities and limitations. Ethical decision-making involves setting realistic expectations and considering the evolving nature of the metaverse technologies, anticipating future advancements that may address current limitations.
(b) Realism and limitations of virtual simulations in medical training:
Virtual simulations in medical training offer unique opportunities but are bound by certain limitations. Ethical considerations involve acknowledging the realism of virtual simulations and understanding their scope and boundaries in providing effective medical training. Balancing the benefits of virtual simulations with the hands-on experience required in health-care education is crucial.

Human Factors The human elements in virtual health-care interactions are essential, and understanding their nuances is crucial for ethical metaverse integration.

(a) Emotional nuances in virtual patient interactions:
Virtual patient interactions may lack certain emotional nuances present in face-to-face encounters. Acknowledging this limitation is vital for ethical practice. Health-care professionals engaging in virtual interactions must be trained to interpret and respond to emotional cues effectively, ensuring empathetic and patient-centered care.
(b) Trust-building in virtual health-care settings:
Building trust between health-care providers and patients is foundational. In virtual health-care settings, establishing and maintaining trust becomes a critical ethical consideration. Strategies for transparent communication, secure data practices, and demonstrating the reliability of virtual health-care technologies are essential for fostering trust in these innovative platforms.

Economic Considerations The economic aspects of the metaverse adoption in health care require careful consideration to ensure sustainable and ethical practices.

(a) Cost implications of the metaverse adoption in health care:
The economic viability of integrating the metaverse into health care must be assessed with attention to cost implications. Ethical decision-making involves evaluating the financial feasibility of adopting the metaverse technologies while ensuring that the associated costs do not compromise the accessibility and quality of health-care services.
(b) Balancing investment with tangible outcomes:
Ethical economic considerations involve striking a balance between investment in the metaverse technologies and the tangible outcomes they deliver. Investments should align with the goals of improving patient care, enhancing medical training, and advancing research. Ethical decision-makers prioritize investments that yield meaningful and sustainable benefits for the health-care industry and its stakeholders.

2 Conclusion

As the health-care industry embarks on the transformative journey into the metaverse, understanding and addressing the challenges, ethical considerations, and limitations becomes imperative. This chapter provides a comprehensive exploration of these facets, aiming to guide practitioners, researchers, and policymakers in navigating the complex intersection of the metaverse and health care.

Navigating the ethical challenges and limitations of integrating the metaverse into the health-care industry requires a concerted effort from stakeholders. By addressing privacy concerns, ensuring inclusivity, and overcoming technological barriers, the health-care sector can harness the transformative potential of the metaverse responsibly. Subsequent discussions and case studies in the book will further explore strategies for successful implementation and ethical considerations within this evolving landscape.

References

1. Kilic, F. (2024). Revolutionizing healthcare – The integration of virtual worlds, AR, and metaverse technology. *Open Journal of Applied Sciences, 14*(01), 27–37.
2. Petrigna, L., & Musumeci, G. (2022). The metaverse: A new challenge for the healthcare system: A scoping review. *Journal of Functional Morphology and Kinesiology, 7*(3), 63.
3. Asif, H., Zahid, R., Bashir, U., Afzal, W., Firdous, M., Zahid, A., & Hasnain, M. (2024). Metaverse for healthcare: Possible potential applications (virtual reality technologies), opportunities, challenges, and future directions. *Metaverse Applications for Intelligent Healthcare*, 274–305.
4. Damaševičius, R., & Abayomi-Alli, O. O. (2024). The future of telemedicine: Emerging technologies, challenges, and opportunities. *Metaverse Applications for Intelligent Healthcare*, 306–338.
5. Moodley, K. (2024). Artificial intelligence (AI) or augmented intelligence? How big data and AI are transforming healthcare: Challenges and opportunities. *South African Medical Journal, 114*(1), 22–26.
6. Shwedeh, F. (2024). Harnessing digital issue in adopting metaverse technology in higher education institutions: Evidence from the United Arab Emirates. *International Journal of Data and Network Science, 8*(1), 489–504.
7. Anthwal, A., Uniyal, A., Gairolla, J., Singh, R., Gehlot, A., Abbas, M., & Akram, S. V. (2024). Industry 4.0 technologies adoption for digital transition in drug discovery and development: A review. *Journal of Industrial Information Integration*, 100562.
8. El-Kady, R. M. (2024). Investigating forensic evidence in metaverse: A comparative analytical study. In *Forecasting cyber crimes in the age of the metaverse* (pp. 227–258). IGI Global.
9. Qu, Q., Hatami, M., Xu, R., Nagothu, D., Chen, Y., Li, X. E., et al. (2024). Microverse: A task-oriented edge-scale metaverse. *Future Internet, 16*(2), 60. https://doi.org/10.3390/fi16020060
10. Ahmed, Y., Reddy, M., Mederos, J., McDermott, K. C., Varma, D. K., Ludwig, C. A., et al. (2024). Democratizing health care in the Metaverse: How video games can monitor eye conditions using the vision performance index: A pilot study. *Ophthalmology Science, 4*(1), 100349.

Index

C. L. Chowdhary (ed.), *The Metaverse for the Healthcare Industry*,
https://doi.org/10.1007/978-3-031-60073-9

Printed by Printforce, the Netherlands